HEMODYNAMICS AND MECHANOBIOLOGY OF ENDOTHELIUM

HEMODYNAMICS AND MECHANOBIOLOGY OF ENDOTHELIUM

Editors

Tzung K Hsiai
University of Southern California, USA

Brett Blackman
University of Virginia, USA

Hanjoong Jo
Georgia Institute of Technology/Emory University, USA

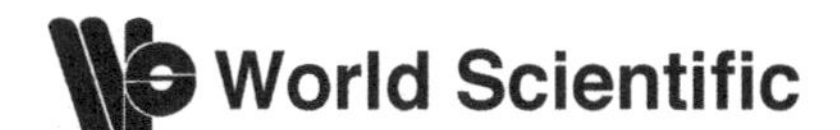

NEW JERSEY • LONDON • SINGAPORE • BEIJING • SHANGHAI • HONG KONG • TAIPEI • CHENNAI

Published by

World Scientific Publishing Co. Pte. Ltd.
5 Toh Tuck Link, Singapore 596224
USA office: 27 Warren Street, Suite 401-402, Hackensack, NJ 07601
UK office: 57 Shelton Street, Covent Garden, London WC2H 9HE

British Library Cataloguing-in-Publication Data
A catalogue record for this book is available from the British Library.

HEMODYNAMICS AND MECHANOBIOLOGY OF ENDOTHELIUM

ISBN-13 978-981-4280-41-9
ISBN-10 981-4280-41-0

Typeset by Stallion Press
Email: enquiries@stallionpress.com

Printed in Singapore.

PREFACE

This book is dedicated to Dr. Bradford Berk who along with many of our colleagues made seminal contributions that promoted the importance of the field of "Hemodynamics & Mechanobiology in Vascular Endothelium". Their contribution has paved the way for the post-genomic era of research in the cardiovascular and mechanobiology community.

The central theme of this book focuses on mechanosignal transduction and vascular disease in response to the dynamics of blood flow. A cadre of leading investigators in this field has contributed to the state-of-the-art topics that have enriched our knowledge with relevance to vascular therapeutics and interventions. The authors have intended to provide an overview, followed by an in-depth analysis as a basis for the emerging vascular fields, including but not limited to redox signaling and inflammatory responses, tissue engineering and regenerative medicine, genomics and bioinformatics, as well and micro- and nanotechnology.

The reader should be able to embark on a vascular journey from molecular and cellular basis to organs and organisms in the context of fluid shear stress and atherosclerosis. The editors welcome reader's critiques that will be critical to enhance the future edition. Your invaluable contribution as the student, academician, clinician, and/or researcher from pharmaceutical and biotechnology industries would further build the foundation for the new generation of vascular biologists and biomedical engineers. Finally, we are grateful for how much our research has been enriched by our ties with our mentors, teachers, colleagues, students, and patients.

Tzung K. Hsiai
Brett R. Blackman
Hanjoong Jo
January, 2010

CONTENTS

Chapter 1

FLOW AND ATHEROSCLEROSIS

IAN CAMPBELL* and W. ROBERT TAYLOR*,†,‡

*The Wallace H. Coulter Department of Biomedical Engineering, Georgia Institute of Technology and Emory University

†The Department of Medicine, Division of Cardiology, Emory University
wtaylor@emory.edu

‡The Atlanta VA Medical Center, Atlanta, Ga

Atherosclerosis, the pathological formation of fibrous and lipid-rich plaques in large arteries, is a disease modulated in part by patterns of blood flow. Although all arteries tend to change in composition and become more fibrous with age, a process known as arteriosclerosis, atherosclerosis is a focal disease with unique pathology wherein the arterial wall thickens in distinct sites. Numerous studies have noted that atherosclerotic plaques form preferentially in specific locations, suggesting that the mechanics of flowing blood regulates such biological remodeling.[1] Wall shear stress resulting from the frictional force of blood dragging against its surrounding arteries has been shown *in vitro* and *in vivo* to modulate atherogenic processes.[2] Atherosclerosis is a multifactorial disease that is present in nearly all persons in the modern world, but biomechanics influences the location, progression, and resulting morbidity.

1. Overview and Clinical Significance

Among the most commonly-cited risk factors for atherosclerosis are hyperlipidemia, hypercholesterolemia, and hypertension, all chronic problems in the modern world. Consequently, atherosclerosis is the leading cause of death and mortality in North America and is associated with more than 12 million deaths worldwide each year.[3,4] Despite the prevalence of the disease in modern society, atherosclerosis is no modern phenomenon — advanced lesions have been observed in Egyptian mummies from thousands of years ago, when diet and lifestyle were notably different from what a person would likely experience today.[5] Because a complex array of risk factors influences the formation and progression of plaques, atherosclerosis cannot be prevented by simple maintenance of one's cholesterol, lipid levels, and blood pressure. Biomechanical factors that are innate to all humans also contribute to the formation of lesions.

The formation of atherosclerotic plaques begins during childhood, but morbidity and mortality resulting from atherosclerosis typically does not occur until adulthood.[3] Negative outcomes associated with atherosclerotic lesions are the result of reduced blood flow, which leads to ischemia and infarction of tissue downstream from the site of occluded flow. Extremely advanced plaques form significant stenoses. Such stenoses may result in reduced blood flow, especially noteworthy in the coronary arteries, where myocardial infarction can cause scar formation and heart failure leading to cardiac death. Highly stenotic plaques may also cause a drop in blood pressure across the stenosis that may alter blood flow patterns and reduce velocity, yielding an entirely different hemodynamic environment when compared to nonstenotic vessels.[6]

Plaques can restrict blood flow indirectly if they form a thrombus. A thrombus may partially or completely occlude blood flow through the artery or embolize distally, even if the plaque itself is not stenotic.[6] Traditionally, atherosclerosis-related thrombosis was almost always thought to be result of plaque rupture, when the plaque acutely breaks open and exposes its thrombogenic components.[7] Recently, a second process for atherosclerosis-induced thrombus formation called plaque erosion was described. Like ruptured plaques, eroded plaques form thrombi that partially or completely occlude blood flow, but unlike ruptured plaques, an eroded plaque does not disrupt the fibrous cap or contain a thrombus that communicates with the necrotic core (Fig. 1).[8]

To address the problem of blood flow occlusion or restriction by plaques, the modern clinician may select from several interventional tools to treat atherosclerosis. Popular procedures currently include thrombolysis, stent implantation, angioplasty, endarterectomy, and bypass grafting.[9] Statin therapy has also been shown effective at reducing serum cholesterol, hindering the progression of atherosclerotic lesions and perhaps even causing regression of plaques or stabilizing plaques likely to rupture.[10] However effective these tools might be, clinicians still require better techniques to identify and treat, or, better yet, prevent, atherosclerotic plaques.[11] Such techniques might only be derived by a comprehensive understanding of the interplay between vascular biology and mechanics.

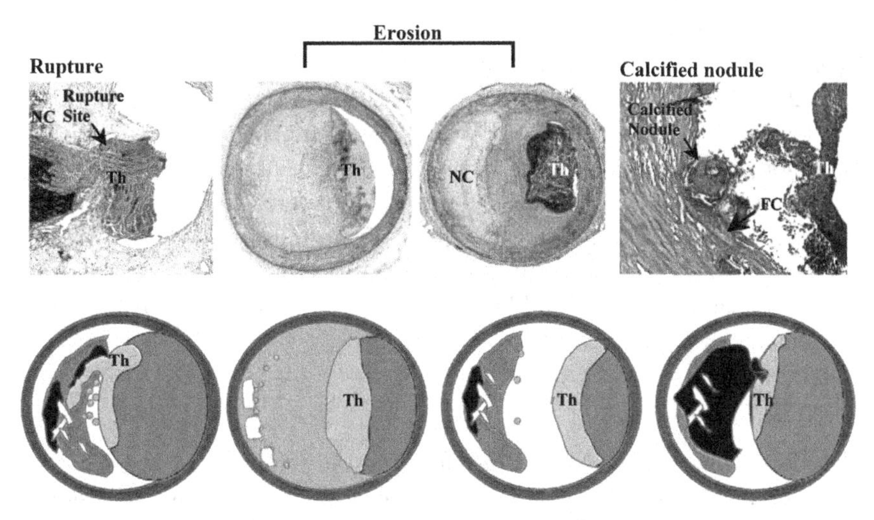

Fig. 1. Histological cross-sections demonstrate different types of lumenal thrombus (Th) formation. Diagrams below each section demonstrate how the thrombus is located relative to the rest of the lesion, particularly the necrotic core (NC). Ruptured plaques (left) have a thin fibrous cap over the necrotic core, and the thrombus communicates with this necrotic core. In eroded samples, the fibrous cap is intact, and the thrombus does not communicate with the necrotic core. In the lesion at right, a calcified nodule has erupted from the fibrous cap, and a thrombus has formed.[12]

1.1. *Composition and Progression of Atherosclerotic Plaques*

A healthy artery consists of three layers: the intima, a monolayer of endothelial cells that lines the lumen of the vessel, the media, a layer of smooth muscle cells and elastic lamina, and the adventitia, an outer layer of fibrous tissue that stabilizes the artery against the surrounding organs. In atherosclerosis, tissue called neointima forms underneath the endothelial monolayer and, in more advanced lesions, replaces the media. This neointima typically will develop a lipid-rich core of necrotic tissue, surrounded by a cap of predominantly fibrous tissue.[13,14] In very advanced lesions, calcification occurs inside the plaque.[15] Macrophages engorged with low-density lipoprotein (LDL) and cholesterol, called foam cells, may enter the plaque through extravasation, undergo apoptosis, and deposit cholesterol inside the core.[16]

Because atherosclerotic plaques develop over a period of decades, investigators may encounter plaques with distinct morphological features in varying stages of development. The American Heart Association (AHA) appointed a Committee on Vascular Lesions to formulate a classification scheme to describe atherosclerotic plaques in each phase of development (Fig. 2). Although atherosclerosis can be described as a "continuum of histological changes in the arterial wall", this committee's reports describe six major phenotypes of plaques, each at a distinct phase in the progression of atherosclerosis.[10,17,18] Lesions begin as fatty streaks in the walls of arteries, typically in children. Macrophage foam cells invade these streaks and become necrotic, creating a lipid-laden necrotic core underneath a fibrous cap that may grow and become stenotic, rupture or erode and form a thrombus, or become calcified.[12,19]

1.1.1. *Early Lesions*

The exact mechanism for lesion initiation in humans is not known. The dominant hypotheses regarding the formation of initial lesions, classified as AHA Type I, involve cholesterol accumulation in the matrix of vessel walls or endothelial injury. Under these conditions, isolated foam cells, macrophages containing lipid droplets, enter the region.[18] Injured endothelial cells are known to produce surface proteins such as intracellular adhesion molecule (ICAM-1) and vascular cell adhesion molecule (VCAM-1) to signal for inflammatory cells, lending plausibility to this hypothesis.[20,21] Whatever the underlying pathology, isolated foam cells appear within a small but distinct region. AHA Type I lesions are most frequently observed in infants and very young children, although they may be present in adults in vascular regions thought to be resistant to plaque formation as result of local flow mechanics.[18]

When these isolated regions grow to macroscopically visible fatty streaks, they are classified as AHA Type II lesions, also known as xanthomas (defined as "focal accumulations of fat-laden macrophages").[12] Larger clusters of foam cells are present, and lipid droplets are additionally present in smooth muscle cells. These lesions are subclassified into progression-prone (Type IIa) and progression-resistant (Type IIb) lesions based on propensity to advance to Type III. Slight morphological differences exist between these two subclasses (progression-prone lesions contain more foam cells and smooth muscle cells, for example), but the greatest determinant of progression at this point is the dynamic of blood flow across the lesion. The location in the vasculature determines the relative level of wall shear stress the plaque will experience, and regions of low and oscillatory wall shear stress tend to be atherogenic, which is to say that the lesion will

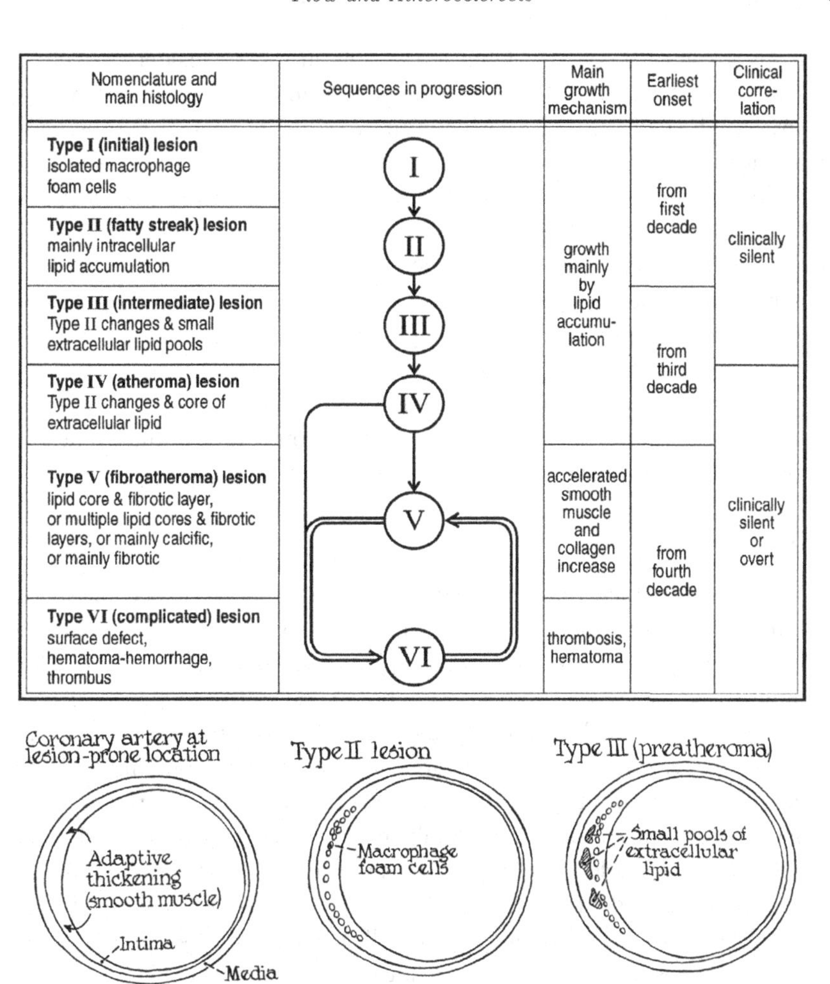

Nomenclature and main histology	Sequences in progression	Main growth mechanism	Earliest onset	Clinical corre-lation
Type I (initial) lesion isolated macrophage foam cells	I	growth mainly by lipid accumu-lation	from first decade	clinically silent
Type II (fatty streak) lesion mainly intracellular lipid accumulation	II			
Type III (intermediate) lesion Type II changes & small extracellular lipid pools	III		from third decade	
Type IV (atheroma) lesion Type II changes & core of extracellular lipid	IV			clinically silent or overt
Type V (fibroatheroma) lesion lipid core & fibrotic layer, or multiple lipid cores & fibrotic layers, or mainly calcific, or mainly fibrotic	V	accelerated smooth muscle and collagen increase	from fourth decade	
Type VI (complicated) lesion surface defect, hematoma-hemorrhage, thrombus	VI	thrombosis, hematoma		

Fig. 2. The American Heart Association Committee on Vascular Lesions of the Council on Arteriosclerosis defined six types of distinct atherosclerotic lesions. The classification scheme is described at top, and sketches of characteristic lesions for each type are drawn at bottom.[17]

likely progress to Type III. Type IIb lesions are not considered likely to advance. In general, Type II lesions emerge around puberty in humans.[18]

Although slight intimal thickening may occur in Type II lesions, more pronounced, pathological intimal thickening is observed in AHA Type III lesions, also known as "intermediate" or "preatheromas". Pools of extracellular lipid exist between smooth muscle cells, replacing the matrix that typically holds these cells together. However, these lipid pools are not organized into a large, confluent lipid core characteristic of a traditional plaque. The increased amount of lipid over that observed in Type II lesions is complimented by an increase in the amount of free cholesterol, as well. Pathological intimal thickening and accumulation of extracellular lipid pools and cholesterol frequently occurs in young adults and eventually progresses into an AHA Type IV developed plaque.[18]

1.1.2. *Advanced Lesions*

After the first 3 stages of progression, plaque development becomes more divergent and unpredictable, likely because so many mechanical and biological factors are involved in the pathogenesis of plaque formation. Advanced lesions, AHA Types IV, V, and VI, describe plaques with large confluent lipid pools that may or may not be associated with significant fibrous tissue, calcification, or thrombus formation. The most fundamental of these types is the Type IV lesion, also known as the "atheromatous plaque", which progresses from a Type III lesion after the lipid pools merge to form a single large lipid core. Typically, the atheroma is located eccentrically towards the wall of the vessel where intimal thickening occurred in stages I-III. Smooth muscle cells become dispersed and replaced with fibrous tissue, and vascularity increases within the plaque around the periphery of the lipid pool to supply blood to the thick wall of the artery.[17]

All arteries become more fibrous with age as result of arteriosclerosis, and atherosclerotic plaques are no exception. As the plaque ages, it becomes more fibrous and may diverge into one of several types of advanced plaques, and thus the AHA has defined three subclassifications for Type V lesions. If the plaque forms new fibrous tissue but retains a large lipid core (or cores if fibrous tissue subdivides lipid regions), it is an AHA Type Va (or simply a Type V) lesion. If calcification replaces part of the plaque, it is a Type Vb (sometimes called a Type VII) lesion, and if the lipid core is mostly replaced with fibrous tissue, leaving a predominantly fibrous region, the

AHA classification denotes these as Type Vc (also called a Type VIII) lesion.[17]

When plaques experience mechanical stresses past the threshold sustainable by their material components, fissuring occurs.[7] The AHA recognizes histological consequences of three types of plaque disruption: hematoma (Type VIa), hemorrhage (Type VIb), and thrombus formation (Type VIc). The former two pathologies likely result from disruption of blood vessels within the lesion supplying blood to the plaque tissue itself, while thrombus formation occurs when blood flowing through the lumen of the artery clots over the plaque, occluding blood flow. All three subclassifications of Type VI plaque disruption events are frequently subclinical, and pathologists have observed disrupted plaques that have healed and re-ruptured multiple times.[17]

Not formally recognized under the AHA classification scheme as a distinct type of plaque is the thin-cap fibroatheroma, sometimes called the "vulnerable plaque". Such a plaque would be classified by the AHA as a Type IV or Type Va lesion, but these categories fail to distinguish between plaques based on cap thickness. Observational and experimental evidence suggest that plaques with fibrous caps thinner than 65 nm are most prone to rupture and form a thrombus, while plaques with fibrous caps thicker than this threshold tend to remain clinically silent and not become disrupted.[12] While classification of plaques based on cap thickness presumes that plaque rupture is the cause of thrombosis and ignores other thrombogenic events such as plaque erosion and calcified nodule eruption, such a classification can help investigators identify a portion of plaques that are likely to cause a thrombus. Erosion may occur in lesions with thicker fibrous caps or even without a lipid pool (Type IV, Va, and Vc), although it has not been established as such a common cause of thrombosis as rupture.[22]

1.1.3. *Outward Remodeling and Plaque Stenosis*

Flow may also be disrupted by stenotic plaques that reduce the cross-sectional area of the lumen, increasing resistance and reducing blood flow across the stenosis. Although plaque formation is a vascular remodeling process that results in a thickened wall, paradoxically, many plaques do not result in any lumenal stenosis. According to theoretical framework developed by Glagov *et al.*, plaques initially expand the vessel wall outward, preserving the diameter of the lumen. Most lesions classified as Type IV under the AHA scheme exhibit minimal, if any, degree of stenosis. Only after the lesion has increased to occupy about 40% of the area inside the internal elastic lamina (the elastic layer between the media and intima) does it begin to remodel inward and form a stenosis.[23] While some plaques do eventually form significant stenosis and occlude blood flow, these plaques are quite advanced.[24]

2. Methods for Studying the Role of Flow in the Pathogenesis of Atherosclerosis

Cardiovascular flows can be quite intricate. Tortuous vascular geometry, narrowing in more distal vessels, and bifurcating vessels all create a complex environment where flow conditions can vary widely between seemingly similar vessels. Flow is pulsatile, and both heart rate and stroke volume, metrics affecting total cardiac output, can vary in response to a plethora of external stimuli and affect the amount of blood traveling through vessels. Upstream as well as downstream conditions can affect pressures and velocities of flow.[25] Vessels are compliant, lending capacitance to the arterial tree. The no-slip condition mandates that blood velocity is always zero immediately at the arterial wall, but velocity is nonzero inside the lumen away from the wall, leading to parabolic or more complicated velocity profiles across the area of the lumen (Fig. 3). Blood itself is complex, as it is a suspension of solid erythrocytes and other cells suspended in plasma.[26] All of these factors affect the flow environment that endothelial cells sense and to which they respond through the process of mechanotransduction. For this reason, investigators interested in the biomechanics of flow and atherosclerosis may use *in vitro*, *in vivo*, or *in silico* (computational) methods to understand biological responses to mechanical stimuli.

2.1. *Tools for Studying Biological Responses to Mechanical Stimuli in Vitro*

Among the most direct methods of studying atherogenic or atheroprotective responses to mechanical stimuli is through *in vitro* cell culture work. Under very controlled conditions, an investigator can modulate flow across plated vascular cells such as endothelium or smooth muscle. Polymerase chain reaction (PCR), immunohistochemistry, and other assays performed on these cells can reveal how biological function is modulated by shearing flow. Because of the established link between atherosclerosis and both

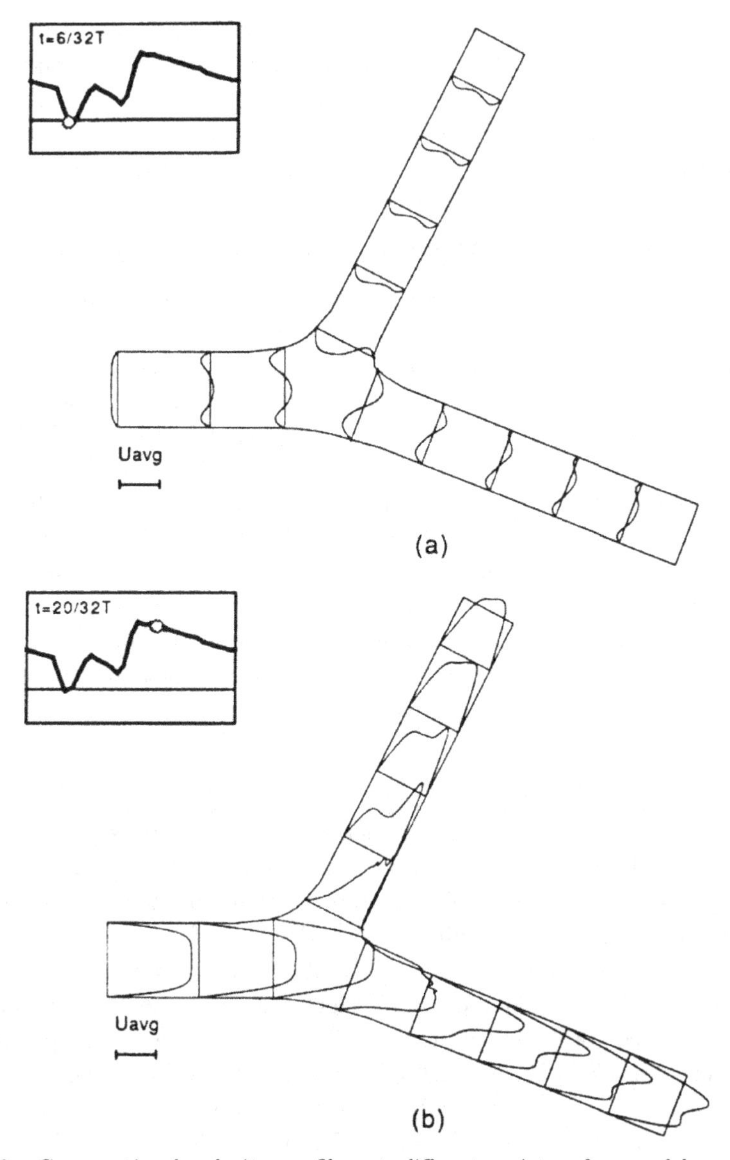

Fig. 3. Cross-sectional velocity profiles at different points of a model coronary branch site during (a) systole and during (b) diastole. Blood velocity is always zero at the walls as result of the no-slip condition, but velocity away from the wall may demonstrate parabolic, "M-shaped", or other profiles depending on flow conditions and geometry.[1]

magnitude and direction of shear stress, investigators often study gene expression in response to low, high, and oscillatory shearing flow conditions. Unidirectional steady flow, pulsatile flow, and spinning disc chambers all mimic specific aspects of cardiac-driven flow of interest in the pathogenesis of atherosclerosis.[27]

2.2. *Animal Models of Atherosclerosis and Relation to Flow*

Animal models provide a direct means for investigators to study the pathogenesis of atherosclerosis *in vivo*. While *in vitro* studies reveal how isolated endothelium modulates its biological response to flow conditions, an *in vivo* system contains additional tissue types and provides a more accurate picture of how different tissues interact to form atherosclerotic plaques. An *in vivo* animal model is more physiologically relevant towards investigation of human pathology, but isolating specific causal mechanisms may be more difficult than *in vitro*. In addition to the extra degrees of freedom resulting from the presence of other organ systems, investigators must consider differences between human and animal physiology such as heart rate, blood pressure, and protein differences. Despite the presence of confounding physiological processes, several animal models are routinely employed in cardiovascular research.[28]

2.2.1. *Genetically-manipulated Mouse Models*

Among the most common animal model is the atherosclerosis-prone mouse. Traditional laboratory rodents are naturally resistant to plaque formation except under extreme high-fat dietary conditions or when genes related to lipid metabolism are manipulated.[29] Because of the relative ease of manipulating the mouse genome, two of the most popular and best-characterized animal models of atherosclerosis are in mice. The low-density lipoprotein receptor knockout mouse ($LDLr^{-/-}$) and the Apolipoprotein E knockout mouse ($ApoE^{-/-}$) both reliably and rapidly form atherosclerotic plaques that are morphologically similar to those observed in humans, particularly when fed a high-fat diet.[30] Both animals have lost the ability to produce proteins essential for lipoprotein metabolism and clearance from the bloodstream, although the $LDLr^{-/-}$ mouse is considered a more moderate model than its $ApoE^{-/-}$ counterpart. Consequently, these mice become hyperlipidemic and hypercholesterolemic, and advanced lesions can appear within several weeks when fed an atherogenic diet.[30]

Popularity of the atherosclerosis-prone mouse model is due in part to its propensity to form plaques in similar anatomic locations as in humans. Plaques tend to form at the aortic sinus, the inner curvature of the aortic arch, on the upstream edge of the brachiocephalic and left common carotid arteries proximal to branching from the arch, and in the descending aorta; all occur at sites of relatively low wall shear stress when compared to nearby sections of artery or in regions of disturbed flow.[31,32] Using assays of mRNA expression and immunostaining on tissue harvested from mice, investigators have identified many signaling proteins involved in plaque formation that are also present in human plaques, such as inflammatory proteins like ICAM-1 and VCAM-1 and the production of reactive oxygen species in the endothelium (Fig. 4).[20]

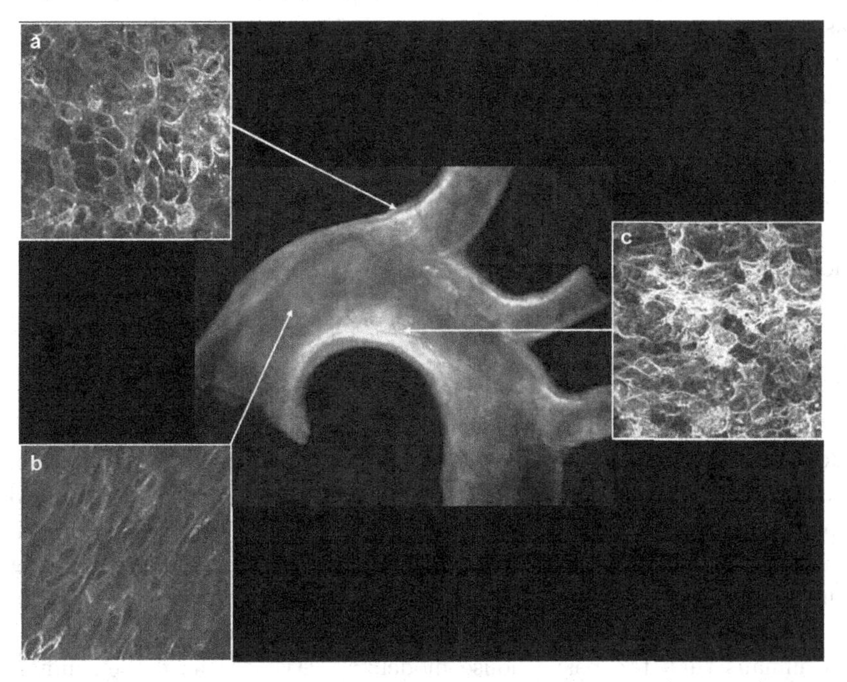

Fig. 4. Fluorescent expression of vascular cell adhesion molecule-1 (VCAM-1) labeled with quantum dots in the aortic arch of a mouse. Epifluorescent whole mount (center) and *en face* confocal microscopy (inlays a-c) reveal that VCAM-1 is expressed mostly on the upstream sides of branching vessels (a) and the inner curvature of the arch (c) as compared to other regions of the vessel (b). Computational fluid dynamic analysis of blood flow through the aorta found that regions of lowest mean wall shear stress (WSS) corresponded with regions of highest VCAM-1 fluorescent expression.[20]

2.2.2. *Mechanical Induction of Stenosis in Animals*

To eliminate the possibility that plaque localization is due to biological differences in the walls of arteries where lesions tend to form, several investigators have directly altered flow dynamics by inducing a coarctation in animal models. By placing a clip or a cast with a narrow inner diameter around an otherwise astenotic artery, researchers can alter flow conditions to study vascular response to a specific mechanical environment. Often, a large coarctation will create a zone of relatively high wall shear stress upstream of the stenotic region and low or oscillatory shear stress distal from the stenosis.[33,34,35]

In rats, organisms naturally resistant to plaque formation, animals subjected to aortic coarctation and a high-fat diet developed intimal thickening specifically in regions of aorta experiencing low wall shear stress as result of the clip. Areas exposed to relatively higher wall shear stress did not exhibit any evidence of atherosclerosis.[33] A similar study in mice placed constricting casts on carotid arteries and found that lesions formed in regions of low and oscillatory wall shear stress but not high wall shear stress. The authors also noted that the frequency of intraplaque hemorrhage was highest in regions of low but not oscillatory shear stress, suggesting that flow-modulated processes may be related to atherosclerotic morbidity and not merely to plaque occurrence.[35]

2.2.3. *Larger Animal Models of Atherosclerosis*

Although mice are popular animal models in atherosclerosis research, larger animal species may provide additional insight into human pathology. Because many small rodents are naturally resistant to plaque formation, investigators must carefully control genetic, dietary, and biomechanical conditions in order to induce atherosclerosis. As with any animal model, cautious characterization of the model must be performed before applying any insights gained from animal research towards humans. Larger animals such as rats, rabbits, swine, and primates are metabolically more similar to humans than the basic mouse model.[28,29] Also, because the animals are larger, their blood vessel diameters and heart rates are closer to that of humans, and consequently flow conditions more closely mimic human hemodynamics. However, larger animals require more space and food to house than do mice, increasing the cost to use these models. Pigs and primates live much longer than most standard laboratory rodents and develop atherosclerotic lesions more slowly, so the time course of larger animal experiments may be extended over that required for an experiment using mice. Additionally, as must be considered in any animal research, use of larger animal models such as primates carries a larger ethical burden.[29]

2.3. *Flow in Humans and Its Role in Atherosclerosis*

Atherosclerotic plaques in humans, which develop according to the phases classified by the American Heart Association Committee on Vascular Lesions, form preferentially in specific locations in the human vascular tree.[36] While no artery is immune from the possibility of plaque formation, regions experiencing relatively lower levels of wall shear stress and regions experiencing oscillatory flow reversal tend to be most at risk to form lesions (AHA Type IIa lesions in these areas are considered "progression-prone"). AHA Type IIb ("progression-resistant") lesions are usually located where wall shear stress is relatively higher.[18] The inner edges of curving vessels and branching vessels immediately distal to bifurcation are most prone to lesion formation.[37]

A retrospective survey of 13,827 patients from one hospital determined that nearly all lesions occur in four primary regions in the body. The coronary arteries, major branches of the aortic arch such as the carotid arteries, the visceral branches of the abdominal aorta such as the renal arteries, and the terminal branches of the abdominal aorta such as the femoral arteries are the principal regions where plaques form in humans.[38] Other regions, such as the thoracic aorta where minimal branching occurs, tend not to form lesions.[6] The coronary arteries, which supply blood to the myocardium, branch frequently and often form plaques immediately distal to divisions.[39] Similar patterning of atherosclerotic plaques is observed in the abdominal aorta, where less branching occurs but lesions tend to form immediately distal to branch locations.[40,41] The internal mammary artery, a long, straight vessel with few bifurcations and consequently minimal flow disturbance, rarely forms lesions, even in patients exhibiting advanced atherosclerosis in other vessels.[42]

Blood flow in humans can be very complex because of the tortuous, branching geometry of the arterial tree and because the cardiac pulse wave must propagate through compliant vessels whose diameter decreases distally from the heart. Consequently, different regions of the arterial

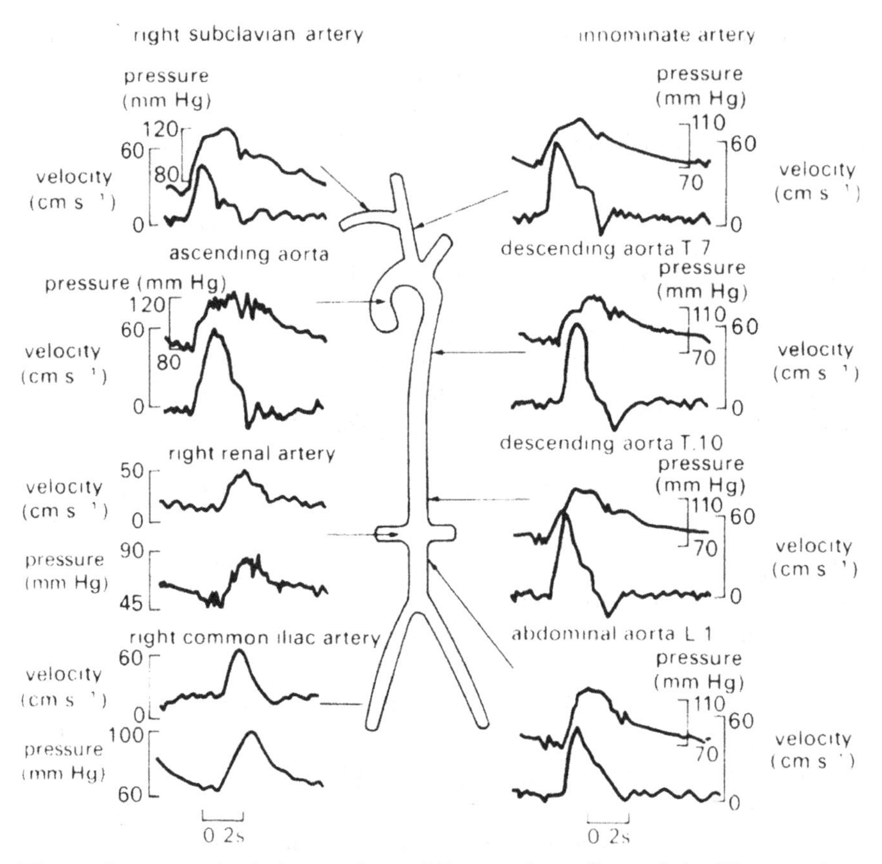

Fig. 5. Pressure and velocity waveforms differ over the cardiac cycle in different regions of the human aortic tree. Local geometric and flow parameters such as vessel diameter and vascular compliance all impact the phase and magnitude of the velocity and pressure of blood at each site.[1]

tree will experience different waveforms of flow across the cardiac cycle (Fig. 5).[1,6] An example of the impact of complex vascular geometry is found in the carotid arteries, which supply blood to the brain and also frequently form atherosclerotic plaques, where flow will often reverse directions during the cardiac cycle. The carotid bulb, a pouching on the internal carotid artery immediately distal to the carotid bifurcation, can form secondary flows due to its size, shape, and branching angles. While the external carotid artery typically remains plaque-free, the internal carotid artery routinely forms plaques (Fig. 6).[43,44] In the abdominal aorta, the geometry

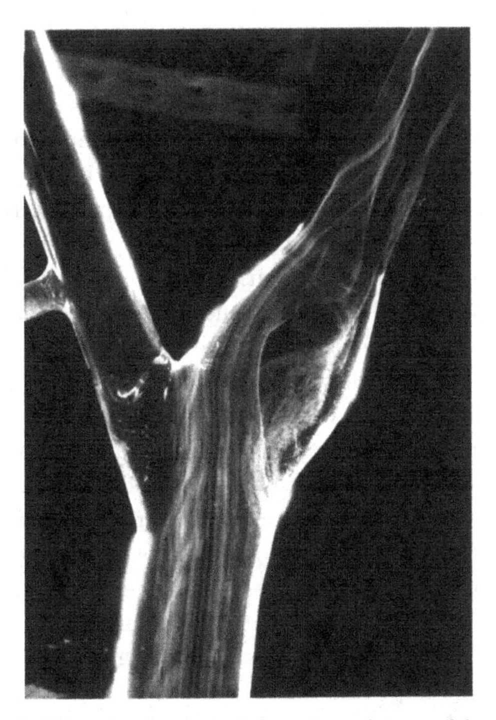

Fig. 6. Hydrogen bubble visualization of flow through a model carotid bifurcation. Secondary flows are present in the carotid bulb (middle right of bifurcation), creating a region of low-magnitude oscillatory shear stress where atherosclerotic lesions are known to form preferentially.[1]

of branching does not regularly create secondary flows, but the low wall shear stress regions still preferentially form plaques.[40] In the coronary arteries, blood flow occurs primarily during diastole rather than during systole. Although the flow waveform in the coronary arteries is temporally out of sync with other arteries, atherosclerotic plaques still form in regions modulated by flow.[1,6]

2.4. *Computational Fluid Dynamics*

When researchers study biological responses to flow conditions *in vivo* or *in vitro*, analysis of experimental results often requires an understanding of the system's flow conditions. The speed and direction of flow, as well as the wall shear stress (WSS), are flow parameters of interest that are extremely difficult to measure directly at high resolution without significantly disturbing the flow system.[45] Instead, numerical values are often calculated via solutions to the Navier-Stokes equations, a mathematical framework that describes the motion of fluids. Traditionally, to make such calculations manageable, simplifying assumptions about the nature of the flow had to be employed.[25] Consequently, researchers were only able to determine approximate values for flow and were typically limited to studying idealized systems such as cylindrical tubes or non-pulsatile hemodynamics. With the advent of more powerful computers and more efficient algorithms, researchers have become able to eliminate some of these assumptions in order to study the more complicated nature of realistic *in vivo* flows.

Currently, among the most popular tools for studying vascular flows involves the use of computational fluid dynamics (CFD), a technique for simulating flow with computers. Especially when coupled with *in vivo* or *in vitro* experimentation, CFD enables researchers to analyze flow conditions in any location of a physiologically realistic vessel at any point during the cardiac cycle.[46] While traditional engineering analysis of vasculature simplifies arteries to cylindrical tubes containing steady laminar flow, an acceptable first-order approximation for the geometry of vessels, wall shear stress can only be computed for the entire region:

$$\tau = \frac{32\mu Q}{\pi D^3} \tag{2.1}$$

where τ is the wall shear stress, μ is the dynamic viscosity of blood, Q is the blood velocity and D is the diameter of the cylinder.[6] Using CFD techniques, calculation of WSS in more complex environments becomes possible, such as in curving vessels which experience different WSS magnitudes on the inner edge and outer edge of curvature. A more accurate formula for WSS allows evaluation of its magnitude at any point within the geometry:

$$\tau = \mu \frac{\partial v}{\partial n} \tag{2.2}$$

where

$$\frac{\partial v}{\partial n} \tag{2.3}$$

is the near-wall velocity gradient.[25]

2.4.1. *Imaging Data for Lesion-specific Geometry*

To create more complicated computer models of vascular flow, especially patient-specific models, investigators must use imaging techniques to obtain data on flow and geometry through atherosclerosis-prone regions. While early CFD analysis of blood flow mostly simplified the vasculature to geometric, smooth cylinders, modern imaging and computation technology allows simulation of patient-specific blood flow.[47] Currently, most CFD analysis remains within research labs. Patient-specific CFD may soon become feasible within a clinical setting, allowing rapid identification of WSS conditions favorable for atherogenesis so that rapid, targeted interventions may prevent atherosclerosis-related morbidity and mortality.[46]

Currently, the only means of real-time *in vivo* flow visualization is with color Doppler vascular ultrasound. This technique detects the velocity of flowing blood through an axial cross-section of the artery at relatively low resolution and, assuming the wall shear stress equation for cylinders (Eqn. 2.1), can approximate the wall shear stress in that region.[47] This technique can identify general regions of oscillatory flow and has been used to predict sites of atherogenesis in coarcted mice.[35] A more powerful means for imaging vascular flow is through magnetic resonance imaging (MRI). While more expensive to operate and more time-consuming to acquire, MRI can image the borders of the lumen of large arteries with MR angiography (MRA) techniques such as a time-of-flight (TOF) scan.[48,49,50] Using phase-contrast MR (PCMR) imaging, investigators can record the velocity of blood through cross-sectional slices of an artery across the cardiac cycle.[51] CFD models derived from MRA geometry and PCMR velocity boundary conditions are being used to correlate arterial wall thickening due to atherosclerosis with magnitude of wall shear stress.[52,53,54]

Other popular imaging techniques in cardiovascular research are angiography and intravascular ultrasound (IVUS). These techniques are invasive but can provide high-resolution imaging of stenotic plaques and vascular flow rate. Angiography is not effective at detecting non-stenotic plaques, but IVUS analysis coupled with ultrasound phase delay processing can identify components of the arterial wall itself.[55,56] Computed tomography (CT) scanning of vasculature can produce very high-resolution imaging of vascular walls, especially of calcifications within plaques, but CT cannot image flow.[57] Because each imaging methodology offers both benefits and drawbacks as input for CFD models, atherosclerosis researchers sometimes piggyback several imaging modalities to create a CFD model, although combination of image sources presents the additional challenge of image registration.

2.4.2. *Modeling Assumptions*

As in any type of research, experimental design requires the investigator to make simplifying assumptions. A good study should involve a well-characterized model system, and careful interpretation of conclusions based on accepted limitations is a necessity. In computational fluid dynamics, modelers simulate a discretely digitized environment that is only a representation of the true continuous physiological geometry. While an optimal computer model would be robust to all such simplifying assumptions, in reality such a model would be computationally infeasible. Therefore, researchers must keep in mind that a model is exactly that — a model, and a model is only as good as its assumptions. CFD calculation of precise WSS magnitudes may be impractical, as simplifying assumptions could significantly affect exact magnitudes.[26,58,59,60] Fortunately, evidence suggests that relative levels of WSS may be more important for plaque formation than exact magnitudes.[20,61] Humans experience a wide range of WSS magnitudes, and these magnitudes may vary greatly between individuals depending on factors like vascular diameter, cardiac output, and blood pressure.[1] Despite these differences, nearly all people develop some atherosclerosis, and arteries that experience relatively lower levels of WSS than others may be more likely to form plaques, regardless of the precise magnitude of WSS.[37]

3. Wall Shear Stress is a Potent Modulator of Plaque Formation and Localization

Endothelial mechanotransduction regulates metabolic processes and production of signaling molecules within the intima of arteries. Some of these processes cause atherogenesis, the formation of atherosclerotic plaques. The most potent of these modulators is wall shear stress, the result of the frictional force of blood dragging across the endothelium as it flows. As wall shear stress is uneven throughout the vasculature as result of complex flow patterns, so too are plaques unevenly distributed throughout the arterial tree. Specific anatomic features of arteries such as branch points and curving vessels tend to create similar wall shear stress patterns among individuals, and consequently, atherosclerotic plaques tend to form preferentially in specific locations.[62]

3.1. *Low and Oscillatory Wall Shear Stress Promote Atherosclerotic Plaque Formation*

Arteries experiencing relatively low or oscillatory wall shear stress tend to be most prone to form atherosclerotic plaques. In humans, the coronary arteries, the carotid bulb, and the branches of the abdominal aorta tend to experience such flow conditions and consequently form lesions.[1,37] Such sites are particularly of clinical interest because, although advanced lesions only form in humans over a period of decades, these arteries supply the heart, the brain, and other organs essential for homeostasis. Any lesion that could disrupt blood flow to such organs may result in significant morbidity or mortality.

The molecular mechanism of atherogenesis begins in the endothelium, which senses flow by means of mechanoreceptors and begins to produce molecules like reactive oxygen species (Fig. 7).[21] A complex array of downstream effectors are produced with antioxidant, anti-apoptotic, pro-differentiative, and anti-proliferative effects that interact to regulate vascular remodeling in response to such mechanical stimulus.[27] Among these effectors are tissue growth factor β (TGFβ) that regulates proliferation and inflammatory surface proteins such as ICAM-1 and VCAM-1 (Fig. 4).[21] These inflammatory proteins, when exposed on endothelial cells to the blood pool, recruit inflammatory cells and promote monocyte and leukocyte extravasation. These monocytes can become macrophages, and if they enclose a large quantity of lipid droplets, may become the foam cells necessary to initiate lesion formation.[63] Dozens of proteins and molecules interact in this process of mechanotransduction, forming a tightly regulated and highly complex network that results in lesion formation over a time scale of several decades.[21,27,36]

3.2. *High Wall Shear Stress Protects Arteries from Atherosclerosis*

Conversely, while low or oscillatory shear stress upregulate atherogenic processes, relatively high levels of wall shear stress tend to be athero-protective, which is to say that lesions are less likely to form in these

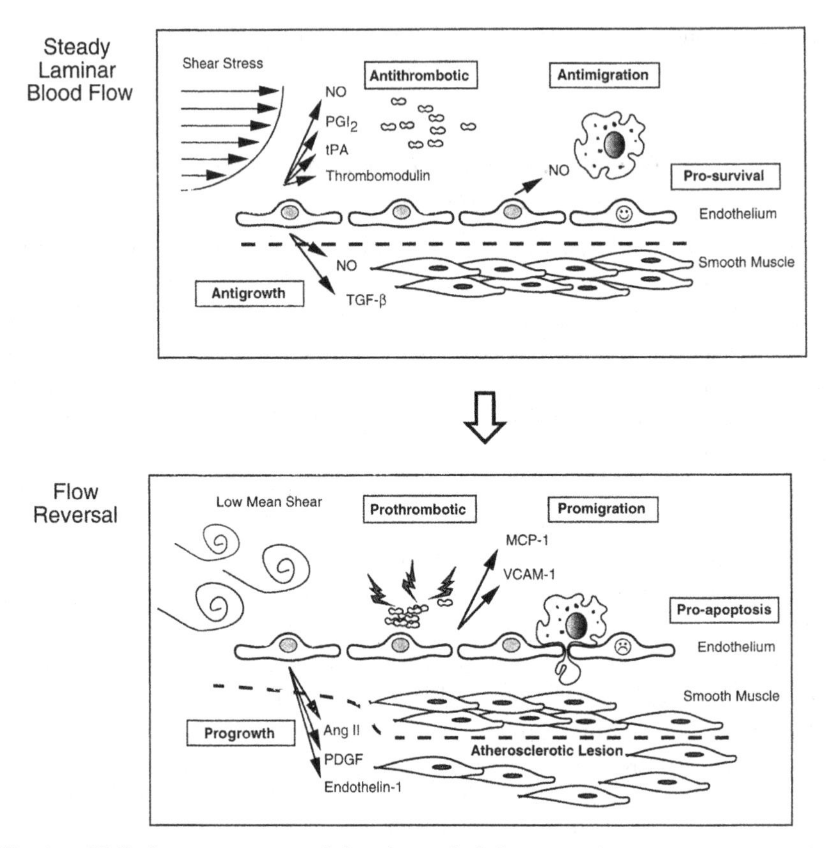

Fig. 7. Wall shear stress sensed by the endothelium regulates numerous vascular biological processes through mechanotransduction. Many of these processes, such as apoptosis, the production of inflammatory proteins, and macrophage recruitment, are associated with atherogenesis.[64]

regions. Rather than producing reactive oxygen species that cause oxidative damage to cells and upregulate inflammatory processes, endothelial cells experiencing higher levels of wall shear stress remain more stable.[37] However, definitions of "high" and "low" wall shear stress are relative terms, and a quantitative threshold between atheroprotective and atherogenic regions of WSS is difficult to define. WSS magnitudes in the aortic arch of mice are significantly higher than in humans, and yet plaques commonly form at this location in mice.[20] If atherogenesis was a binary process dependent purely upon WSS magnitude, which is to say that plaques form when WSS is below a certain threshold and do not form above that threshold, then atherosclerosis likely would not occur in mice. Rather, such a localized dependence on WSS for the presence or absence of atherosclerosis allows investigators to identify high-risk areas in humans as well as in animal or *in vitro* model systems.[20,46] In addition to WSS magnitude, directionality of flow may contribute to atherogenesis (Section 3.3, Section 5.3, and Fig. 8).[40]

3.3. *Hemodynamic Parameters Related to Plaque Formation*

Because the direct action of flowing blood across the endothelium elicits a biological response, investigators have identified several metrics to quantify patterns of flow. The most commonly-reported parameter is wall shear stress, the mechanical stimulus thought essential to form advanced plaques.[37] Because physiologic flow is rapid, pulsatile and cyclic while atherosclerosis develops gradually over a much longer timescale, investigators have derived additional parameters to collapse the properties of wall shear stress and flow into non-temporal metrics for comparison with vascular biology. Mean and maximum wall shear stress over the cardiac cycle are both popular metrics because of their simplicity to calculate and ease of interpretation. Both have been correlated with atherogenic response in model systems.[44]

However, more robust flow analysis should include broader consideration of temporal and spatial changes in wall shear stress. The wall shear stress gradient (WSSg) is a measure of spatial changes in WSS and may offer additional insight if one considers that relative levels of WSS might more significantly determine atherosclerosis than direct WSS magnitude. WSSg can be computed at any time during the cardiac cycle, so mean and maximum WSSg are both commonly-computed parameters as well.[65] Oscillatory shear index (OSI) is a measure of how much flow changes direction over the cardiac cycle. Several competing definitions for OSI exist, but all assess essentially the same phenomenon.[66] Perhaps the most straightforward definition of OSI is that proposed by Moore *et al.*:[67]

$$\mathrm{OSI} = \frac{\int_0^T |\tau \cdot \bar{\tau}| \; H(\tau \cdot \bar{\tau}) dt}{\int_0^T |\tau \cdot \bar{\tau}| \, dt} \tag{3.1}$$

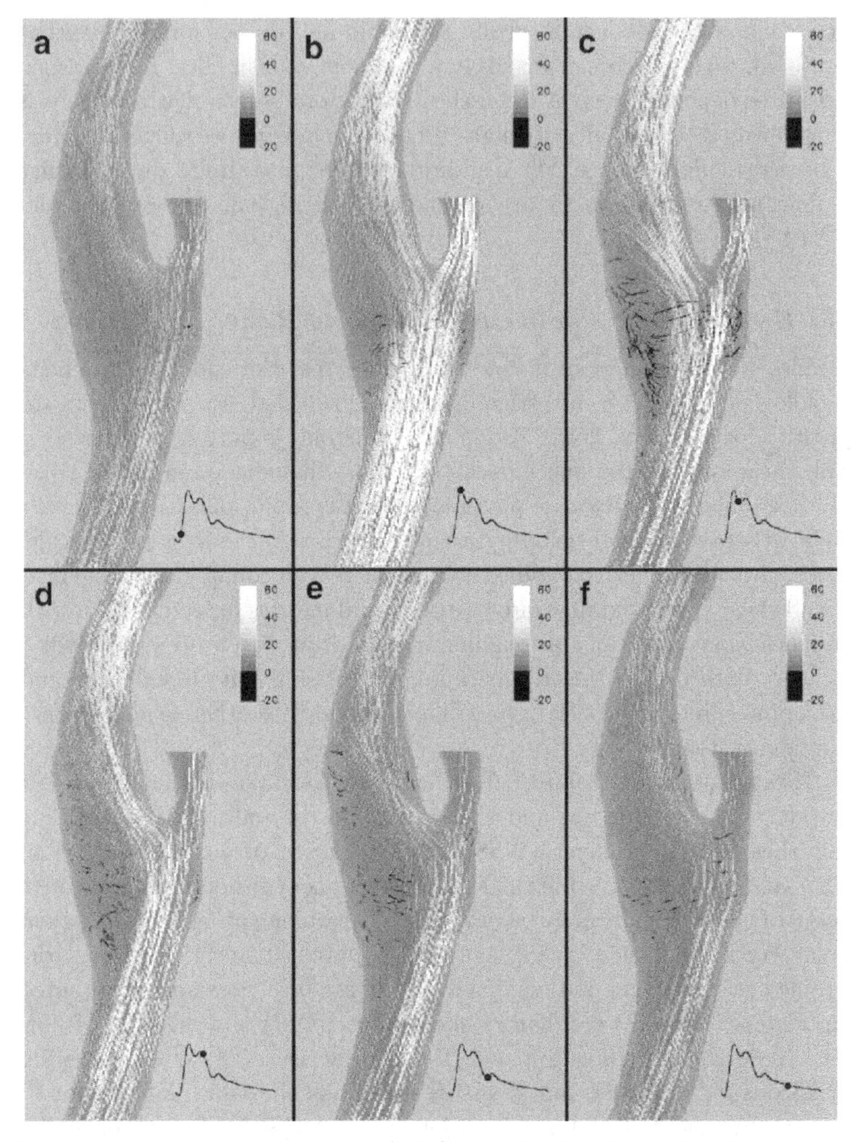

Fig. 8. Computational fluid dynamics (CFD) simulation of pulsatile blood flow through the bifurcation of the carotid artery reveals both the magnitude and direction of blood velocity throughout the lumen. Hemodynamic wall parameters such as wall shear stress (WSS) and oscillatory shear index (OSI) based on these velocity vectors may be correlated with the progression of atherosclerosis. Here, swirling flow with relatively low velocity magnitude (resulting in high OSI and low WSS) are observed in the carotid bulb, a site known to develop atherosclerotic plaques.[52]

where τ represents WSS at any time t during the total cardiac cycle of time T, $\bar{\tau}$ represents the mean shear direction:

$$\bar{\tau} = \int_0^T \frac{\tau}{\|\tau\|} dt \tag{3.2}$$

and H is the Heaviside unit function, a binary parameter which takes value 1 whenever the instantaneous shear direction exceeds an investigator-determined threshold between 0 and $\pi/2$. In other words, OSI measures the percent of the cardiac cycle when flow is going a different direction than the mean flow direction. OSI could be especially important in locating regions of oscillatory flow, which are known to be atherogenic but may not be identified by flow parameters like maximum wall shear stress (Fig. 9).

3.4. *Wall Shear Stress and Plaque Rupture*

Hemodynamic wall parameters may also be useful in predicting sites of plaque rupture.[69,70] When a plaque ruptures, the fibrous cap covering the lipid core fissures and opens, exposing the blood pool in the lumen to thrombogenic components inside the plaque.[7,24] Although it is not known why certain plaques rupture and others do not, a phenotype of plaques with a thin fibrous cap over a large lipid core is considered most "vulnerable" to rupture.[13,24] Hemodynamic disturbance may be linked to the plaque rupture event — case reports employing both MRI and IVUS imaging techniques paired with CFD have colocalized regions of very high wall shear stress with sites of plaque rupture.[69,70] Although relatively higher levels of wall shear stress are known to be atheroprotective, very high magnitudes of WSS could result in endothelial damage and weakening of the fibrous components comprising the caps of plaques.

4. Flow is Not the Only Biomechanical Determinant of Plaque Formation and Disruption

The biomechanics of blood flowing through arteries is linked to every phase of atherosclerosis, as wall shear stress is known to modulate plaque growth, and in some cases it may be more tightly linked to disruption. However, the biomechanics of atherosclerosis extends beyond wall shear stress and flow. Blood flowing through the lumen of arteries exerts pressure against vessel walls, which translates to solid mechanical stresses within the tissues

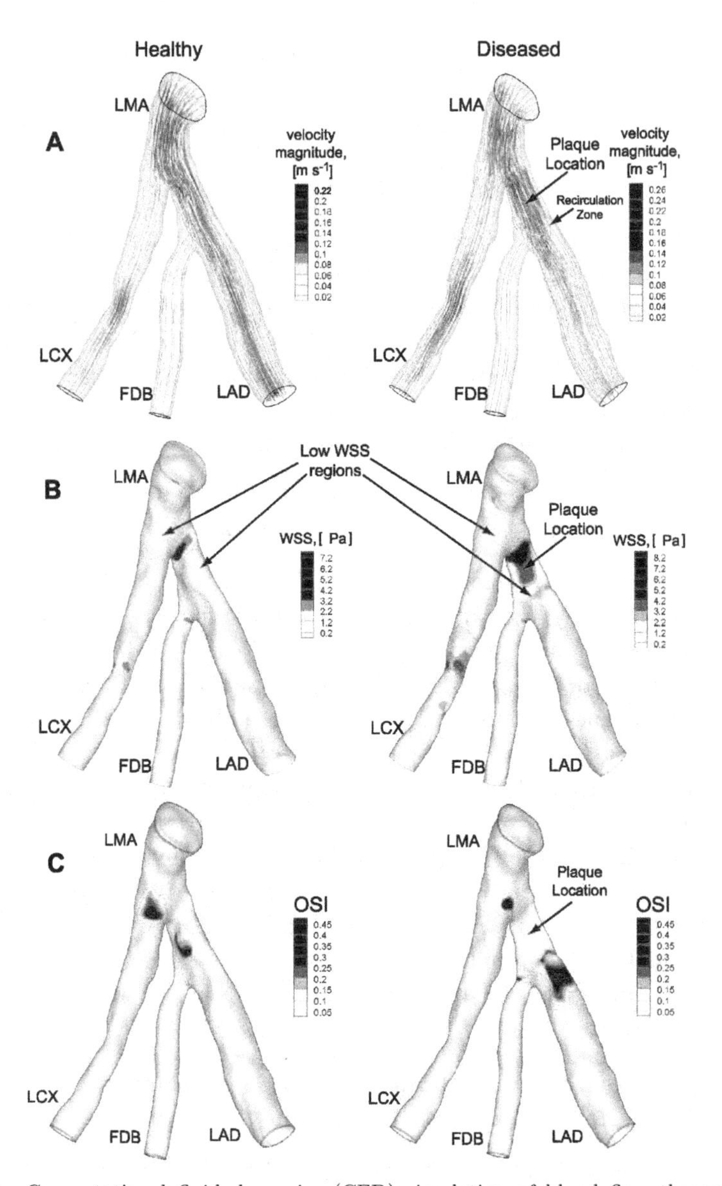

Fig. 9. Computational fluid dynamics (CFD) simulation of blood flow through the coronary artery of a patient with an atherosclerotic lesion (right column) and where the plaque has been digitally removed (left column). (A): Streamlines show increased blood velocity across a stenotic lesion. (B): In a healthy patient, wall shear stress (WSS) magnitude is relatively low where the lesion is known to form but is higher over a stenotic plaque. (C): Oscillatory shear index (OSI) reveals a region of oscillatory flow over the cardiac cycle in a healthy patient that is colocalized with the site of a lesion. Adapted from Ref. 68.

composing the walls as well. These internal stresses have been shown to modulate cell proliferation and vascular remodeling, and a comprehensive examination of the biomechanics of atherosclerosis is not complete without consideration of solid mechanics.[71]

4.1. *Solid Wall Mechanics and Atherosclerotic Responses to Stretch*

As vessels become distended by the pressure pulse from each heart beat, wall tissues sense and respond to strains.[62] While arteries are naturally compliant, lesion formation replaces components of the media and intima with new tissue, typically made of less compliant materials.[72] Consequently, biological processes regulated by stretch become dysregulated, especially when a plaque is located eccentrically towards one side of the artery.[73] The distribution of stresses and strains within the wall of the artery resulting from blood pressure becomes uneven as result of the heterogeneous arrangement of wall components.[56,72] Such dysregulation further contributes to asymmetric remodeling of arteries. Among other targets, an association between activated NF-κB, which is a marker of inflammation, and mechanical stress has been described.[71]

The relationship between mechanical stresses within the walls of arteries and the progression of atherosclerosis may be more complex than a simple monotonic relationship between stress and protein regulation, however. As each stage of plaque formation carries a unique set of morphological properties, so too may each stage correspond to a particular biological response to mechanical stress.[71] As described by Glagov and colleagues, arteries tend to remodel outward and preserve lumenal diameter until the vessel reaches a threshold of plaque burden, after which point inward remodeling commences and the plaque becomes stenotic.[23]

An additional mechanical consideration in vascular research is the effect of cyclic loading. Much as a rubber band becomes weakened after repeated stretching, so too might the walls of blood vessels become weakened in response to repeated distension from pulsing blood. While the difference between a rubber band and an artery is that the artery can heal itself and regenerate its walls, such cyclic effects might still weaken areas of the vessel over human timescales. A heart beating once per second will cause nearly one billion pulses in 30 years, and human lifetimes are often three times this amount. Computational studies of fatigue in lipid-rich plaques suggest that geometric shapes and locations of lipid pools under fibrous caps increase the likelihood of fissuring under cyclic loading.[74]

4.2. *Plaque Composition Influences Solid Wall Mechanics and Risk for Rupture*

Besides the remodeling response to stresses within vessel walls, cardiovascular researchers also take interest in the solid mechanics of plaques because of its role in plaque rupture. When stresses become too great, mechanical failure may occur and result in fissuring of the plaque.[75,76] Although blood vessels are coated with antithrombotic proteins on the surface of endothelial cells, fissuring of the fibrous cap over a lipid core will expose blood in the lumen to thrombogenic components inside the plaque and may form a thrombus.[7,24] Thrombosis that results in occluded blood flow will likely cause morbidity or mortality, so it is of clinical interest to identify such lesions for intervention before a clinical event.

Vascular researchers have identified a specific phenotype of plaques that tends to rupture most frequently: lesions with a thin fibrous cap over a large necrotic core, also known as the thin-cap fibroatheroma.[13] Ruptured lesions also tend to exhibit minimal stenosis but notable outward remodeling.[12,13] However, not all thin-cap fibroatheromas rupture, and many plaques remodel outward and subsequently inward without ever rupturing, suggesting that differences beyond gross phenotype influence vulnerability to rupture. Computer modeling of mechanical stresses within plaques has revealed that the size, shape, and geometric distribution of lesion components all impact the magnitude and location of stress concentrations within the wall (Fig. 10).[77,78] The thin-cap fibroatheroma ruptures more readily than other plaque phenotypes because stresses are concentrated on the fibrous cap, so material failure will expose the lipid core.[79] Typically, the site of greatest stress where rupture occurs is located at the shoulder of the plaque where the thin fibrous cap ends.[80] The thickness of the fibrous cap as well as the area, thickness, and angle of the lipid core all affect the magnitude of the stress experienced within vessel walls containing pressurized blood.[56,75,81] Stresses tend to be highest around calcified nodules, and some have suggested that calcification of advanced lesions is a biological mechanism to redistribute stresses away from the vulnerable fibrous cap and stabilize the plaque.[79] Conversely, others have proposed that microcalcifications within the thin fibrous cap itself may result in material debonding and cause the plaque to rupture.[82,83]

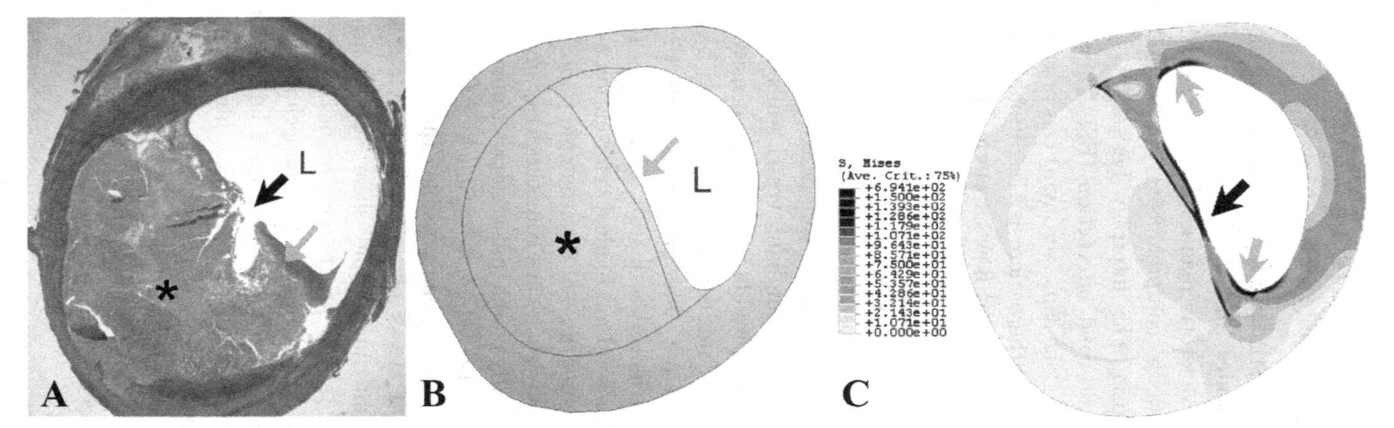

Fig. 10. Solid wall stresses are linked to fibrous cap fissuring that leads to plaque rupture. (A) A histological cross-section of a ruptured plaque demonstrates a break (black arrow) in the fibrous cap (grey arrow) over a large necrotic core (asterisk). When the plaque is digitally reconstructed (B), the stresses within the wall may be calculated using computational structural mechanics techniques (C). A map of wall stresses reveals the greatest stress magnitude almost exactly colocalized with the site of known rupture (black arrow). Two other regions of high stress (grey arrows) are also identified at the shoulders of the plaque, regions where plaques are known to rupture frequently.[78]

4.3. *Fluid-solid Interaction Provides Additional Biomechanical Insight into Atherosclerosis*

Numerous studies have demonstrated the critical nature of both fluid mechanics and solid mechanics in the initiation, progression, and potential disruption of atherosclerotic plaques. However, neither of these properties alone can provide a comprehensive understanding of the biomechanics of atherosclerosis. The interplay between both fluid and solid biomechanics, called fluid-solid interaction (FSI, alternately called fluid-structure interaction using the same acronym) can provide additional insight into the pathogenesis of atherosclerosis. Traditional computational fluid dynamic analysis simulates blood flow through a rigid vessel lumen and neglects the effects of compliance on blood flow. Similarly, traditional computational structural mechanics simulates vessel stretch based on average lumen blood pressures rather than pressures that vary with spatial location as result of the complexity of flowing blood. By coupling these computer models in FSI, an investigator can more robustly model the biomechanics within and against compliant vessel walls resulting from pulsatile blood flow.[84,85] FSI can provide more comprehensive insight into plaque disruption events such as rupture or erosion that may be due in large part to mechanical failure of plaque materials. For example, the fibrous cap over a plaque lipid core experiences both wall shear stress from viscous blood flowing over it as well as solid mechanical deformation as pressurized blood pushes on the cap and compresses it into the lipid pool.[86] Each single force alone may not explain why such caps sometimes become disrupted.

Not only does FSI potentially enable investigators to model blood flow with greater physiological accuracy, but also studies of the simultaneous effects of fluid and solid stresses become possible. Tarbell and colleagues have investigated the role of stress phase angle (SPA), a measure of the temporal lag between maximum fluid shear stress and maximum circumferential solid stress, in the progression of atherosclerosis. Such studies indicate that endothelial response to biomechanics varies from responses predicted by either fluid mechanics or by solid mechanics alone.[87] *In vitro* studies have shown that cells experiencing large magnitudes of SPA produce less nitrous oxide (NO) in endothelium, a condition linked to atherogenesis. Atherosclerosis-prone regions of the human vasculature such as the coronary arteries, the outer edge of the carotid artery, and the descending aorta all characteristically experience relatively larger SPA, and

FSI studies have shown that under hypertension, a traditional risk factor for atherosclerosis, SPA magnitude increases further.[88,89] This colocalization of high SPA with atherosclerosis and its related processes suggests that fluid mechanics and solid mechanics alone are not sufficient to characterize the details of atherogenesis. However, the complexity of implementing FSI models has prevented more widespread use at present, and further understanding of the role of properties like SPA is currently an unmet need in cardiovascular research.

5. Current Dilemmas and Future Directions for Atherosclerotic Research

Because morbidity and mortality resulting from cardiovascular disease affect so many people in the modern world, a large volume of research has investigated the causes, progression, and potential thrombogenic disruption of atherosclerotic plaques. Despite such focused effort by the research community, uncertainty remains about details in the pathology of atherosclerosis. Current techniques to identify and treat lesions thought likely to present clinical symptoms can benefit from further consideration and optimization. Future research will improve our ability to target vulnerable lesions by means of a better understanding of the role of fluid and solid stresses in atherosclerosis.

5.1. *Need for Better Understanding of Plaque Disruption Events*

Retrospective clinical studies and computer modeling analyses have identified a phenotype of atherosclerotic plaque most vulnerable to rupture, the thin-cap fibroatheroma. However, clinicians still lack the ability to predict exactly when or where such plaques will become disrupted. More selective identification of vulnerable lesions will eliminate unnecessary interventions and better target plaques not currently recognized as potential problems. As fluid and solid mechanics are both implicated in the pathogenesis of plaque disruption, further research exploring how FSI impacts rupture is necessary. Lesser-studied thrombogenic events like plaque erosion and formation of calcified nodules may also be influenced by the biomechanics of flow, but the mechanisms for these events are not well understood.

5.2. *How Do Flow-mediated Mechanisms of Atherogenesis Occur on Human Timescales?*

A large body of *in vitro* work has explained how mechanoreceptors in vascular tissue regulate atherogenic biological processes in response to flow conditions. In culture conditions, formation of reactive oxygen species results in molecular signaling cascades that are detectable within hours of onset of low or oscillatory shearing flow conditions. Expression of proteins directly associated with atherogenesis occurs inside of very short and precisely measurable timescales in response to flow stimuli. However, in humans, development and progression of lesions to full atherosclerotic plaques takes decades — AHA Type IV plaques are rarely observed in individuals less than 40 years of age, although Type I and Type II initial lesions are often observed in children.[17] Why does flow modulate macrophage recruitment within days *in vitro*, while large necrotic cores resulting from lipid-laden macrophage invasion only appear over a period of years *in vivo*, even when flow conditions are seemingly identical? Why do other atherogenic processes, when isolated *in vitro*, not produce the same effects in humans on the same timescale? Are other processes, undetectable within *in vitro* timescales and currently undiscovered as result, essential for atherosclerotic lesion formation? Future research must reconcile the orders of magnitude difference in timescale of response to flow conditions between *in vitro* and *in vivo* systems.

5.3. *How Much Does Directionality of Flow Contribute to Atherosclerosis?*

Evidence suggests that both low and oscillatory wall shear stress are atherogenic conditions. However, oscillatory flow can expose arteries to higher instantaneous magnitudes of WSS than in unidirectional low WSS regions. These higher magnitudes can reach levels experienced in atheroprotected regions of vasculature, and yet plaques form anyways. Because flow direction is changing in regions of oscillatory flow, the average wall shear stress endothelial cells experience over the cardiac cycle may be very low, and yet instantaneously it may be quite high. How do mean WSS and instantaneous WSS affect plaque formation and localization? Is one factor more important than the other? In both *in vitro* and *in vivo* work, different phenotypes of endothelial cells have been shown to grow under laminar flow and oscillatory flow conditions. Do these phenotypic differences translate to different types of plaques? More research is needed to study plaques that form under oscillatory and under laminar flow conditions and answer questions such as: Do plaques form more readily in one flow environment? Are plaques experiencing certain types of flow more likely to become disrupted and form a thrombus? Does flow modulate calcification or formation of additional fibrous tissue?

6. Conclusion

Atherosclerosis is a multifactorial disease that is related to over 12 million deaths annually and affects nearly all people in the modern world. In 2009, estimated direct and indirect costs for clinical care of cardiovascular disease in the United States alone are $475.3 billion.[9] As obesity, hypertension, and diabetes become more prevalent, so too will the need for care for atherosclerosis-related morbidity. Although atherosclerosis is a heavily-researched disease, more work remains. Clinicians require still better tools to identify and treat plaques that are likely to cause morbidity or mortality. While much is now understood about how mechanical flow conditions modulate biological responses that result in atherogenesis, investigators should strive for an increasingly comprehensive understanding of vascular biomechanics in order to further improve treatment. Vessels may be biological tissues, but in cardiology, one must always consider the effects of flow.[61]

References

1. Ku, D. N. (1997) Blood flow in arteries. *Annual Reviews of Fluid Mechanics* **29**, pp. 399–434.
2. Malek, A. M., Alper, S. L., and Izumo, S. (1999) Hemodynamic shear stress and its role in atherosclerosis. *JAMA: the journal of the American Medical Association* **282** (21), pp. 2035–42.
3. Kavey, R. W., Daniels, S. R., Lauer, R. M., Atkins, D. L., and Hayman, L. L. (2003) American Heart Association Guidelines for Primary Prevention of Atherosclerotic Cardiovascular Disease Beginning in Childhood. *Circulation* **107**(11), pp. 1562–1566.
4. Lopez, A. D., Mathers, C. D., Ezzati, M., Jamison, D. T., and Murray, C. J. (2001) Global and regional burden of disease and risk factors, 2001: systematic analysis of population health data. *The Lancet* **367**(9524), pp. 1747–1757.
5. Cockburn, E., and Reyman, T. A. (1998) *Mummies, Disease, & Ancient Cultures*, Cambridge University Press, Cambridge.

6. Wootton, D. M., and Ku, D. N. (1999) Fluid Mechanics of Vascular Systems, Diseases, and Thrombosis. *Annual Reviews of Biomedical Engineering* **1**, pp. 299–329.
7. Davies, M. J., and Thomas, A. C. (1985) Plaque fissuring–the cause of acute myocardial infarction, sudden ischaemic death, and crescendo angina. *British heart journal* **53**(4), pp. 363-73.
8. Farb, A., Burke, A. P., Tang, A. L., Liang, T. Y., Mannan, P., Smialek, J., and Virmani, R. (1996) Coronary plaque erosion without rupture into a lipid core. A frequent cause of coronary thrombosis in sudden coronary death. *Circulation* **93**(7), pp. 1354–63.
9. Lloyd-Jones, D., Adams, R., Carnethon, M., De Simone, G., Ferguson, T. B., Flegal, K., Ford, E., Furie, K., Go, A., Greenlund, K., Haase, N., Hailpern, S., Ho, M., Howard, V., Kissela, B., Kittner, S., Lackland, D., Lisabeth, L., Marelli, A., McDermott, M., Meigs, J., Mozaffarian, D., Nichol, G., O'Donnell, C., Roger, V., Rosamond, W., Sacco, R., Sorlie, P., Stafford, R., Steinberger, J., Thom, T., Wasserthiel-Smoller, S., Wong, N., Wylie-Rosett, J., and Hong, Y. (2009) Heart disease and stroke statistics–2009 update: a report from the American Heart Association Statistics Committee and Stroke Statistics Subcommittee. *Circulation* **119**(3), pp. e21–181.
10. Insull, W. (2009) The pathology of atherosclerosis: plaque development and plaque responses to medical treatment. *The American journal of medicine* **122**(1 Suppl), pp. S3–S14.
11. Ricotta, J. J., Pagan, J., Xenos, M., Alemu, Y., Einav, S., and Bluestein, D. (2008) Cardiovascular disease management: the need for better diagnostics. *Medical & biological engineering & computing* **46**(11), pp. 1059–68.
12. Virmani, R., Kolodgie, F. D., Burke, A. P., Farb, A., and Schwartz, S. M. (2000) Lessons from sudden coronary death: a comprehensive morphological classification scheme for atherosclerotic lesions. *Arteriosclerosis, thrombosis, and vascular biology* **20**(5), pp. 1262–75.
13. Virmani, R., Burke, A. P., Farb, A., and Kolodgie, F. D. (2006) Pathology of the vulnerable plaque. *Journal of the American College of Cardiology* **47**(8 Suppl), pp. C13–8.
14. Fuster, V., and Chesebro, J. H. (1996) Atherosclerosis — A. Pathogenesis: initiation, progression, acute coronary syndromes, and regression, Mayo Clinic Practice of Cardiology, E. Giuliani, B. Gersh, M. McGoon, D. Hayes, and H. Schaff, Mosby, St. Louis, pp. 1056–1081.
15. Huang, H., Virmani, R., Younis, H., Burke, A. P., Kamm, R. D., and Lee, R. T. (2001) The impact of calcification on the biomechanical stability of atherosclerotic plaques. *Circulation* **103**(8), pp. 1051–6.
16. Shah, P. K. (2009) Inflammation and plaque vulnerability. *Cardiovascular drugs and therapy/sponsored by the International Society of Cardiovascular Pharmacotherapy* **23**(1), pp. 31–40.
17. Stary, H. C., Chandler, A. B., Dinsmore, R. E., Fuster, V., Glagov, S., Insull, W., Rosenfeld, M. E., Schwartz, C. J., Wagner, W. D., and Wissler, R. W. (1995) A definition of advanced types of atherosclerotic

lesions and a histological classification of atherosclerosis. A report from the Committee on Vascular Lesions of the Council on Arteriosclerosis, American Heart Association. *Arteriosclerosis, thrombosis, and vascular biology* **15**(9), pp. 1512–31.
18. Stary, H. C., Chandler, A. B., Glagov, S., Guyton, J. R., Insull W., Rosenfeld, M. E., Schaffer, S. A., Schwartz, C. J., Wagner, W. D., and Wissler, R. W. (1994) A definition of initial, fatty streak, and intermediate lesions of atherosclerosis. A report from the Committee on Vascular Lesions of the Council on Arteriosclerosis, American Heart Association. *Circulation* **89**(5), pp. 2462–78.
19. Burke, A. P., Farb, A., Malcom, G. T., Liang, Y. H., Smialek, J., and Virmani, R. (1997) Coronary risk factors and plaque morphology in men with coronary disease who died suddenly. *The New England journal of medicine* **336**(18), pp. 1276–82.
20. Suo, J., Ferrara, D. E., Sorescu, D., Guldberg, R. E., Taylor, W. R., and Giddens, D. P. (2007) Hemodynamic shear stresses in mouse aortas: implications for atherogenesis. *Arteriosclerosis, thrombosis, and vascular biology* **27**(2), pp. 346–51.
21. Chatzizisis, Y. S., Coskun, A. U., Jonas, M., Edelman, E. R., Feldman, C. L., and Stone, P. H. (2007) Role of endothelial shear stress in the natural history of coronary atherosclerosis and vascular remodeling: molecular, cellular, and vascular behavior. *Journal of the American College of Cardiology* **49**(25), pp. 2379–93.
22. Arbustini, E., Dal Bello, B., Morbini, P., Burke, A. P., Bocciarelli, M., Specchia, G., and Virmani, R. (1999) Plaque erosion is a major substrate for coronary thrombosis in acute myocardial infarction. *Heart (British Cardiac Society)* **82**(3), pp. 269–72.
23. Glagov, S., Weisenberg, E., Zarins, C. K., Stankunavicius, R., and Kolettis, G. J. (1987) Compensatory enlargement of human atherosclerotic coronary arteries. *The New England Journal of Medicine* **316**(22), pp. 1371–5.
24. Fishbein, M. C. (2008) The vulnerable and unstable atherosclerotic plaque. *Cardiovascular pathology: the official journal of the Society for Cardiovascular Pathology.*
25. Panton, R. L. (2005) Incompressible Flow, Wiley.
26. Lee, S., and Steinman, D. A. (2007) On the relative importance of rheology for image-based CFD models of the carotid bifurcation. *Journal of biomechanical engineering* **129**(2), pp. 273–8.
27. Wasserman, S. M., and Topper, J. N. (2004) Adaptation of the endothelium to fluid flow: in vitro analyses of gene expression and in vivo implications. Vascular medicine (London, England), **9**(1), pp. 35–45.
28. Ni, M., Chen, W. Q., and Zhang, Y. (2009) Animal models and potential mechanisms of plaque destabilization and disruption. Heart (British Cardiac Society), (March).
29. Russell, J. C., and Proctor, S. D. (2006) Small animal models of cardiovascular disease: tools for the study of the roles of metabolic syndrome, dyslipidemia,

and atherosclerosis. *Cardiovascular pathology: the official journal of the Society for Cardiovascular Pathology* **15**(6), pp. 318–30.

30. Zadelaar, S., Kleemann, R., Verschuren, L., de Vries-Van der Weij, J., van der Hoorn, J., Princen, H. M., and Kooistra, T. (2007) Mouse models for atherosclerosis and pharmaceutical modifiers. *Arteriosclerosis, thrombosis, and vascular biology* **27**(8), pp. 1706–21.
31. Rosenfeld, M. E., Polinsky, P., Virmani, R., Kauser, K., Rubanyi, G., and Schwartz, S. M. (2000) Advanced atherosclerotic lesions in the innominate artery of the ApoE knockout mouse. *Arteriosclerosis, thrombosis, and vascular biology* **20**(12), pp. 2587–92.
32. Seo, H. S., Lombardi, D. M., Polinsky, P., Powell-Braxton, L., Bunting, S., Schwartz, S. M., and Rosenfeld, M. E. (1997) Peripheral vascular stenosis in apolipoprotein E-deficient mice. Potential roles of lipid deposition, medial atrophy, and adventitial inflammation. *Arteriosclerosis, thrombosis, and vascular biology* **17**(12), pp. 3593–601.
33. Prado, C. M., Ramos, S. G., Elias, J., and Rossi, M. A. (2008) Turbulent blood flow plays an essential localizing role in the development of atherosclerotic lesions in experimentally induced hypercholesterolaemia in rats. *International journal of experimental pathology* **89**(1), pp. 72–80.
34. Willett, N., Oshinski, J., Giddens, D., Guldberg, R., and Taylor, W. R. (2009) Redox Signaling in an In Vivo Murine Model of Tailored Wall Shear Stress. American Society of Mechanical Engineers 2009 Summer Bioengineering Conference, Lake Tahoe, CA.
35. Cheng, C., Tempel, D., van Haperen, R., van Der Baan, A., Grosveld, F., Daemen, M. J., Krams, R., and de Crom R. (2006) Atherosclerotic lesion size and vulnerability are determined by patterns of fluid shear stress. *Circulation* **113**(23), pp. 2744–53.
36. Slager, C. J., Wentzel, J. J., Gijsen, F. J., Thury, A., van Der Wal, A. C., Schaar, J. A., and Serruys, P. W. (2005) The role of shear stress in the destabilization of vulnerable plaques and related therapeutic implications. *Nature clinical practice. Cardiovascular medicine* **2**(9), pp. 456–64.
37. Slager, C. J., Wentzel, J. J., Gijsen, F. J., Schuurbiers, J. C., van Der Wal, A. C., van Der Steen, A. F., and Serruys, P. W. (2005) The role of shear stress in the generation of rupture-prone vulnerable plaques. *Nature clinical practice. Cardiovascular medicine* **2**(8), pp. 401–7.
38. DeBakey, M. E., Lawrie, G. M., and Glaeser, D. H. (1985) Patterns of atherosclerosis and their surgical significance. *Annals of surgery* **201**(2), pp. 115–31.
39. Mancini, G. B., Ryomoto, A., Kamimura, C., Yeoh, E., Ramanathan, K., Schulzer, M., Hamburger, J., and Ricci, D. (2007) Redefining the normal angiogram using population-derived ranges for coronary size and shape: validation using intravascular ultrasound and applications in diverse patient cohorts. *The international journal of cardiovascular imaging* **23**(4), pp. 441–53.
40. Moore, J. E., Xu, C., Glagov, S., Zarins, C. K., and Ku, D. N. (1994) Fluid wall shear stress measurements in a model of the human abdominal

aorta: oscillatory behavior and relationship to atherosclerosis. *Atherosclerosis* **110**(2), pp. 225–40.

41. Taylor, C. A., Hughes, T. J., and Zarins, C. K. (1998) Finite element modeling of three-dimensional pulsatile flow in the abdominal aorta: relevance to atherosclerosis. *Annals of biomedical engineering* **26**(6), pp. 975–87.
42. Abad, C., Santana, C., Diaz, J., and Feijoo, J. (1995) Arteriosclerotic histologic evaluation of the internal mammary artery in patients undergoing coronary artery bypass grafting. *European journal of cardio-thoracic surgery: official journal of the European Association for Cardio-thoracic Surgery* **9**(4), pp. 198–201.
43. Ku, D. N., and Giddens, D. P. (1983). Pulsatile flow in a model carotid bifurcation. Arteriosclerosis (Dallas, Tex.), **3**(1), pp. 31–9.
44. Ku, D. N., Giddens, D. P., Zarins, C. K., and Glagov, S. (1985) Pulsatile flow and atherosclerosis in the human carotid bifurcation. Positive correlation between plaque location and low oscillating shear stress. Arteriosclerosis (Dallas, Tex.), **5**(3), pp. 293–302.
45. Johnson, K., Sharma, P., and Oshinski, J. (2008) Coronary artery flow measurement using navigator echo gated phase contrast magnetic resonance velocity mapping at 3.0 T. *Journal of biomechanics* **41**(3), pp. 595–602.
46. Steinman, D. A. (2004) Image-based computational fluid dynamics: a new paradigm for monitoring hemodynamics and atherosclerosis. *Current drug targets. Cardiovascular & haematological disorders* **4**(2), pp. 183–97.
47. Steinman, D. A. (2002) Image-based computational fluid dynamics modeling in realistic arterial geometries. *Annals of biomedical engineering* **30**(4), pp. 483–97.
48. Glor, F. P., Ariff, B., Hughes, A. D., Crowe, L. A., Verdonck, P. R., Barratt, D. C., McG Thom, S. A., Firmin, D. N., and Xu, X. Y. (2004) Image-based carotid flow reconstruction: a comparison between MRI and ultrasound. *Physiological measurement* **25**(6), pp. 1495–509.
49. Redaelli, A., Rizzo, G., Arrigoni, S., Di Martino, E., Origgi, D., Fazio, F., and Montevecchi, F. (2002) An assisted automated procedure for vessel geometry reconstruction and hemodynamic simulations from clinical imaging. *Computerized medical imaging and graphics: the official journal of the Computerized Medical Imaging Society* **26**(3), pp. 143–52.
50. Suri, J. S., Pattichis, C. S., Li, C., Macione, J., Yang, Z., Fox, M. D., Wu, D., and Laxminarayan, S. (2005) Plaque imaging using ultrasound, magnetic resonance and computer tomography: a review. *Studies in health technology and informatics* **113**, pp. 1–25.
51. Yim, P., Demarco, K., Castro, M. A., and Cebral, J. (2005) Characterization of shear stress on the wall of the carotid artery using magnetic resonance imaging and computational fluid dynamics. *Studies in health technology and informatics* **113**, pp. 412–42.
52. Steinman, D. A., Thomas, J. B., Ladak, H. M., Milner, J. S., Rutt, B. K., and Spence, J. D. (2002) Reconstruction of carotid bifurcation hemodynamics

and wall thickness using computational fluid dynamics and MRI. *Magnetic resonance in medicine: official journal of the Society of Magnetic Resonance in Medicine/Society of Magnetic Resonance in Medicine* **47**(1), pp. 149–59.
53. Tang, D., Yang, C., Mondal, S., Liu, F., Canton, G., Hatsukami, T. S., and Yuan, C. (2008) A negative correlation between human carotid atherosclerotic plaque progression and plaque wall stress: in vivo MRI-based 2D/3D FSI models. *Journal of biomechanics* **41**(4), pp. 727–36.
54. Stone, P. H., Coskun, A. U., Kinlay, S., Popma, J. J., Sonka, M., Wahle, A., Yeghiazarians, Y., Maynard, C., Kuntz, R. E., and Feldman, C. L. (2007) Regions of low endothelial shear stress are the sites where coronary plaque progresses and vascular remodelling occurs in humans: an in vivo serial study. *European heart journal* **28**(6), pp. 705–10.
55. Wu, H., Chen, S. Y., Shroff, S. G., and Carroll, J. D. (2003) Stress analysis using anatomically realistic coronary tree. *Medical physics* **30**(11), pp. 2927–36.
56. Ohayon, J., Finet, G., Gharib, A. M., Herzka, D. A., Tracqui, P., Heroux, J., Rioufol, G., Kotys, M. S., Elagha, A., and Pettigrew, R. I. (2008) Necrotic core thickness and positive arterial remodeling index: emergent biomechanical factors for evaluating the risk of plaque rupture. *American journal of physiology. Heart and circulatory physiology* **295**(2), pp. H717–27.
57. Suo, J., Oshinski, J. N., and Giddens, D. P. (2008) Blood flow patterns in the proximal human coronary arteries: relationship to atherosclerotic plaque occurrence. *Molecular & cellular biomechanics: MCB* **5**(1), pp. 9–18.
58. Moyle, K. R., Antiga, L., and Steinman, D. A. (2006) Inlet conditions for image-based CFD models of the carotid bifurcation: is it reasonable to assume fully developed flow? *Journal of biomechanical engineering* **128**(3), pp. 371–9.
59. Berthier, B., Bouzerar, R., and Legallais, C. (2002) Blood flow patterns in an anatomically realistic coronary vessel: influence of three different reconstruction methods. *Journal of biomechanics* **35**(10), pp. 1347–56.
60. Wake, A. K., Oshinski, J. N., Tannenbaum, A. R., and Giddens, D. P. (2009) Choice of in vivo versus idealized velocity boundary conditions influences physiologically relevant flow patterns in a subject-specific simulation of flow in the human carotid bifurcation. *Journal of biomechanical engineering* **131**(2), p. 021013.
61. Richter, Y., and Edelman, E. R. (2006) Cardiology is flow. *Circulation* **113**(23), pp. 2679–82.
62. Davies, P. F., Spaan, J. A., and Krams, R. (2005) Shear stress biology of the endothelium. *Annals of biomedical engineering* **33**(12) pp. 1714–8.
63. Kovanen, P. T. (2007) Mast cells: multipotent local effector cells in atherothrombosis. *Immunological reviews* **217**(1), pp. 105–22.
64. Traub, O., and Berk, B. C. (1998) Laminar shear stress: mechanisms by which endothelial cells transduce an atheroprotective force. *Arteriosclerosis, thrombosis, and vascular biology* **18**(5), pp. 677–85.

65. Lee, S., Antiga, L., and Steinman, D. a. (2009) Correlations among indicators of disturbed flow at the normal carotid bifurcation. *Journal of biomechanical engineering* **131**(6), p. 061013.
66. Passerini, T. (2009) Computational hemodynamics of the cerebral circulation: multiscale modeling from the circle of Willis to cerebral aneurysms, Biomedical Engineering.
67. Moore, J. A., Steinman, D. A., Prakash, S., Johnston, K. W., and Ethier, C. R. (1999) A numerical study of blood flow patterns in anatomically realistic and simplified end-to-side anastomoses. *Journal of biomechanical engineering* **121**(3), pp. 265–72.
68. Olgac, U., Poulikakos, D., Saur, S. C., Alkadhi, H., and Kurtcuoglu, V. (2009) Patient-specific three-dimensional simulation of LDL accumulation in a human left coronary artery in its healthy and atherosclerotic states. *American journal of physiology. Heart and circulatory physiology* **296**(6), pp. H1969–82.
69. Fukumoto, Y., Hiro, T., Fujii, T., Hashimoto, G., Fujimura, T., Yamada, J., Okamura, T., and Matsuzaki, M. (2008) Localized elevation of shear stress is related to coronary plaque rupture: a 3-dimensional intravascular ultrasound study with in-vivo color mapping of shear stress distribution. *Journal of the American College of Cardiology* **51**(6), pp. 645–50.
70. Groen, H. C., Gijsen, F. J., van Der Lugt, A., Ferguson, M. S., Hatsukami, T. S., van Der Steen, A. F., Yuan, C., and Wentzel, J. J. (2007) Plaque rupture in the carotid artery is localized at the high shear stress region: a case report. *Stroke; a journal of cerebral circulation* **38**(8), pp. 2379–81.
71. Hallow, K. M., Taylor, W. R., Rachev, A., and Vito, R. P. (2009) Markers of inflammation collocate with increased wall stress in human coronary arterial plaque. *Biomechanics and modeling in mechanobiology*, (Liu 1999).
72. Kilpatrick, D., Goudet, C., Sakaguchi, Y., Bassiouny, H. S., Glagov, S., and Vito, R. (2001) Effect of plaque composition on fibrous cap stress in carotid endarterectomy specimens. *Journal of biomechanical engineering* **123**(6), pp. 635–8.
73. Varnava, A. M., Mills, P. G., and Davies, M. J. (2002) Relationship between coronary artery remodeling and plaque vulnerability. *Circulation* **105**(8), pp. 939–43.
74. Versluis, A., Bank, A. J., and Douglas, W. H. (2006) Fatigue and plaque rupture in myocardial infarction. *Journal of biomechanics* **39**(2), pp. 339–47.
75. Loree, H. M., Kamm, R. D., Stringfellow, R. G., and Lee, R. T. (1992). Effects of fibrous cap thickness on peak circumferential stress in model atherosclerotic vessels. *Circulation research* **71**(4), pp. 850–8.
76. Loree, H. M., Tobias, B. J., Gibson, L. J., Kamm, R. D., Small, D. M., and Lee, R. T. (1994) Mechanical properties of model atherosclerotic lesion lipid pools. *Arteriosclerosis and thrombosis: a journal of vascular biology/American Heart Association* **14**(2), pp. 230–4.

77. Li, Z., Tang, T., U-King-Im, J., Graves, M., Sutcliffe, M., and Gillard, J. H. (2008) Assessment of carotid plaque vulnerability using structural and geometrical determinants. *Circulation journal: official journal of the Japanese Circulation Society* **72**(7), pp. 1092–9.
78. Li, Z., Howarth, S., Trivedi, R. A., U-King-Im, J. M., Graves, M. J., Brown, A., Wang, L., and Gillard, J. H. (2006) Stress analysis of carotid plaque rupture based on in vivo high resolution MRI. *Journal of biomechanics* **39**(14), pp. 2611–22.
79. Glagov, S., Bassiouny, H. S., Sakaguchi, Y., Goudet, C. A., and Vito, R. P. (1997) Mechanical determinants of plaque modeling, remodeling and disruption. *Atherosclerosis* **131 Suppl**, pp. S13–4.
80. Lee, R. T. (2000) Atherosclerotic lesion mechanics versus biology. *Zeitschrift für Kardiologie* **89 Suppl 2**, pp. 80–4.
81. Finet, G., Ohayon, J., and Rioufol, G. (2004) Biomechanical interaction between cap thickness, lipid core composition and blood pressure in vulnerable coronary plaque: impact on stability or instability. *Coronary artery disease* **15**(1), pp. 13–20.
82. Vengrenyuk, Y., Carlier, S., Xanthos, S., Cardoso, L., Ganatos, P., Virmani, R., Einav, S., Gilchrist, L., and Weinbaum, S. (2006) A hypothesis for vulnerable plaque rupture due to stress-induced debonding around cellular microcalcifications in thin fibrous caps. *Proceedings of the National Academy of Sciences of the United States of America* **103**(40), pp. 14678–83.
83. Bluestein, D., Alemu, Y., Avrahami, I., Gharib, M., Dumont, K., Ricotta, J. J., and Einav, S., (2008) Influence of microcalcifications on vulnerable plaque mechanics using FSI modeling. *Journal of biomechanics* **41**(5), pp. 1111–8.
84. Tang, D., Yang, C., Zheng, J., Woodard, P. K., Sicard, G. A., Saffitz, J. E., and Yuan, C. (2004) 3D MRI-based multicomponent FSI models for atherosclerotic plaques. *Annals of biomedical engineering* **32**(7), pp. 947–60.
85. Kock, S. A., Nygaard, J. V., Eldrup, N., Fründ, E., Klaerke, A., Paaske, W. P., Falk, E., and Yong Kim, W. (2008) Mechanical stresses in carotid plaques using MRI-based fluid-structure interaction models. *Journal of biomechanics* **41**(8), pp. 1651–8.
86. Li, Z., Howarth, S. P., Tang, T., and Gillard, J. H. (2006) How critical is fibrous cap thickness to carotid plaque stability? A flow-plaque interaction model. *Stroke; a journal of cerebral circulation* **37**(5), pp. 1195–9.
87. Tada, S., Dong, C., and Tarbell, J. M. (2007) Effect of the stress phase angle on the strain energy density of the endothelial plasma membrane. *Biophysical journal* **93**(9), pp. 3026–33.
88. Dancu, M. B., and Tarbell, J. M. (2006) Large Negative Stress Phase Angle (SPA) attenuates nitric oxide production in bovine aortic endothelial cells. *Journal of biomechanical engineering* **128**(3), pp. 329–34.
89. Tada, S., and Tarbell, J. M. (2005). A computational study of flow in a compliant carotid bifurcation-stress phase angle correlation with shear stress. *Annals of biomedical engineering* **33**(9), pp. 1202–12.

Chapter 2

SHEAR STRESS-MEDIATED SIGNAL TRANSDUCTION

JUN-ICHI ABE*, SHI PAN†, BROOKE KROVIC and KEIGI FUJIWARA‡
Aab Cardiovascular Research Institute,
University of Rochester, Rochester, NY 14642
**jun-ichi_abe@urmc.rochester.edu*
†shi_pan@urmc.rochester.edu
‡keigi_fujiwara@urmc.rochester.edu

Emerging evidence shows that steady laminar flow is atheroprotective while disturbed flow creates an atheroprone environment in vivo. Chronic inflammation and reactive oxygen species production represent some of the pathogenic features of atherosclerosis formation, and it has become clear that steady laminar flow and disturbed flow or low shear stress have significant roles to modify these atherogenic events via regulating "mechanosignal transduction". In this chapter, first we will discuss the possible pathological role of mechanosignal transduction in cardiovascular disease. Next the possible role of PECAM-1 as a mechanosensor and its regulatory mechanisms will be reviewed. Third, redox regulation induced by flow and its contribution to endothelial inflammation and apotosis will be summarized. Finally, we will discuss the interplay between cytokine-mediated inflammatory and laminar flow-mediated anti-inflammatory signaling in endothelial cells. The emphasis will be the regulatory mechanism between JNK and ERK5 and post-translational modification of ERK5 by SUMOylation. We believe that the clarification of these mechanosignaling pathways will lead us to understand the process of atherosclerosis formation in areas exposed to disturbed flow, especially in its initial phase of chronic inflammation.

1. Introduction

The concept that inflammation plays a key role in the pathogenesis of atherosclerosis is well established.[1–4] For example, fatty streak formation is associated with expression of the monocyte adhesion ligand, vascular cell adhesion molecule-1 (VCAM-1), on endothelial cells (ECs).[5] During plaque progression monocytes present in the plaque proliferate, oxidize LDL, and secrete cytokines that attract other inflammatory cells.[2] Thus multiple recurrent inflammatory events contribute to atherosclerosis initiation and progression. The cell that primarily limits the atherosclerotic processes is the EC. These cells secrete anti-inflammatory molecules such as nitric oxide (NO)[6] and prostacyclin,[7,8] and activate a genetic program of intracellular mediators that counteract inflammation.

Atherosclerosis develops preferentially in regions of branches and curvatures of large arteries, where blood flow is disturbed from a steady laminar pattern. Substantial evidence exists that steady laminar flow (10–20 dyn/cm^2, termed s-flow here) exerts atheroprotective effects on ECs in vivo, since atherosclerosis preferentially occurs in area of disturbed flow or low shear stress (d-flow), whereas regions with steady laminar flow and physiologic shear stress are protected. Many atheroprotective signals are stimulated by s-flow.[9,10] For example, Kruppel-like factor-2 (KLF2) is induced by s-flow, which induces endothelial NO synthase (eNOS) expression and inhibits induction of VCAM-1 and E-selectin.[11,12] KLF2 is also important for the anti-thrombotic effect of s-flow[13] (These issues will be discussed in detail by Dr. M. Jain).

Furthermore, Dr. B. Berk's group has shown that s-flow inhibits TNF-α-mediated VCAM-1 expression by increasing anti-oxidant mechanisms and blocking inflammatory signaling events. One of the mechanisms by which s-flow is atheroprotective involves inhibition of TNF (Tumor necrosis factor)-α-mediated activation of the JNK (c-Jun N-terminal kinase)/p38 kinase pathway.[14] Understanding the mechanism by which s-flow regulates JNK activation by TNF-α will provide insights into the atheroprotective mechanisms induced by s-flow. Here we discuss recent studies on how s-flow and d-flow differentially regulate mechanosignaling pathways and control a variety of cell and tissue behaviors, some of which subsequently lead to atherosclerosis formation. A fundamental issue on studying flow effects on ECs is the question regarding the mechanism of flow sensing. This chapter will begin with a brief discussion on unique features of mechnaosensor research and a molecule that has been proposed to have a mechano-responsive property.

2. Mechanosignal Transduction: From Molecular Sensors to Cellular Responses

The ability of a cell to sense and respond to different mechanical forces plays a central role in normal and pathological biological processes. The process by which a cell converts a mechanical force into a biochemical signal is referred to as mechanotransduction. It requires several key components: a stimulus (the mechanical force), a sensor, comprised of a molecule or molecular complex that converts the mechanical force into a biochemical signal, second messenger molecules to relay the signal downstream within the cell, and a resulting biological response. Mechanical stimuli, second messengers, and the biological responses of cells are fairly straightforward and easy to identify within a particular tissue or organ. However, to identify mechanosensor molecules is arguably the most difficult aspect of the mechanotransduction research. A mechanosensor is a molecule that alters its molecular property in response to mechanical force. For example, it can take the form of an enzyme, whose activity is awaken by a mechanical trigger and directly initiates downstream chemical signaling. It can also be a protein that, upon a force-induced conformational change, reveals cryptic sites to which other proteins may bind or which may be phosphorylated/dephosphorylated, both of which leading to downstream signaling.

It has been postulated that the cytoskeleton acts as a mechanosensor. However, one must consider the possibility that the cytoskeleton only transmits mechanical forces from one part of the cell to another where mechanically responsive molecules are localized. In this case, the cytoskeleton is required for mechanosensing, but does not convert a mechanical stimulus into a biochemical signal. Thus, one must carefully categorize molecules within a mechanosignaling cascade and distinguish between a mechanotransducer, a structural component, and downstream signaling molecules.

Mechanosignaling cascades often parallel or converge with chemical signaling cascades. Both types of pathways can lead to changes in protein localization, gene expression, and cell growth, differentiation, morphology, motility, death, and survival. Imposition of a physical force upon the cell is capable of activating multiple signaling pathways simultaneously. It is through the convergence of these multiple signaling pathways that the cell is able to subtly and appropriately respond to a particular mechanical stimulus.

3. The Role of Mechanotransduction in Cardiovascular Health and Disease

The study of mechanosignaling is particularly relevant to the field of cardiovascular biology. The entire vasculature is exposed to varying degrees of hemodynamic forces, including stretch, fluid shear stress, and hydrostatic pressure. Effects of hydrostatic pressure are considered to be less critical as a large part of this force is converted into stretch. Cardiomyocytes, cardiac and vascular fibroblasts, vascular smooth muscle cells, and ECs are all exposed to stretch while only ECs are exposed to shear stress.

In addition to environmental/soluble factors, hemodynamic forces play a major role in the development of atherosclerosis. Hemodynamic forces alone do not lead to development of the disease per se, but they dictate where atherosclerotic plaques will be localized. While the entire vasculature is exposed to systemic risk factors for the disease, plaques have been observed to form preferentially at artery curvatures and bifurcations.[15,16] In general, blood flow within the vasculature follows a laminar pattern, with little turbulence or changes in direction. Such a flow pattern is considered atheroprotective, because it promotes the expression of bioactive substances and genes that protect against the development of atherosclerotic plaques while also downregulating the expression of genes that promote plaque formation.[17] It is within the areas of curvatures and bifurcations that hemodynamic forces become less well organized, with blood flow patterns changing from laminar to disturbed and disorganized. Such localized plaque development, as a result of highly localized changes in hemodynamics, highlights the importance of mechanical forces in vascular biology as well as the sensitivity and responsiveness of individual ECs to subtle changes in the mechanical microenvironment.

Concerning mechanical forces and cardiovascular disease, much work has been done to study the effects of fluid shear stress on the biology of ECs. A main goal of many of these studies is to identify and characterize signaling cascades involved in the progression of endothelial dysfunction and cardiovascular disease development. From this body of research, several molecules have been proposed to be endothelial mechanosensors, including ion channels, integrins, G protein-coupled receptors, the cytoskeleton, the glycocalyx, and cell-cell adhesion molecules.[18–21] The main reason for these molecules to be called mechanosensors or flow-sensors is that certain flow-induced EC responses are downregulated when the expression or specific functions of these molecules are compromised. The possible role of each in mechanosensation in ECs and various other cell types continues to intrigue and challenge research laboratories around the world.

4. The Unique Role of PECAM-1 in Mechanosensing

4.1. *Forced-induced PECAM-1 Phosphorylation and Mechano-signaling*

Roughly 15 years ago, we reported a rapid (less than 1 min) tyrosine phosphorylation of a 128 kDa glycoprotein in ECs exposed to >4 dyn/cm^2 of laminar shear stress.[22] This protein was later cloned and identified as platelet endothelial cell adhesion molecule-1, or PECAM-1.[23] PECAM-1 phosphorylation by flow was confirmed by other investigators,[24,25] and our further studies revealed that osmotic changes,[26] which can mechanically stimulate the plasma memberane, and stretch[27] also elicited rapid PECAM-1 phosphorylation. PECAM-1 is a member of the immunoglobulin-inhibitory receptor family of proteins, comprised of six extracellular immunoglobulin-like domains, a single transmembrane domain, and a short cytoplasmic domain. Localized primarily to EC-EC contact areas where it functions as a cell adhesion molecule, PECAM-1 contains within its cytoplasmic domain two immunoreceptor tyrosine-based inhibitory motifs (ITIMs). It is thought that these tyrosine residues are phosphorylated upon application of mechanical forces.

Tyrosine phosphorylation of PECAM-1 by mechanical forces was an interesting phenomenon, but what is important is to elucidate if this has any role in mechanosignaling. To see if phosphorylated PECAM-1 specifically interacted with any signaling proteins, we performed immunoprecipitation experiments and found that Src homology 2 domain-containing phosphatase (SHP)-2 bound to tyrosine-phosphorylated PECAM-1.[26] In fact, there are three major SHP-2 binding proteins in ECs; Grb-2-associated binder-1 (Gab1), protein zero related (PZR), and PECAM-1.[28] Because SHP-2 was involved in activating extracellular signal-regulated kinases 1/2 (ERK1/2) and because Dr. Berk's group has shown that ERK1/2 is activated by s-flow,[29] we investigated if s-flow-induced ERK1/2 activation depended on PECAM-1 phosphorylation and found that PECAM-1 expression was required for ERK1/2 activation by s-flow.[30] More recent studies by Tzima *et al.* have showed that PECAM-1 is required in other flow-elicited signaling events and atherogenesis[31] (see chapter by M. Schwartz).

Interestingly, we have recently found that SHP-2 itself becomes tyrosine phosphorylated by mechanical stimuli, such as fluid shear stress. However, this phosphorylation occurs in ECs treated with PECAM-1 siRNA, indicating that the signaling cascade leading to SHP2 phosphorylation is not activated by PECAM-1 phosphorylation, an event we propose to be an EC mechanotransduction (see below). The use of kinase inhibitors is currently being employed to determine the identity of the kinase(s) responsible for this phosphorylation and to elucidate the mechanosignaling cascade responsible for this PECAM-1-independent EC mechanoresponse and its physiological significance.

4.2. *PECAM-1 as a Mechanosensor*

PECAM-1 phosphorylation can be elicited by other means such as stimulation by ligands, but such phosphorylation responses are not as rapid as phosphorylation by mechanical means, suggesting that the mechanism of PECAM-1 phosphorylation by mechanical forces is different from that of ligand-dependent phosphorylation. Although tyrosine phosphorylation of PECAM-1 by mechanical forces is rapid, there are flow-induced EC responses that can be detected in the order of seconds, such as a Ca^{2+} response. We found that the rapid PECAM-1 phosphorylation did not depend on phosphoinositide turnover, increased cytoplasmic Ca^{2+}, or PKC activation,[22] suggesting that PECAM-1 phosphorylation is not a secondary effect of this flow-induced signaling and that it may occur as the result of mechanical force directly acting on the molecule.

To test this hypothesis, we used magnetic beads that were coated with antibodies against the external domain of PECAM-1 to trap PECAM-1 on the cell surface and applied magnetic force to pull on PECAM-1.[30] We found that the fraction of PECAM-1 bound to beads was phosphorylated only when magnetic force was applied. Not all PECAM-1 molecules on the cell surface were trapped by the antibody-coated beads and those not bound to beads were not phosphorylated even after magnetic force was exerted. This suggests that PECAM-1 phosphorylation is regulated locally each molecule at a time (i.e. dependent on whether or not an individual PECAM-1 molecule is mechanically stimulated), not globally in the same manner throughout the whole cell. Our study further demonstrated that when PECAM-1 is directly pulled in this manner, ERK1/2 was also activated.[30] Figure 1 shows our working hypothesis regarding PECAM-1 mechanotransduction. In a confluent EC monolayer, PECAM-1 localized in the cell-cell border is externally anchored to the PECAM-1 of the neighboring cell and internally it is thought to be anchored to actin filaments via β- and α-catenins.[32,33] Thus, we propose that when the relative position of ECs in a monolayer is perturbed by mechanical forces

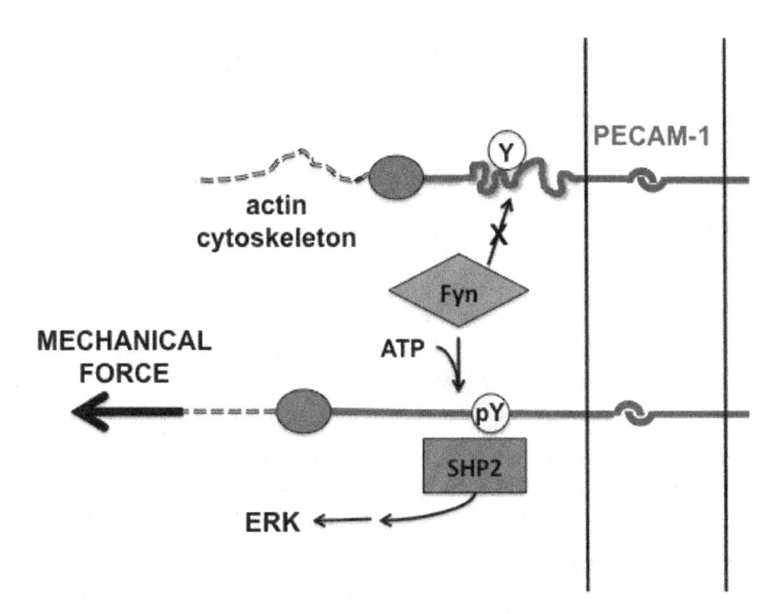

Fig. 1. PECAM-1 phosphorylation and downstream signaling in response to a mechanical force. In the absence of mechanical forces, the cytoplasmic region of PECAM-1 is folded upon itself or other unidentified proteins, thus protecting its tyrosine residues from phosphorylation. When a mechanical force is applied to the cell, the cytoplasmic domain of PECAM-1, attached to actin filaments via catenins (oval), is stretched, exposing the tyrosine residues to be phosphorylated by Fyn kinase. SHP-2 binds to phosphorylated PECAM-1, activating downstream signaling.

(such as shear stress, stretch, and osmotic shock), the cytoplasmic domain of PECAM-1 may be stretched so that the cryptic tyrosine residue(s) may be exposed. The exposed tyrosine then can be phosphorylated, activating mechanosignaling cascades such as the ERK1/2 pathway.

SHP-2 binds to phosphorylated PECAM-1 and this interaction can be used to visualize the part of EC borders where PECAM-1 phosphorylation, thus PECAM-1 mechanosignaling, is taking place following mechanical stimuli.[26] Using fluorescence microscopy, we have found that SHP-2 unevenly localizes to cell-cell borders in cells exposed to 5 minutes of 24 dyne/cm^2 of s-flow (Fig. 2). SHP-2 appears to accumulate preferentially to cell contacts perpendicular to the direction of flow. This indicates heterogeneity in the phosphorylation state of the population of PECAM-1 at cell-cell borders, consistent with the result of the bead experiment described earlier. Such differential PECAM-1 phosphorylation suggests a difference in the profile of mechanical forces being applied across the

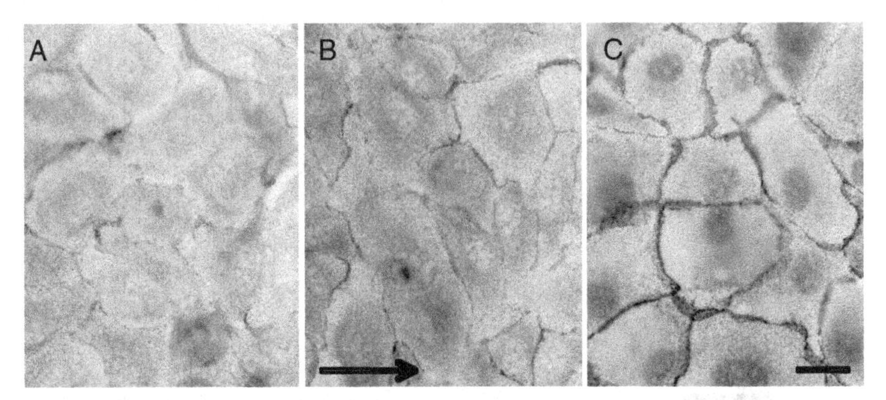

Fig. 2. SHP-2 localization in response to mechanical forces in bovine aortic endothelial cells. SHP2 localization was determined by immunofluorescence in confluent monolayers of bovine aortic endothelial cells. Cells were left unstimulated (A), or exposed to 5 minutes of 24 dyne/cm^2 fluid shear stress (direction of flow indicated by arrow)(B), or 5 minutes of hyperosmotic shock (C), then fixed with ice-cold methanol and stained for SHP-2. SHP-2 rapidly relocalizes to cell-cell borders in response to both types of mechanical stimuli. While hyperosmotic shock stimulated PECAM-1 at the cell border in more or less uniform manner, fluid shear stress tends to act on the cell border that is perpendicular to the direction of flow. Scale: 10 μm.

cell, with the greatest level of force being applied to the cell borders perpendicular to the direction of flow.

4.3. *PECAM-1 Kinase in Mechanotransduction*

To determine if force-induced PECAM-1 phosphorylation is a purely mechanical event and at the same time to tease out the molecular mechanism of converting mechanical force into a biochemical event, we used an in vitro cell model. A "dead" cell system was employed by Sawada and Sheetz[34] to study stretch-dependent molecular associations, and we adapted this technique to study PECAM-1 phosphorylation by mechanical forces.[27] A confluent cell monolayer was extracted with a Triton-containing buffer solution and then exposed to mechanical stretch in the presence or absence of ATP. To our amazement, PECAM-1 was phosphorylated in a stretch- and ATP-dependent manner. This indicates that our cell model, which has lost the plasma membrane barrier (hence all of the ionic regulation of live cells) and the soluble components of the cytoplasm such as second messengers, is still capable of converting mechanical force into a biochemical form that will, in living cells, activate cellular signaling cascades. It also indicates that the molecules necessary to phosphorylate PECAM-1 by mechanical force are preserved in our model, presumably in the form of a mechanosensing molecular complex.

Because PECAM-1 contains no intrinsic enzymatic activity, its phosphorylation is achieved by the action of tyrosine kinase(s) and the kinase must be associated with our cell model. By screening with a series of kinase inhibitors, the list of possible kinases was narrowed to only three candidates, Fyn, Src, and Yes. Using siRNAs specific to each kinase individually, it was determined that Fyn kinase was responsible for stretch-induced PECAM-1 tyrosine phosphorylation in the Triton-extracted ECs.[27] By repeating Fyn-specific siRNA experiments, it was found that Fyn is also responsible for stretch- and fluid shear stress-induced PECAM-1 phosphorylation in intact cells. Other kinases have been reported to phosphorylate PECAM-1,[35,36] but they do not appear to play roles in PECAM-1 mechanotransduction. Our studies reviewed briefly here establish PECAM-1 as a mechanotransduction protein of ECs.

5. S-flow-mediated Redox Regulation and Inflammation

Oxidative stress induced inflammation and endothelial dysfunction play pivotal roles in the development of atherosclerosis. Increased generation of reactive oxygen species (ROS) breaks the oxidation-reduction balance of the endothelium and activates signal transduction that induces adhesion molecule expression and inflammation.

Laminar shear stress is indispensable in EC homeostasis.[10] Along with NO production, s-flow increases the expression and the activity of antioxidant enzymes to detoxify ROS.[37] Furthermore, it suppresses the expression of the proteins that initiate inflammation and subsequently vascular damage through redox-dependent mechanisms.[38] In this sense, studies by Dr. Berk's laboratory have demonstrated that thioredoxin (Trx) and glutaredoxin (Grx) systems are novel regulators of EC redox homeostasis in response to shear stress[38–40] (Fig. 3).

5.1. *TRX and TRX-interacting Protein (TXNIP)*

Increasing evidence indicates that TXNIP plays a role in cardiovascular disorders.[41,42] The role of TXNIP in vascular inflammation has been extensively investigated by Dr. Berk's laboratory. TXNIP, (also termed VDUP-1 for vitamin D3-upregulated protein 1) is an endogenous inhibitor

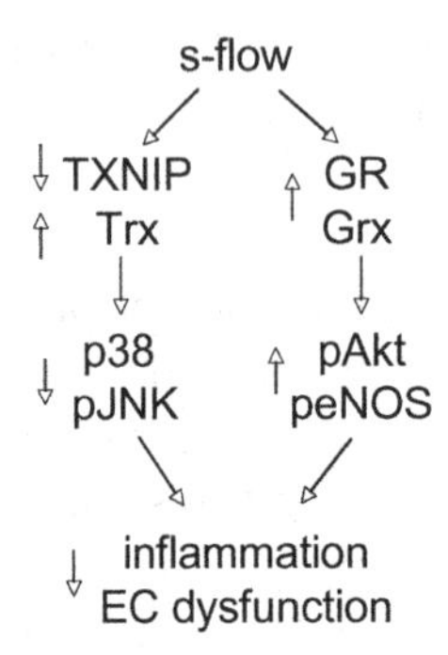

Fig. 3. The role of Trx and Grx on s-flow-mediated signaling in ECs.

of Trx originally isolated by yeast two-hybrid system as a Trx binding protein.[43] Trx is a ubiquitous thiol oxidoreductase that regulates the cellular redox state and promotes cell growth. In addition, Trx directly binds to and inhibits the activation of apoptotic signaling kinase 1 (ASK1).[44]

In order to understand the role of Trx and TXNIP in EC function in response to laminar shear stress, an ex vivo organ culture system was employed in our studies. Chronic exposure of rabbit aortas to laminar flow decreased TXNIP expression, at least partly due to increased Trx activity.[38] Consequently, decreased TXNIP expression attenuated TNF-α-induced inflammation. It was found that knockdown of TXNIP by siRNA increased Trx binding to ASK1 leading to decreased p38, JNK phosphorylation and VCAM-1 expression. Consistent with these results, a decrease in TNF-α-induced VCAM-1 expression was observed in TXNIP deficient mice aortas suggesting a novel mechanism for the atheroprotective effect of laminar shear stress via inhibiting TXNIP[38] (Fig. 3).

5.2. *Thiol Regulation and Glutaredoxin*

Although the molecular mechanisms for shear stress regulation of TXNIP remain elusive, the redox status of intracellular thiol is critical for laminar shear stress inhibition of inflammation. The interplay between Trx and TXNIP, as well as between Trx and ASK1, are dependent on the thiol redox states.[45] For example, TXNIP only binds to reduced Trx through disulfide bond formation. Therefore, C427S mutant of TXNIP does not bind to Trx.[45] Similarly, the interaction between ASK1 and Trx also requires reduced thiols of Trx.[46,47] Trx inhibits ASK1 activation by binding to the

N-terminus of ASK1. When exposed to oxidative stress, Trx forms disulfide bond between its two catalytic cysteines (C32 and C35). That causes its dissociation from ASK1 leading to ASK1 activation.[44]

As the most abundant intracellular antioxidant thiol group, glutathione is regulated by shear stress.[48,49] Studies by Dr. Berk's laboratory have shown that laminar shear stress increases the activity of glutathione reductase, which consequently increases the ratio of reduced glutathione (GSH) to its oxidized form (GSSG). Interestingly, the increased activity of glutathione reductase is responsible for laminar shear stress-mediated inhibition of JNK activation while inhibiting thioredoxin reductase has no such effects.[49]

Because GSH is essential for reducing oxidized Grx, laminar shear stress activation of glutathione reductase has a critical impact on the Grx system.[50] Grx is a thioltransferase involved in many cellular functions. It has been shown to play a role in redox signaling through its ability to reduce the protein thiol-glutathione mixed disulfide bond. Our recent studies suggest a role of Grx in laminar shear stress-mediated protection of EC function.[51] It was found that Grx was activated in a glutathione reductase-dependent manner in response to laminar shear stress, probably due to an increased GSH level.[51] Either knockdown of Grx by siRNA or blocking glutathione reductase by 1,3-bis[2-chloroethyl]-1-nitrosourea attenuated laminar flow-induced eNOS and Akt phosphorylation (Fig. 3). Interestingly, overexpression of Grx mimicked the effect of laminar shear stress on NO production. Further studies on the roles of Trx, and Grx in laminar shear stress-mediated redox regulation will shed light on the antioxidant mechanisms for the atheroprotective effects of laminar shear stress.

6. S-flow Inhibits TNF-α Signaling by Multiple Mechanisms

6.1. *MAP Kinases in Response to s-flow and TNF-α*

Mitogen-activated protein kinases (MAPKs) are highly conserved serine/threonine kinases that are activated in response to a wide variety of stimuli including growth factors, G protein–coupled receptors, and environmental stresses. Consequently, they play a role in numerous cell functions including growth and proliferation. The MAPKs themselves require dual phosphorylation on a Thr-X-Tyr motif to become active. Three major MAPK cascades have been extensively studied in the vessel: extracellular signal–regulated kinases (ERK1 and ERK2), c-Jun N-terminal

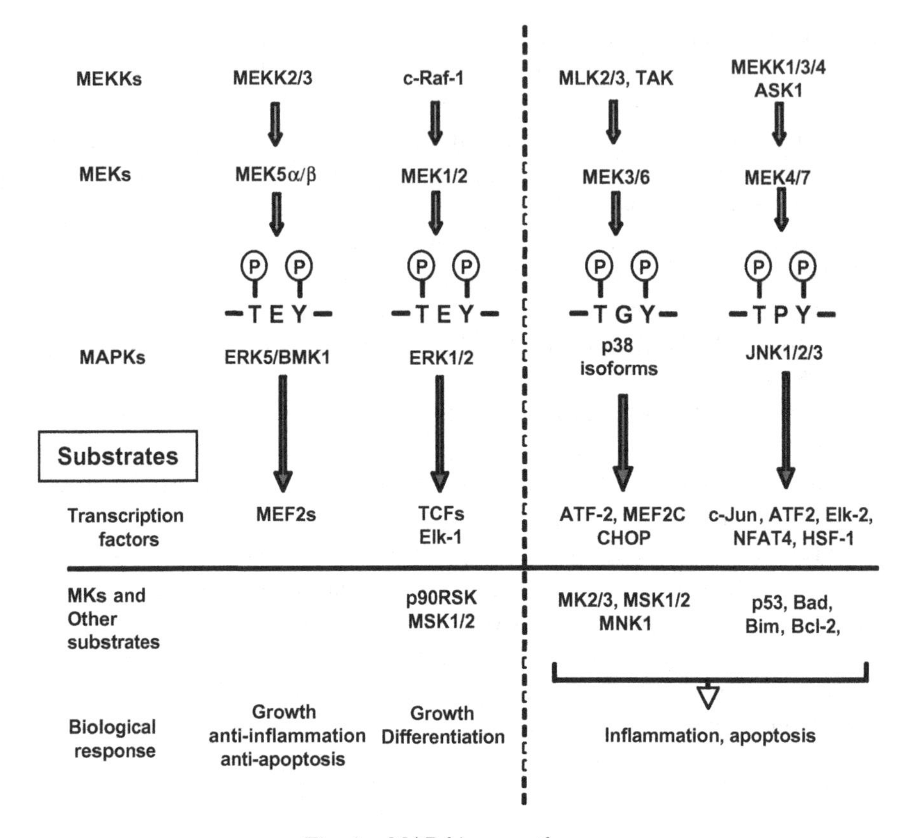

Fig. 4. MAP kinase pathways.

kinases (JNK1 and JNK2), and p38 kinases. A fourth MAPK member, ERK5, also known as big MAPK-1 (BMK1), has been identified in ECs[52–54] (Fig. 4).

The critical role of JNK activation in endothelial inflammation and apoptosis has been reported. JNK can phosphorylate several transcription factors including, c-Jun, ATF2, Elk-2, RXRα, NFAT4, HSF-1, and p53.[55] JNK activation is required for TNF-α-mediated induction of adhesion molecules including VCAM-1, ICAM-1, and E-selectin.[56–58] Furthermore, there is increasing evidence to support the key role of JNK in regulating apoptosis. JNK can promote apoptosis by two different ways. One mechanism is for activated JNK to translocate to the nucleus, where it phosphorylates c-Jun and p53 and promotes apoptosis by increasing the expression of pro-apoptotic genes such as TNF-α, Fas-L, Bak, Bax and PUMA through transactivation of the c-Jun- and p53-dependent mechanism.[59,60] For example, JNK phosphorylates p53 at Ser6, which inhibits ubiquitin-mediated p53 degradation and increases p53 expression level. Subsequently, p53 upregulates several pro-apoptotic genes including Bax and PUMA.[59,61]

The other mechanism is for JNK to translocate to mitochondria and phophorylate Bcl2, Bim, and Bid.[55] BH3-domian only protein Bcl2 can be phosphorylated by JNK at Ser70, which inhibits anti-apoptotic effect of Bcl2.[62] In addition, JNK-mediated phosphorylation of Ser65[63] or Thr56[64] Bim can activate its pro-apoptotic activity via activating Bax and Bak by inhibiting the anti-apoptotic effect of Bcl-2. The involvement of the BH3-domain only protein Bid in JNK-mediated apoptosis has also been reported. The unique side of Bid is that Bid can be cleaved and activated by caspase 8. The truncated Bid (tBid) translocates to mitochondria and induces apoptosis via increasing cytochrome c release.[65,66] Interestingly, JNK also induces cleavage of Bid. However, JNK-mediated cleavage is caspase 8-independent and the cleavage site is different, thus generating a JNK-mediated Bid cleavage product (jBid). Like tBid, jBid translocates to mitochondria and induces apoptosis through releasing Smac/DIABLO, not cytochrome c.[67] JNK may regulate apoptosis by coordinating these two pathways in ECs.

The role of JNK on atherosclerosis likely depends on its isoforms. Ricci *et al.*[68] reported that atherosclerosis-prone ApoE$^{-/-}$ mice simultaneously lacking JNK2 (ApoE$^{-/-}$ JNK2$^{-/-}$ mice), but not ApoE$^{-/-}$ JNK1$^{-/-}$ mice, developed less atherosclerosis than ApoE$^{-/-}$ mice. Pharmacological inhibition of JNK activity efficiently reduced plaque formation. These data suggest the critical role of JNK activity in atherosclerosis although the unique contribution of endothelial JNK2 to atherogenesis needs further analyses in this model.[68,69] The generation of endothelial specific JNKs knock out mice might be necessary to answer this question.

Interestingly, Dr. Berk's group has shown that s-flow stimulates ERK1/2, p38, and ERK5 while it inhibits TNF-α-mediated JNK activation.[14] Therefore, the s-flow-mediated anti-inflammatory and anti-apoptotic effects may be due to inhibition of JNK signaling. Here we will discuss several possible mechanisms of s-flow-mediated JNK signaling inhibition.

6.2. *S-flow Inhibits PKCζ Signaling in ECs*

Protein kinase C (PKC) enzymes are serine/threonine kinases that phosphorylate several effector proteins in a cell- and stimulus-specific manner.[71] Among the PKC family members, the atypical PKCζ has recently emerged as an important isoform in ECs. PKCζ has 3 functional domains: (1) a PB1 domain (Phox and Bem1p) which constitutes a recently recognized protein-protein interaction domain found in the atypical protein kinase C (aPKC) isoenzymes, PKCζ and PKCλ/ι,; members of MAPK modules like MEK5, MEKK2, and MEKK3;[72,73] and in several scaffold proteins involved in cellular signaling; (2) a zinc finger (ZF) domain for nuclear interactions, and (3) a kinase domain. PKCζ promotes the adhesive phenotype of EC, when activated by TNF-α[74] via the regulation of nuclear factor κ-B (NFκ B)-dependent ICAM-1 expression.[74,75] A recent study demonstrated a correlation between PKCζ activity and flow patterns in porcine arteries: lower PKCζ activity in ECs exposed to s-flow than those under d-flow.[76] Prolonged exposure to d-flow induces cell adhesion molecule expression in ECs *in vitro* and *in vivo*.[77] Together, these observations suggest that PKCζ activity, differentially regulated by s-flow versus d-flow and TNF-α, could be an important determinant of atherogenesis susceptibility via regulation of inflammatory pathways.

To date, the role of PKCζ in the apoptotic events induced by TNF-α has not been well defined in ECs. Previous work showed that TNF-α and cycloheximide (CHX) treatment induced PKCζ (72 kDa) processing into a 50 kDa fragment consisting of the catalytic domain (CATζ).[78] This caspase 3-dependent processing occurs at three aspartate residues (Asp 210, 222, and 239) and frees the enzyme from the auto-inhibitory state by separating the kinase domain (aa 268–335) from the pseudosubstrate auto-inhibitory sequence (aa 116–122),[79] thus increasing its kinase activity. CATζ exhibits substantially higher kinase activity than PKCζ, presumably due to loss of endogenous negative regulation.[78]

Recently, we have reported that PKCζ activity was required for TNF-α–mediated activation of JNK and caspase-3 in ECs. Upon stimulation by TNF-α, PKCζ was rapidly converted to CATζ in cultured bovine and human aortic ECs and also in intact rabbit vessels. Interestingly, CATζ not only enhanced JNK and caspase-3 activity but also PKCζ processing was inhibited by inhibitors of PKCζ, JNK, and caspase, suggesting a positive feedback system for these enzymes via regulating CATζ formation in ECs. Finally, we found that s-flow reduced caspase-dependent PKCζ processing

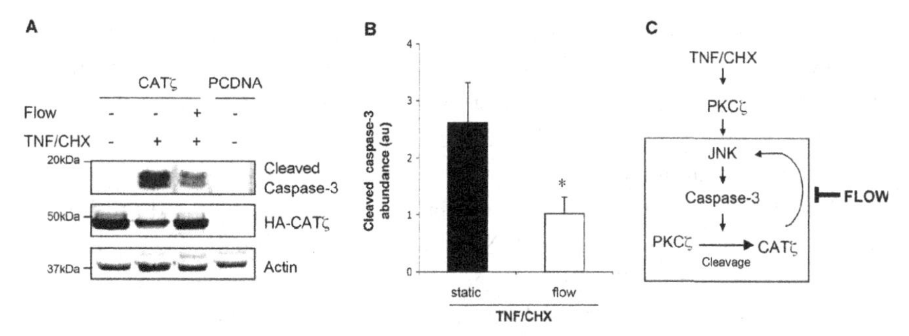

Fig. 5. Flow reduces CATζ proapoptotic effects. BAECs overexpressing CATζ were preexposed or not to flow for 24 hours before TNF/CHX. A, Caspase-3 activity was estimated by the detection of its cleaved form by Western blot. Anti-HA antibody was used to detect the CATζ transfected form. B, Western blots were quantified by densitometry. All figures are representative of 3 to 4 independent experiments. * $P < 0.05$ vs static TNF/CHX-treated cells. C, Model: Flow inhibits PKCζ cleavage and prevents apoptosis. TNF/CHX, via induction of caspase-3 activation, induces PKCζ cleavage to yield CATζ. CATζ enhances TNF-α–induced JNK and caspase-3 activation leading to a death pathway where CATζ stimulates caspase-3 activation and subsequent PKCζ cleavage. In contrast, flow mediates prosurvival effects via inhibiting caspase-3 and JNK, thus decreasing PKCζ cleavage.[70] (Obtained permission to reproduce from Wolters Kluwer Health).

and caspase-3 activation (Fig. 5). These results define a novel role of PKCζ as a shared signaling mediator for flow and TNF-α and indicate its important role in s-flow-mediated inhibition of inflammation and apoptosis in ECs.

6.3. *S-flow Inhibits TNF-α-mediated SHP-2 Phosphatase Activity and MEKK3 Signaling*

Our group and colleagues have found that there are several mechanisms by which s-flow can inhibit TNF-α signaling.[14,80,81] One of the important regulators of the TNF-α pathway is SHP-2, whose activity is required for activation of JNK and NF-κ B.[82,83] SHP-2 is an ubiquitously expressed cytosolic protein that contains 2 amino-terminal tandem SH2 domains and a carboxyl-terminal catalytic domain.[84] It associates with tyrosine-phosphorylated growth factor receptors such as epidermal growth factor receptor and platelet-derived growth factor and with cytokine receptors such as interferon α/β receptors.[85–87] MEKK3 was required for this TNF-α-induced c-Jun and NF-κ B transcriptional activity.[81,88] We investigated the role of SHP-2 phosphatase activity in regulating MEKK3 signaling.

We transfected HUVECs with SHP-2C/S (phosphatase inactive mutant with cysteine 495 mutated to serine) and a constitutively active form of MEKK3 (CA-MEKK3). We found that CA-MEKK3 increased c-Jun and NF-κ B tranactivation, and SHP-2C/S inhibited this transactivation in a dose-dependent manner.[80]

We also found that Gab1 associated with MEKK3 and inhibited the MEKK3-induced c-Jun and NF-kB transactivation.[81] Therefore, we investigated if SHP-2 phosphatase activity regulated this association. The binding between Gab1 and MEKK3 in vitro was enhanced by the presence of SHP-2C/S. Overexpresssion of wild type SHP-2 did not affect the Gab1/MEKK3 association, but this association was enhanced by SHP-2C/S expression, suggesting that SHP-2 phosphatase activity regulates Gab1-MEKK3 association and consequently TNF-α signaling in ECs (Fig. 6).

Yang *et al.*[88] and we have found that MEKK3 is a critical mediator for regulating the TNF-α-induced c-Jun and NF-κB transcriptional activity and that Gab1 has an inhibitory effect on their transcriptional activity induced by TNF-α as well as by MEKK3. As we have discussed, SHP-2 activity regulates MEKK3-Gab1 interaction and signaling by TNF-α and MEKK3, and in addition, SHP-2 also regulates the MEKK3-induced c-Jun

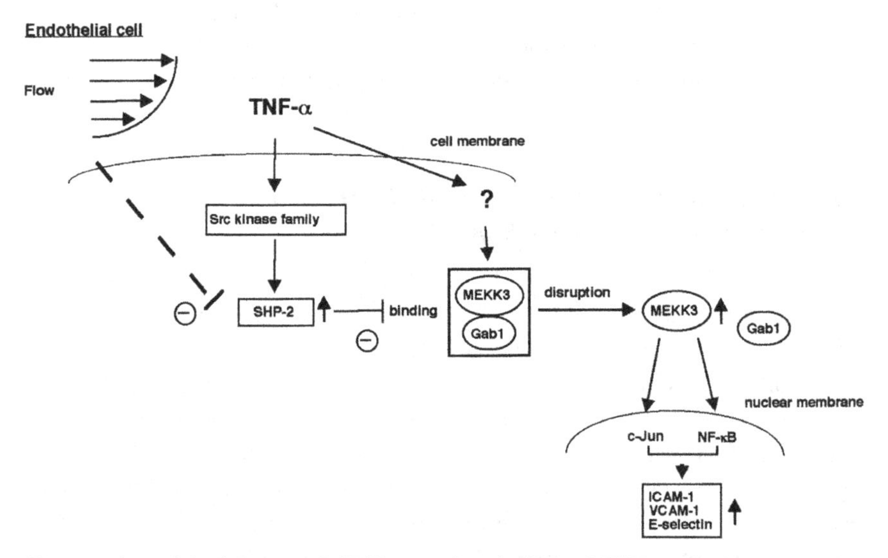

Fig. 6. A model of flow- and TNF-α–mediated SHP-2-MEKK3 signal transduction pathways that regulate adhesion molecule expression in endothelial cells.[80] (Obtained permission to reproduce from Wolters Kluwer Health).

and NF-κB transactivation. These observations suggest the critical role of the SHP-2/Gab1/MEKK3 complex in regulating TNF-α signaling (Fig. 6). Since s-flow significantly inhibited TNF-α–induced SHP-2 phosphatase activity,[80] this could maintain the MEKK3-Gab1 interaction and inhibit the TNF-α-mediated c-Jun and NF-κB activation and subsequent induction of adhesion molecules expression.

6.4. *ERK5 Inhibits TNF-α-mediated JNK Activation*

As explained above, Dr. Berk's group has shown that s-flow decreases TNF-α-mediated VCAM1 expression in ECs in a JNK-dependent manner.[89] A key role of ERK5, but not ERK1/2 was demonstrated: (1) PD184352 at concentrations that blocked ERK1/2, but not ERK5, had no effect on flow inhibition of TNF-mediated JNK activation, and (2) BIX02188, a MEK5 inhibitor, completely reversed the inhibitory effects of flow. These findings indicate that s-flow inhibits TNF-α-mediated signaling in ECs by a mechanism dependent on activation of MEK5-BMK1, but not MEK1-ERK1/2. The mechanisms by which MEK5-BMK1 inhibit TNF signaling remain to be elucidated fully. Intriguingly, both MEK5 and PKC-ζ are PB1 domain containing proteins. Thus, it is possible that competition between MEK5 and PKC-ζ influences the relative activation of these pathways. In fact, we found that association between PKCζ and ERK5 and PKCζ activation inhibited ERK5 transcriptional activity. However, the exact role of PKCζ on ERK5 remains unclear.

7. ERK5 and Shear Stress

7.1. *s-flow Mediated ERK5 Activation*

ERK5 (Fig. 7) is a unique MAPK with transcriptional activity.[90,91] It is activated by redox and hyperosmotic stresses, growth factors, and pathways involving certain G-protein-coupled receptors.[92] It has a TEY sequence in its dual phosphorylation site, like ERK1/2, but has a unique carboxyl (C)-terminus and a loop-12 domain, suggesting that its regulation and function are different from ERK1/2. MEK5 is the upstream kinase that phosphorylates ERK5.[93,94] Like other MAPKs, it plays a significant role in cell growth and differentiation although emerging evidence suggests other unique functions. Redox activation of ERK5 is tied to an anti-apoptotic effect[95] and ERK5 knockout mice have impaired cardiac and

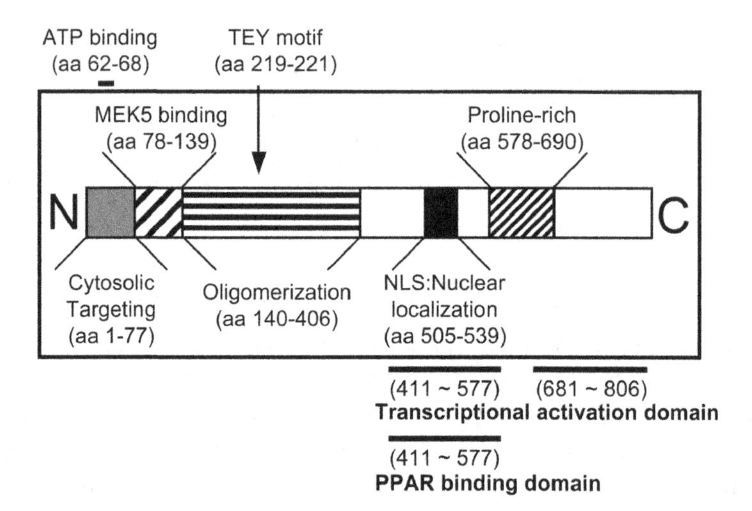

Fig. 7. ERK5 kinase structure.

vascular development.[96] In addition, ERK5 not only is a kinase but also has transcriptional activity. Its C-terminal region has two transactivation domains, and one of them (aa684–806) is active without activation by MEK5a. However, when activated, the amino (N)-terminal self-inhibitory effect is released and becomes a fully activated transcription factor. Thus, ERK5 transactivation is regulated by an intramolecular interaction[90] (Fig. 7).

There is a strong correlation between EC dysfunction and areas of d-flow. It is well known that vessel bifurcation is a pro-atherogenic area, where low eNOS expression and high adhesion molecule expression are observed and this particular area experiences d-flow.[97,98] It is also important to state that steady laminar flow can increase the secretion of NO, PGI_2, tPA from ECs, which downregulate coagulation and leukocyte adhesions.[6–8,99] In contrast, d-flow including low flow increases secretion of proinflammatory molecules such as MCP-1, PDGFs, and endothelin-1 and increases leukocyte infiltration and smooth muscle proliferation, leading to development of atherosclerosis.[100–102] We have reported that s-flow stimulation of PPARγ1 activity via activation of ERK5 contributes to the anti-inflammatory and atheroprotective effects of s-flow. S-flow potently activates ERK5[103] and inhibits leukocyte binding as well as adhesion molecule expression.[104]

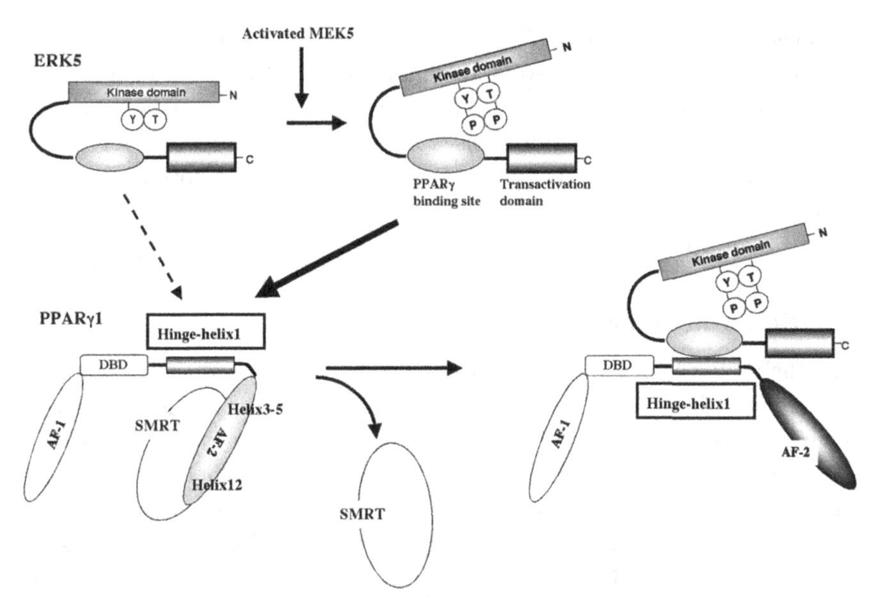

Fig. 8. Model of the ERK5-PPARγ interaction-mediated PPARγ transactivation. The position of Helix 12 is regulated by ligand binding. When the PPARγ ligand binds to the receptor, Helix 12 folds back to form part of the co-activator binding surface, and inhibits co-repressor (such as SMRT) binding to PPARγ.[107] The co-repressor interaction surface requires Helix 3–5.[108] We found a critical role of the PPARγ hinge-helix 1 domain on ERK5-mediated PPARγ transactivation. The inactive N-terminal kinase domain of ERK5 inhibits its own transactivation and PPARγ binding. After ERK5 activation the inhibitory effect of N-terminal domain of ERK5 decreases, and subsequently the middle region of ERK5 can fully interact with the hinge-helix 1 region of PPARγ. The association of ERK5 with the hinge-helix 1 region of PPARγ releases co-repressor of SMRT and induces full activation of PPARγ,[90] AF-1/2: Activating function (AF)-1/2 transactivation domain, DBD: DNA binding domain. (Obtained permission to reproduce from American Society for Microbiology).

We have explored the molecular mechanism of ERK5-mediated PPARγ activation. Kasler *et al.*[91] reported that the ERK5 C-terminal region contained a MEF2-interacting domain and also a potent transactivation domain. We found that the middle region of ERK5, but not the C-terminus of ERK5, associated with PPARγ1[90] (Fig. 8). We also found that the inactive N-terminal kinase domain acted as a negative regulator of the C-terminal region and that activation by CA-MEK5a disrupted this inhibitory effect.[90] Importantly, ERK5 kinase activity was necessary for ERK5-PPARγ1 association and full activation of PPARγ transcriptional activity.[90] We as well as others have found that ERK5 activation initiates its nuclear translocation.[105,106] It appears that both disruption of the inhibitory effect of the N-terminal region and nuclear translocation are required for ERK5 to fully activate PPARγ1. Furthermore, since we found that the ERK5-PPARγ1 binding disrupted the interaction of SMRT (a co-repressor that silences the mediator of retinoid and thyroid hormone action) with PPARγ, we believe that one of the mechanisms for ERK5 to activate PPARγ1 is to disrupt this interaction.[90]

7.2. *ERK5 in Diabetes: ERK5-SUMOylation*

Endothelial inflammation is one of the major initiators of atherosclerosis, and diabetes significantly affects this process. However, what is lacking is a plausible relationship between diabetes and any of the known regulators of endothelial inflammation that play a significant role in accelerating atherosclerosis formation. Recently, we and others have found that s-flow but not d-flow acts as an anti-inflammatory modulator by increasing the ERK5 and PPARγ transcriptional activity and decreasing adhesion molecule expression in ECs. S-flow-induced ERK5 activation has a critical role in regulating PPARγ and KLF2, a recently identified transcriptional inhibitor of endothelial inflammation, as well as inhibiting TNF-α-mediated adhesion molecule expression, suggesting a critical anti-inflammatory role of ERK5 in ECs.[90,109] Increased expression of adhesion molecules and inflammation under diabetic conditions has been reported in vitro and in vivo.[110,111] In this section, we will discuss the involvement of ERK5 SUMOylation, one of the post-transcriptional modifications, on diabetes-mediated endothelial dysfunction.

7.2.1. *SUMOylation*

SUMO (Small Ubiquitin-like Modifier) covalently attaches to certain residues of specific target proteins and alters their functions such as their cellular localization, protein partnering, and the DNA-binding and/or transactivation functions of transcription factors.[112] SUMOylation may also affect protein turnover as it is a decoy mechanism for ubiquitination and subsequent proteosomal degradation.[113] Such a pathway has been studied with regards to inflammatory gene transcriptional regulation. For example, SUMOylated IκB escapes from ubiquitination and degradation, which then negatively regulates NF-κB.[114] It is clear that SUMO influences many different biological processes, but of particular importance in the

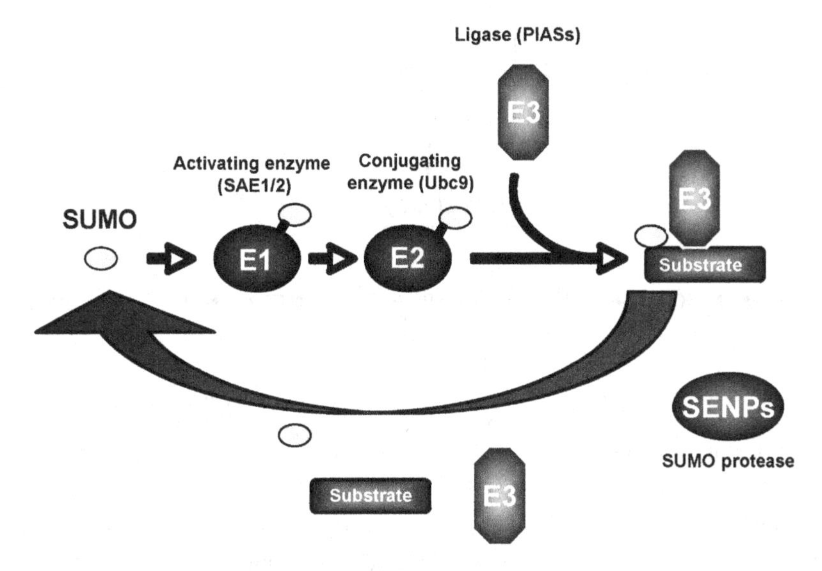

Fig. 9. SUMOylation system.

present context is regulation of transcription. It has been reported that the attachment of SUMO can inhibit the activity of several transcription factor including Elk-1 and STAT-1.[115] The SUMOylation pathway is analogous to that of ubiquitination, but a different set of enzymes is involved (Fig. 9). First, the El-activating enzyme such as SAE1-SAE2 heterodimer (activating enzyme) activates the SUMO cycle in an ATP-dependent manner. Second, the E2-conjugating enzyme of Ubc9 (ubiquitin-conjugating enzyme 9, conjugating enzyme) is recruited for the activated SUMO to be attached to the e-amino group of specific residues in the target substrate.[116] Finally, the SUMO E3-ligating enzyme such as the PIAS (protein inhibitor of activated STAT) family of proteins finalizes the SUMOylation process by ligating SUMO to the targeted molecule efficiently and properly.

7.2.2. *ERK5-SUMOylation*

The formation of ROS and advanced glycation end products (AGE) are the major mechanisms that play a role in the pathogenesis of diabetic vascular dysfunction resulting from hyperglycemia.[118–121] Previously, we found that H_2O_2 and AGE significantly inhibited ERK5/MEF2 transcriptional activity as well as the subsequent increases in KLF2 promoter activity and

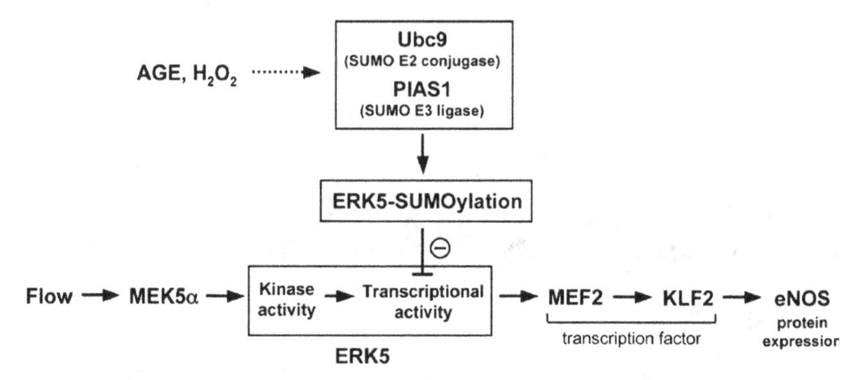

Fig. 10. A signaling scheme describing the relationship between the laminar flow–mediated ERK5/MEF2/KLF2/eNOS pathway and H_2O_2 or AGE-mediated ERK5 SUMOylation.[117] (Obtained permission to reproduce from Wolters Kluwer Health).

in the KLF2 and eNOS expression by shear stress via ERK5 SUMOylation, although H_2O_2 and AGE increased ERK5 phosphorylation and kinase activity (Fig. 10). We first showed that ROS and AGE lead to ERK5-SUMOylation at Lys6 and Lys22 sites and inhibited ERK5 transcriptional activity. To investigate functional correlation between these two events, we compared the extent of inhibition of ERK5 transcriptional activity by H_2O_2 between the wild type ERK5 and the K6/22R mutant and found that inhibition was significantly less in the mutant. We further tested if transfection of DN-Ubc9, a dominant negative form of Ubc9 (conjugating enzyme), could inhibit the H_2O_2-mediated reduction of ERK5 transcriptional activity and we confirmed this inhibition. Because ERK5 can be activated by s-flow, we tested if H_2O_2 or AGE could inhibit ERK5 activation induced by laminar flow. We transfected HUVECs with Gal4-tagged wild type or K6/22R ERK5 constructs, stimulated cells with vehicle or H_2O_2, or BSA or AGE-BSA, exposed them to s-flow or static conditions, and assayed for luciferase activity. H_2O_2 and AGE significantly inhibited flow-induced ERK5 wild type transcriptional activity, but this inhibition was less in the K6/22R mutant (Fig. 11A and B). In addition, we found increased ERK5 SUMOylation in the vessels of diabetic mice. We propose that inhibition of ERK5 SUMOylation may be a new therapeutic target for the treatment of diabetes-mediated endothelial dysfunction and inflammation.

Although it is unclear how H_2O_2 and AGE increase ERK5-SUMOylation, involvement of phosphorylation or association with other

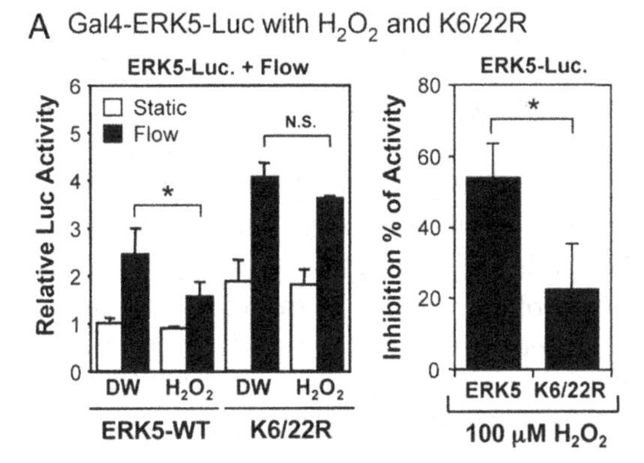

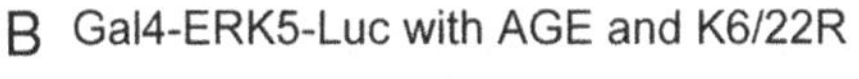

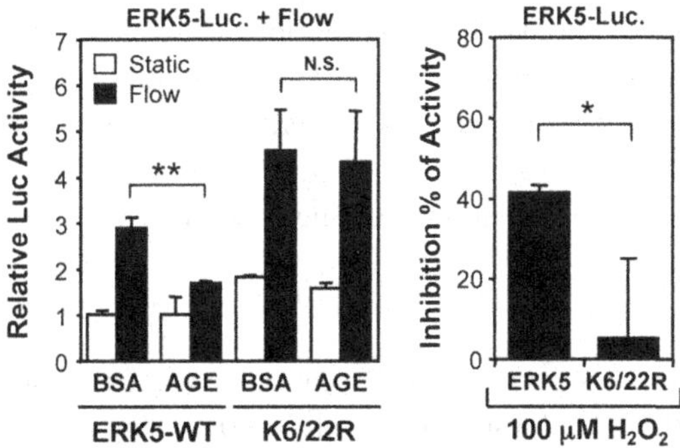

Fig. 11. H_2O_2 and AGE inhibit laminar flow–induced ERK5 transcriptional activity through SUMOylation in ECs. Laminar flow–induced ERK5 transcriptional activity was measured with wild-type ERK5 or ERK5-K6/22R mutant (A and B) in the presence of H_2O_2 (A) or AGE (B) in HUVECs (left). The right graphs in A and B show percentages of inhibition of reporter activity, calculated from the activity of the reporter under each condition in the presence and absence (taken as 100%) of H_2O_2 or AGE as indicated. Subconfluent HUVECs were cotransfected with Gal4 wild-type ERK5 or ERK5-K6/22R mutant. Twenty-four hours after transfection, cells were treated with H_2O_2 (A) or AGE (B) for 1 hour before challenging with shear stress at 12 dyne/cm^2 for 24 hours. ERK5 transcriptional activity was determined by luciferase activity as described in Materials and Methods. Data are expressed as mean percentages ±S.D. from 3 independent experiments. * $P < 0.05$, ** $P < 0.01$.[117] (Obtained permission to reproduce from Wolters Kluwer Health).

adapter molecules may be involved. For example, Gregoire *et al.*[122] have reported that class IIa HDACs stimulate MEF2 SUMOylation. Interestingly, this SUMOylation depended on residues 118 to 488 of MEF2D not on the C-terminal catalytic domain of HDAC4, suggesting that the deacetylase activity of HDAC4 was not required. It is possible that HDACs inhibit transcriptional activity via increasing SUMOylation of transcription factors. Furthermore, they found that ERK5, which is known to phosphorylate Ser179 of MEF2D, negatively regulated MEF2 SUMOylation.[122] Although it is not known whether or not H_2O_2 and AGE induce phosphorylation in these proteins or direct interaction between HDAC and ERK5, it is well known that both H_2O_2 and AGE can activate many kinases, some of which may contribute to the regulation of ERK5 SUMOylation. Further investigation is necessary to clarify the regulatory mechanism of H_2O_2- or AGE-mediated ERK5-SUMOylation.

In summary, determining flow-mediated signal transduction pathways has once again become a hot topic. The ability to make distinctions between d- and s-flow-mediated signaling may provide critical information on initial mechanism of endothelial dysfunction, which leads to atherosclerosis formation. In addition, the interplay between inflammatory molecules such as cytokines and s/d-flow-mediated signaling needs careful evaluation for which identification of mechanosensors and post-translational modification of various molecules in mechanosignaling cascades is critical.

Acknowledgments

This work is supported by grants from the National Institute of Health to J. A. (GM-071485, HL-088637 and HL-077789). J. A. is a recipient of an Established Investigator Award of the American Heart Association (0740013N). We would like to thank Dr. Hakjoo Lee, Carolyn McClain and Thomas Spangenberg for the critical reading of this manuscript.

References

1. Hansson, G. K., Robertson, A. K., and Soderberg-Naucler, C. (2006) *Annu Rev Pathol* **1**, 297–329.
2. Ross, R. (1999) *N Engl J Med* **340**(2), 115–126.
3. Tedgui, A., and Mallat, Z. (2006) *Physiol Rev* **86**(2), 515–581.
4. Libby, P. (2002) *Nature* **420**(6917), 868–874.
5. Cybulsky, M. I., Fries, J. W., Williams, A. J., Sultan, P., Davis, V. M., Gimbrone, M. A., Jr., and Collins, T. (1991) *Am J Pathol* **138**(4), 815–820.
6. Korenaga, R., Ando, J., Tsuboi, H., Yang, W., Sakuma, I., Toyo, O. T., and Kamiya, A. (1994) *Biochem Biophys Res Commun* **198**(1), 213–219.
7. Di Francesco, L., Totani, L., Dovizio, M., Piccoli, A., Di Francesco, A., Salvatore, T., Pandolfi, A., Evangelista, V., Dercho, R. A., Seta, F., and Patrignani, P. (2009) *Circ Res* **104**(4), 506–513.

8. Frangos, J. A., Eskin, S. G., McIntire, L. V., and Ives, C. L. (1985) *Science* **227**, 1477–1479.
9. Gimbrone, M. A., Jr., Nagel, T., and Topper, J. N. (1997) *J Clin Invest* **99**(8), 1809–1813.
10. Traub, O., and Berk, B. C. (1998) *Arterioscler Thromb Vasc Biol* **18**(5), 677–685.
11. SenBanerjee, S., Lin, Z., Atkins, G. B., Greif, D. M., Rao, R. M., Kumar, A., Feinberg, M. W., Chen, Z., Simon, D. I., Luscinskas, F. W., Michel, T. M., Gimbrone, M. A., Jr., Garcia-Cardena, G., and Jain, M. K. (2004) *J Exp Med* **199**(10), 1305–1315.
12. Dekker, R. J., van Soest, S., Fontijn, R. D., Salamanca, S., de Groot, P. G., VanBavel, E., Pannekoek, H., and Horrevoets, A. J. (2002) *Blood* **100**(5), 1689–1698.
13. Lin, Z., Kumar, A., Senbanerjee, S., Staniszewski, K., Parmar, K., Vaughan, D. E., Gimbrone, M. A., Jr., Balasubramanian, V., Garcia-Cardena, G., and Jain, M. K. (2005) *Circ Res.*
14. Berk, B. C. (2008) *Circulation* **117**(8), 1082–1089.
15. Ku, D. N., Giddens, D. P., Zarins, C. K., and Glagov, S. (1985) *Arteriosclerosis* **5**(3), 293–302.
16. Cornhill, J. F., and Roach, M. R. (1976) *Atherosclerosis* **23**(3), 489–501.
17. Brookes, P. S., Digerness, S. B., Parks, D. A., and Darley-Usmar, V. (2002) *Free Radic Biol Med* **32**(11), 1220–1228.
18. Chiu, Y. J., Kusano, K., Thomas, T. N., and Fujiwara, K. (2004) *Endothelium* **11**(1), 59–73.
19. Chachisvilis, M., Zhang, Y. L., and Frangos, J. A. (2006) *Proc Natl Acad Sci U S A* **103**(42), 15463–15468.
20. Shyy, J. Y., and Chien, S. (2002) *Circ Res* **91**(9), 769–775.
21. Ohno, M., Gibbons, G. H., Dzau, V. J., and Cooke, J. P. (1993) *Circulation* **88**(1), 193–197.
22. Harada, N., Masuda, M., and Fujiwara, K. (1995) *Biochem Biophys Res Commun* **214**(1), 69–74.
23. Osawa, M., Masuda, M., Harada, N., Bruno Lopes, R., and Fujiwara, K. (1997) *European J Cell Biol* **72**, 229–237.
24. Kaufman, D. A., Albelda, S. M., Sun, J., and Davies, P. F. (2004) *Biochem Biophys Res Commun* **320**(4), 1076–1081.
25. Fleming, I., Fisslthaler, B., Dixit, M., and Busse, R. (2005) *J Cell Sci* **118**(Pt 18), 4103–4111.
26. Masuda, M., Osawa, M., Shigematsu, H., Harada, N., and Fujiwara, K. (1997) *FEBS Lett* **408**(3), 331–336.
27. Chiu, Y. J., McBeath, E., and Fujiwara, K. (2008) *J Cell Biol* **182**(4), 753–763.
28. Kusano, K., Thomas, T. N., and Fujiwara, K. (2008) *Endothelium* **15**(3), 127–136.
29. Tseng, H., Peterson, T. E., and Berk, B. C. (1995) *Circ Res* **77**(5), 869–878.

30. Osawa, M., Masuda, M., Kusano, K., and Fujiwara, K. (2002) *J Cell Biol* **158**(4), 773–785.
31. Tzima, E., Irani-Tehrani, M., Kiosses, W. B., Dejana, E., Schultz, D. A., Engelhardt, B., Cao, G., DeLisser, H., and Schwartz, M. A. (2005) *Nature* **437**(7057), 426–431.
32. Ilan, N., Cheung, L., Pinter, E., and Madri, J. A. (2000) *J Biol Chem* **275**(28), 21435–21443.
33. Ilan, N., Mahooti, S., Rimm, D. L., and Madri, J. A. (1999) *J Cell Sci* **112**, 3005–3014.
34. Sawada, Y., and Sheetz, M. P. (2002) *J Cell Biol* **11**, 11.
35. Kogata, N., Masuda, M., Kamioka, Y., Yamagishi, A., Endo, A., Okada, M., and Mochizuki, N. (2003) *Mol Biol Cell* **14**(9), 3553–3564.
36. Cao, M. Y., Huber, M., Beauchemin, N., Famiglietti, J., Albelda, S. M., and Veillette, A. (1998) *J Biol Chem* **273**(25), 15765–15772.
37. Dimmeler, S., Hermann, C., Galle, J., and Zeiher, A. M. (1999) *Arterioscler Thromb Vasc Biol* **19**(3), 656–664.
38. Yamawaki, H., Pan, S., Lee, R. T., and Berk, B. C. (2005) *J Clin Invest* **115**(3), 733–738.
39. Yamawaki, H., Haendeler, J., and Berk, B. C. (2003) *Circ Res* **93**(11), 1029–1033.
40. Yamawaki, H., and Berk, B. C. (2005) *Curr Opin Nephrol Hypertens* **14**(2), 149–153.
41. Schulze, P. C., Yoshioka, J., Takahashi, T., He, Z., King, G. L., and Lee, R. T. (2004) *J Biol Chem* **279**(29), 30369–30374.
42. Yoshioka, J., Schulze, P. C., Cupesi, M., Sylvan, J. D., MacGillivray, C., Gannon, J., Huang, H., and Lee, R. T. (2004) *Circulation* **109**(21), 2581–2586.
43. Junn, E., Han, S. H., Im, J. Y., Yang, Y., Cho, E. W., Um, H. D., Kim, D. K., Lee, K. W., Han, P. L., Rhee, S. G., and Choi, I. (2000) *J Immunol* **164**(12), 6287–6295.
44. Saitoh, M., Nishitoh, H., Fujii, M., Takeda, K., Tobiume, K., Sawada, Y., Kawabata, M., Miyazono, K., and Ichijo, H. (1998) *Embo J* **17**(9), 2596–2606.
45. Nishiyama, A., Matsui, M., Iwata, S., Hirota, K., Masutani, H., Nakamura, H., Takagi, Y., Sono, H., Gon, Y., and Yodoi, J. (1999) *J Biol Chem* **274**(31), 21645–21650.
46. Nadeau, P. J., Charette, S. J., and Landry, J. (2009) *Mol Biol Cell* **20**(16), 3628–3637.
47. Nadeau, P. J., Charette, S. J., Toledano, M. B., and Landry, J. (2007) *Mol Biol Cell* **18**(10), 3903–3913.
48. Hermann, C., Zeiher, A. M., and Dimmeler, S. (1997) *Arterioscler Thromb Vasc Biol* **17**(12), 3588–3592.
49. Hojo, Y., Saito, Y., Tanimoto, T., Hoefen, R. J., Baines, C. P., Yamamoto, K., Haendeler, J., Asmis, R., and Berk, B. C. (2002) *Circ Res* **91**(8), 712–718.

50. Holmgren, A. (1976) *Proc Natl Acad Sci U S A* **73**(7), 2275–2279.
51. Wang, J., Pan, S., and Berk, B. C. (2007) *Arterioscler Thromb Vasc Biol* **27**(6), 1283–1288.
52. Abe, J., Baines, C. P., and Berk, B. C. (2000) *Circ Res* **86**(6), 607–609.
53. Abe, J., and Berk, B. C. (1998) *Trends Cardiovasc Med* **8**(2), 59–64.
54. Yan, C., Takahashi, M., Okuda, M., Lee, J. D., and Berk, B. C. (1999) *J Biol Chem* **274**(1), 143–150.
55. Dhanasekaran, D. N., and Reddy, E. P. (2008) *Oncogene* **27**(48), 6245–6251.
56. De Cesaris, P., Starace, D., Starace, G., Filippini, A., Stefanini, M., and Ziparo, E. (1999) *J Biol Chem* **274**(41), 28978–28982.
57. Ahmad, M., Theofanidis, P., and Medford, R. M. (1998) *J Biol Chem* **273**(8), 4616–4621.
58. Min, W., and Pober, J. S. (1997) *J Immunol* **159**(7), 3508–3518.
59. Wong, H. K., Fricker, M., Wyttenbach, A., Villunger, A., Michalak, E. M., Strasser, A., and Tolkovsky, A. M. (2005) *Mol Cell Biol* **25**(19), 8732–8747.
60. Fan, G., Merritt, S. E., Kortenjann, M., Shaw, P. E., and Holzman, L. B. (1996) *J Biol Chem* **271**(40), 24788–24793.
61. Oleinik, N. V., Krupenko, N. I., and Krupenko, S. A. (2007) *Oncogene* **26**(51), 7222–7230.
62. Yamamoto, K., Ichijo, H., and Korsmeyer, S. J. (1999) *Mol Cell Biol* **19**(12), 8469–8478.
63. Putcha, G. V., Le, S., Frank, S., Besirli, C. G., Clark, K., Chu, B., Alix, S., Youle, R. J., LaMarche, A., Maroney, A. C., and Johnson, E. M., Jr. (2003) *Neuron* **38**(6), 899–914.
64. Lei, K., and Davis, R. J. (2003) *Proc Natl Acad Sci U S A* **100**(5), 2432–2437.
65. Luo, X., Budihardjo, I., Zou, H., Slaughter, C., and Wang, X. (1998) *Cell* **94**(4), 481–490.
66. Li, H., Zhu, H., Xu, C. J., and Yuan, J. (1998) *Cell* **94**(4), 491–501.
67. Deng, Y., Ren, X., Yang, L., Lin, Y., and Wu, X. (2003) *Cell* **115**(1), 61–70.
68. Ricci, R., Sumara, G., Sumara, I., Rozenberg, I., Kurrer, M., Akhmedov, A., Hersberger, M., Eriksson, U., Eberli, F. R., Becher, B., Boren, J., Chen, M., Cybulsky, M. I., Moore, K. J., Freeman, M. W., Wagner, E. F., Matter, C. M., and Luscher, T. F. (2004) *Science* **306**(5701), 1558–1561.
69. Sumara, G., Belwal, M., and Ricci, R. (2005) *Cell Mol Life Sci* **62**(21), 2487–2494.
70. Garin, G., Abe, J. I., Mohan, A., Lu, W., Yan, C., Newby, A. C., Rhaman, A., and Berk, B. C. (2007) *Circ Res.*
71. Dekker, L. V., and Parker, P. J. (1994) *Trends Biochem Sci* **19**(2), 73–77.
72. Lamark, T., Perander, M., Outzen, H., Kristiansen, K., Overvatn, A., Michaelsen, E., Bjorkoy, G., and Johansen, T. (2003) *J Biol Chem* **278**(36), 34568–34581.
73. Hirano, Y., Yoshinaga, S., Ogura, K., Yokochi, M., Noda, Y., Sumimoto, H., and Inagaki, F. (2004) *J Biol Chem* **279**(30), 31883–31890.
74. Rahman, A., Anwar, K. N., and Malik, A. B. (2000) *Am J Physiol Cell Physiol* **279**(4), C906–914.

75. Javaid, K., Rahman, A., Anwar, K. N., Frey, R. S., Minshall, R. D., and Malik, A. B. (2003) *Circ Res* **92**(10), 1089–1097.
76. Magid, R., and Davies, P. F. (2005) *Circ Res* **97**(5), 443–449.
77. World, C. J., Garin, G., and Berk, B. (2006) *Curr Atheroscler Rep* **8**(3), 240–244.
78. Smith, L., Chen, L., Reyland, M. E., DeVries, T. A., Talanian, R. V., Omura, S., and Smith, J. B. (2000) *J Biol Chem* **275**(51), 40620–40627.
79. Smith, L., Wang, Z., and Smith, J. B. (2003) *Biochem J* **375**(Pt 3), 663–671.
80. Lerner-Marmarosh, N., Yoshizumi, M., Che, W., Surapisitchat, J., Kawakatsu, H., Akaike, M., Ding, B., Huang, Q., Yan, C., Berk, B. C., and Abe, J. I. (2003) *Arterioscler Thromb Vasc Biol* **23**(10), 1775–1781.
81. Che, W., Lerner-Marmarosh, N., Huang, Q., Osawa, M., Ohta, S., Yoshizumi, M., Glassman, M., Lee, J. D., Yan, C., Berk, B. C., and Abe, J. (2002) *Cir. Res.* **Accepted.**
82. You, M., Yu, D. H., and Feng, G. S. (1999) *Mol Cell Biol* **19**(3), 2416–2424.
83. Fukunaga, K., Noguchi, T., Takeda, H., Matozaki, T., Hayashi, Y., Itoh, H., and Kasuga, M. (2000) *J Biol Chem* **275**(7), 5208–5213.
84. Neel, B. G. (1993) *Semin Cell Biol* **4**(6), 419–432.
85. David, M., Zhou, G., Pine, R., Dixon, J. E., and Larner, A. C. (1996) *J Biol Chem* **271**(27), 15862–15865.
86. Gadina, M., Stancato, L. M., Bacon, C. M., Larner, A. C., and O'Shea, J. J. (1998) *J Immunol* **160**(10), 4657–4661.
87. Case, R. D., Piccione, E., Wolf, G., Benett, A. M., Lechleider, R. J., Neel, B. G., and Shoelson, S. E. (1994) *J Biol Chem* **269**(14), 10467–10474.
88. Yang, J., Lin, Y., Guo, Z., Cheng, J., Huang, J., Deng, L., Liao, W., Chen, Z., Liu, Z., and Su, B. (2001) *Nat Immunol* **2**(7), 620–624.
89. Li, L., Tatake, R. J., Natarajan, K., Taba, Y., Garin, G., Tai, C., Leung, E., Surapisitchat, J., Yoshizumi, M., Yan, C., Abe, J., and Berk, B. C. (2008) *Biochem Biophys Res Commun* **370**(1), 159–163.
90. Akaike, M., Che, W., Marmarosh, N. L., Ohta, S., Osawa, M., Ding, B., Berk, B. C., Yan, C., and Abe, J. (2004) *Mol Cell Biol* **24**(19), 8691–8704.
91. Kasler, H. G., Victoria, J., Duramad, O., and Winoto, A. (2000) *Mol Cell Biol* **20**(22), 8382–8389.
92. Gutkind, J. S. (2000) *Sci STKE* **2000**(40), RE1.
93. Zhou, G., Bao, Z. Q., and Dixon, J. E. (1995) *J Biol Chem* **270**(21), 12665–12669.
94. Lee, J. D., Ulevitch, R. J., and Han, J. (1995) *Biochem Biophys Res Commun* **213**(2), 715–724.
95. Suzaki, Y., Yoshizumi, M., Kagami, S., Koyama, A. H., Taketani, Y., Houchi, H., Tsuchiya, K., Takeda, E., and Tamaki, T. (2002) *J Biol Chem* **277**(11), 9614–9621.
96. Regan, C. P., Li, W., Boucher, D. M., Spatz, S., Su, M. S., and Kuida, K. (2002) *Proc Natl Acad Sci U S A* **99**(14), 9248–9253.

97. Won, D., Zhu, S. N., Chen, M., Teichert, A. M., Fish, J. E., Matouk, C. C., Bonert, M., Ojha, M., Marsden, P. A., and Cybulsky, M. I. (2007) *Am J Pathol* **171**(5), 1691–1704.
98. Jongstra-Bilen, J., Haidari, M., Zhu, S. N., Chen, M., Guha, D., and Cybulsky, M. I. (2006) *J Exp Med* **203**(9), 2073–2083.
99. Diamond, S. L., Eskin, S. G., and McIntire, L. V. (1989) *Science* **243**(4897), 1483–1485.
100. Bao, X., Lu, C., and Frangos, J. A. (1999) *Arterioscler Thromb Vasc Biol* **19**(4), 996–1003.
101. Wang, G. X., Cai, S. X., Wang, P. Q., Ouyang, K. Q., Wang, Y. L., and Xu, S. R. (2002) *Microvasc Res* **63**(2), 209–217.
102. Hsiai, T. K., Cho, S. K., Reddy, S., Hama, S., Navab, M., Demer, L. L., Honda, H. M., and Ho, C. M. (2001) *Arterioscler Thromb Vasc Biol* **21**(11), 1770–1776.
103. Surapisitchat, J., Hoefen, R. J., Pi, X., Yoshizumi, M., Yan, C., and Berk, B. C. (2001) *Proc Natl Acad Sci U S A* **98**(11), 6476–6481.
104. Collins, A. R., Meehan, W. P., Kintscher, U., Jackson, S., Wakino, S., Noh, G., Palinski, W., Hsueh, W. A., and Law, R. E. (2001) *Arterioscler Thromb Vasc Biol* **21**(3), 365–371.
105. Yan, C., Luo, H., Lee, J. D., Abe, J., and Berk, B. C. (2001) *J Biol Chem* **276**(14), 10870–10878.
106. Kato, Y., Kravchenko, V. V., Tapping, R. I., Han, J., Ulevitch, R. J., and Lee, J. D. (1997) *Embo J* **16**(23), 7054–7066.
107. Schulman, I. G., Juguilon, H., and Evans, R. M. (1996) *Mol Cell Biol* **16**(7), 3807–3813.
108. Hu, X., and Lazar, M. A. (1999) *Nature* **402**(6757), 93–96.
109. Parmar, K. M., Larman, H. B., Dai, G., Zhang, Y., Wang, E. T., Moorthy, S. N., Kratz, J. R., Lin, Z., Jain, M. K., Gimbrone, M. A., Jr., and Garcia-Cardena, G. (2006) *J Clin Invest* **116**(1), 49–58.
110. Rohrer, L., Hersberger, M., and von Eckardstein, A. (2004) *Curr Opin Lipidol* **15**(3), 269–278.
111. Alexander, R. W. (1998) *Trans Am Clin Climatol Assoc* **109**, 129–145; discussion 145–126.
112. Hilgarth, R. S., Murphy, L. A., Skaggs, H. S., Wilkerson, D. C., Xing, H., and Sarge, K. D. (2004) *J Biol Chem* **279**(52), 53899–53902.
113. Verger, A., Perdomo, J., and Crossley, M. (2003) *EMBO Rep* **4**(2), 137–142.
114. Desterro, J. M., Rodriguez, M. S., and Hay, R. T. (1998) *Mol Cell* **2**(2), 233–239.
115. Johnson, E. S. (2004) *Annu Rev Biochem* **73**, 355–382.
116. Melchior, F. (2000) *Annu Rev Cell Dev Biol* **16**, 591–626.
117. Woo, C. H., Shishido, T., McClain, C., Lim, J. H., Li, J. D., Yang, J., Yan, C., and Abe, J. I. (2008) *Circ Res.*
118. Hudson, B. I., Wendt, T., Bucciarelli, L. G., Rong, L. L., Naka, Y., Yan, S. F., and Schmidt, A. M. (2005) *Antioxid Redox Signal* **7**(11–12), 1588–1600.

119. Rask-Madsen, C., and King, G. L. (2007) *Nat Clin Pract Endocrinol Metab* **3**(1), 46–56.
120. Ting, H. H., Timimi, F. K., Boles, K. S., Creager, S. J., Ganz, P., and Creager, M. A. (1996) *J Clin Invest* **97**(1), 22–28.
121. Park, L., Raman, K. G., Lee, K. J., Lu, Y., Ferran, L. J., Jr., Chow, W. S., Stern, D., and Schmidt, A. M. (1998) *Nat Med* **4**(9), 1025–1031.
122. Gregoire, S., and Yang, X. J. (2005) *Mol Cell Biol* **25**(6), 2273–2287.

Chapter 3

ENDOTHELIAL GLYCOCALYX STRUCTURE AND ROLE IN MECHANOTRANSDUCTION

JOHN M. TARBELL* and ENO E. EBONG†

**Biomedical Engineering Department,*
The City College of New York, New York, NY
tarbell@ccny.cuny.edu

†Biomedical Engineering Department,
The City College of New York, New York, NY
Neuroscience Department,
Albert Einstein College of Medicine, Bronx, NY
eno.ebong@einstein.yu.edu

The endothelial cell (EC) surface is coated with a glycocalyx (GCX) layer that is composed of a wide variety of membrane-bound macromolecules: sulfated proteoglycans, hyaluronic acid, sialic acids, glycoproteins, and plasma proteins. The GCX surface layer has been estimated to be from 20 nm to several microns thick in a static fluid environment, depending on cell/tissue preservation and microscopic visualization techniques that are reviewed in detail. Recently, there has been growing recognition that the GCX is a mechanotransducer and plays an important role in transmitting force to the cell's actin cytoskeleton and in initiating intracellular signaling. GCX thinning and shedding have been demonstrated to occur in diseases associated with mechanotransduction dysfunction. Recognizing the association of GCX degradation with disease, this chapter will provide an overview and synthesis of current knowledge concerning GCX molecular and physical structure and its function in endothelial mechanotransduction.

1. Introduction

The concept that a thin endocapillary layer might cover the entire endothelial surface was first proposed by Danielli[1] and Chambers and Zweifach[2] and subsequently reexamined by Copley[3] who suggested that the layer was an immobile sheet of plasma and macromolecules. However, this layer evaded observation by light and electron microscopy (EM) until Luft[4] used ruthenium red staining to detect a thin layer (~20 nm thick) in mouse capillaries.

While early studies of the glycocalyx (GCX) were limited largely to microvessels, the association of altered GCX characteristics with atherosclerosis-prone locations in arteries was recognized back in the early 1980s. Lewis *et al.*[5] observed the coronary arteries of White Carneau pigeons and noted that the GCX, as assessed by ruthenium red staining, was thinnest in areas with high disease predilection, and that upon cholesterol challenge, the GCX thickness was reduced in all arterial zones. This idea of association between GCX abundance and arterial disease has been revisited recently by van den Berg *et al.*[6] who showed that low density lipoprotein (LDL) accumulation was enhanced and GCX thickness reduced in the disease prone sinus region of the mouse internal carotid artery relative to the nearby common carotid artery that is spared of disease. Van den Berg *et al.*[7] reported that the GCX is diminished upon systemic atherogenic challenge by a high-fat, high cholesterol diet. Nieuwdorp *et al.*[8] reported that hyperglycemia results in a pronounced 50% loss of GCX volume in humans. Similar reductions in systemic GCX volume found in patients with Type 1 diabetes and in animal models of ischemia-reperfusion injury were reported in a review by van den Berg *et al.*[9] These observations are consistent with studies demonstrating rapid shedding of the GCX from the endothelial surface upon acute stimulation with elevated plasma levels of oxidized LDL or acute exposure to inflammatory agents, reviewed by Gouverneur *et al.*[10]

Recognizing the association of GCX degradation with disease, the present review focuses on the structure of the GCX and its role in mechanotransduction. Clearly the structure is altered in disease states and as we will describe, the capacity of the GCX to function as a mechanotransducer is also impaired by its degradation. Dysfunction of endothelial mechanotransduction, therefore, may be an important mechanism by which disease progresses.

We begin the review by describing the molecular and physical structure of the GCX by providing an overview of the composition, organization, and thickness of the GCX. This section serves as background for an extensive discussion of endothelial mechanotransduction and remodeling. We conclude with a brief summary where we highlight future challenges for our understanding of the structure of the GCX and its function as a mechanotransducer. There have been three previous reviews of the endothelial GCX that have influenced the present one. Pries *et al.*[11] provided an excellent introduction to the GCX and overview of the earlier literature. Tarbell and Pahakis[12] provided an extensive discussion of the biomolecular structure of the GCX with emphasis on mechanotransduction. Weinbaum *et al.*,[13] provided a more comprehensive review including discussion of mechanical and transport properties and the role of the GCX in cell adhesion. The present review draws on these previous works, but introduces the most recent literature and attempts, in particular, to synthesize what is known about the molecular and physical structure of the GCX and its function as a mechanotransducer.

2. Structure of the Glycocalyx

2.1. *Molecular Composition and Organization of the Glycocalyx*

The surface of endothelial cells (ECs) is decorated with a wide variety of membrane-bound macromolecules, which constitute the glycocalyx (GCX). A cartoon that integrates all of the components of the GCX that are described in more detail below is shown in Fig. 1, adapted from Tarbell

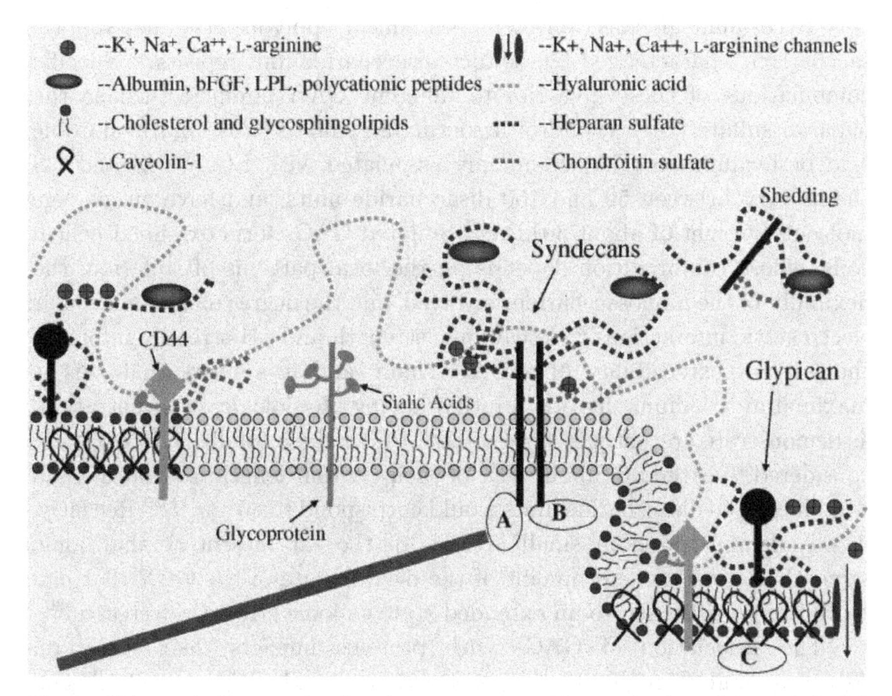

Fig. 1. Schematic diagram showing the components and organization of the endothelial glycocalyx layer. All components are labeled on the diagram. *Adapted from Fig. 1, Tarbell and Pahakis.*[12]

and Pahakis.[12] From glycoproteins bearing acidic oligosaccharides and terminal sialic acids (SA), to proteoglycans along with their associated glycosaminoglycan (GAG) side chains, the polyanionic nature of its constituents imparts to it a net negative charge. Under physiological conditions, an extended endothelial surface layer arises from the association of components of the GCX with blood-borne molecules.[11,14] Plasma proteins, enzymes, enzyme inhibitors, growth factors and cytokines, through cationic sites in their structure, as well as cationic amino acids, cations, and water, all associate with this matrix of biopolyelectrolytes.[15,16] An additional level in the complexity of this biological structure arises from its dynamic nature. The interactions between GAGs and proteins are highly dependent on the conditions of their local microenvironment, such as cation content and concentration, and pH.[17–12] Furthermore, ECs actively regulate the content and physicochemical properties of GAGs on their surface by having high rates of continuous metabolic turnover that allow adaptation to changes in the local environment.[22–24]

Glycosaminoglycans (GAGs) are linear polydisperse heteropolysaccharides, characterized by distinct disaccharide unit repeats.[25] Specific combinations of these give rise to different GAG families, such as the heparan sulfate (HS), chondroitin/dermatan sulfate (CS), and hyaluronic acid or hyaluronan (HA) commonly associated with ECs.[26] HS and CS chains vary between 50 and 150 disaccharide units, and have an average molecular weight of about 30 kDa.[27] Sulfated GAGs form extended helical coils, whose conformation depends on the local patterns of sulfation, the flexibility of the monosaccharides involved, and the degree of intramolecular electrostatic interactions.[28] Local ionic strength and pH strongly influence the level of extensibility of a GAG chain, and it appears that this is maximal in a sodium chloride solution having physiological concentration, as demonstrated recently by Seog *et al.*[29] Under these conditions, GAGs are considered to extend to about 80% of their contour length, so that a chain containing 100 disaccharide units would correspond to 80 nm.[11,29] Recently, it was demonstrated in small arteries of the rat mesentery that ionic strength is a major determinant of the overall state of the GCX that can move from a collapsed to an extended state as ionic strength decreases.[30]

The association of GAGs with proteins impacts their structure. Adamson and Clough[14] demonstrated how, in the absence of plasma proteins, addition of a solution of a large charged marker protein (cationized ferritin, 440 kDa, 12 nm) reveals a collapsed GCX in frog mesenteric capillaries. Addition of a 2% frog plasma solution was enough to significantly lift the layer of ferritin above the endothelial surface, while a 5% albumin solution had a less striking effect.[14] The "preferential" behavior that the GCX displayed for the less oncotic native plasma over albumin alone makes it evident that specific interactions are essential to the physiological structure of the GCX.

HS is the most prominent GAG on the surface of ECs and accounts for 50–90% of the total GAG pool, the rest being comprised of CS and HA.[26] Owing to its structural analogy with heparin, HS and associated proteoglycans (PGs) have been more extensively studied than other GAGs and their associated PGs, with attention recently shifting towards their ability to function as signal transduction molecules.[31,32] PGs are proteins that contain specific sites where sulfated GAGs are covalently attached[25]. Relevant to this review, the transmembrane syndecans and membrane bound glypicans are among the three major protein core families of heparan sulfate proteoglycans (HSPGs) found on ECs (along with the basement matrix associated perlecans).[33]

From the syndecan family of core proteins, syndecans −1 (33 kDa), −2 (22 kDa), and −4 (22 kDa) that are expressed on ECs have three GAG attachment sites close to their N-terminus and distal to the apical surface, substituted primarily but not exclusively by HS.[33,34] Syndecan-1 contains two additional sites which are close to the membrane and reserved for CS.[35] On the other side of the plasma membrane, their cytoplasmic tails associate with the cytoskeleton and assist in its organization, through molecules such as tubulin, dynamin, and alpha-actinin.[36,37] Active participation in signaling stems from the phosphorylation of certain intracytoplasmic residues, which act as switches controlling the oligomerization state and altering the binding properties of syndecans.[31,32,36]

Of the glypican core protein family, glypican-1 (64 kDa) is the only one expressed on ECs.[33] Close to the membrane, its three to four GAG attachment sites are exclusively substituted with HS.[38] Glypican-1 is bound directly to the plasma membrane through a C-terminal glycosylphosphatidylinositol (GPI) anchor.[38] Most importantly, the GPI anchor localizes this proteoglycan to lipid rafts, which are cholesterol and sphingolipid rich membranous domains involved in vesicular transport and cell signaling.[38–40] Caveolae can be considered a subset of lipid rafts, which arise from the incorporation of the protein caveolin-1, a cholesterol carrier, into the membrane, where they may form characteristic cave-like structures (∼100 nm) that are supported by the cytoskeleton.[41]

In contrast with CS and HS, HA is a much longer disaccharide polymer, on the order of 1000 kDa, which is synthesized on the cell surface and is not covalently attached to a core protein.[42] It is not sulfated, but obtains its negative charge from carboxyl groups that endow it with exceptional hydration properties.[42] HA weaves into the GCX through its interaction with surface HA receptors, such as the transmembrane CD44, and CS chains.[43] CD44, which contains CS GAGs, localizes along with HA in caveolae where it has various functional interactions.[44]

Completing the picture, glycoproteins with short branched oligosaccharides attached to their core are also found on the surface of ECs. These oligosaccharides are capped by sialic acid (SA), the 9-carbon monosaccharides that contribute to the net negative charge of the GCX, through their ionization at physiological pH.[45] Many important receptors on the cell surface, such as selectins, integrins, and members of the immunoglobulin superfamily, have oligosaccharides attached to them and are classified as glycoproteins.[11]

2.2. *Glycocalyx Thickness*

The first visualization of the endothelial surface layer revealed a 20-nm thick GCX by using electron microscopy (EM) together with the ruthenium red cationic dye that binds to acidic mucopolysaccharides and generates electron density in the presence of osmium tetroxide.[4] Adamson and Clough[14] later used a large charged marker protein, cationized ferritin, to label the edge of the GCX in frog microvessels. They demonstrated that GCX thickness was several times greater than the 20 nm observed with ruthenium red, and that the GCX would collapse in the absence of plasma proteins, presumably due to elimination of stabilizing intramolecular interactions with plasma proteins. These early methods suffered from dehydration artifacts associated with conventional EM and the aqueous fixatives that likely dissolved much of the proteoglycan GAG structure. Later studies used fixation methods designed to preserve water soluble structures employing fluorocarbons as non-aqueous carriers of osmium tetroxide. This fluorocarbon-glutaraldehyde fixation method was applied to rat capillaries by Rostgaard and Qvortrup[46] to reveal a filamentous brush-like surface coating of thickness 50–100 nm. Another fixation method used in conjunction with EM involves treatment with Alcian Blue that stabilizes anionic carbohydrate structures. This method produced estimates of rat myocardial capillary GCX thickness of 200 to 500 nm.[47] Squire *et al.*[48] prepared samples of fresh, unfixed tissue (frog mesenteric capillaries) rapidly frozen and processed by freeze-fracture, deep-etching, and heavy metal shadowing prior to EM. They observed a GCX thickness of order 200 nm. Using computed autocorrelation functions and Fourier transform analysis they were able to deduce characteristic 20 nm spacing in the GCX structure and a clustering of fibrous elements that are spaced about 100 nm apart and arranged in a quasi-regular hexagonal array suggestive of a submembranous cytoskeletal scaffold.

The experiments described above were obtained by studying the GCX on ECs in fixed vascular explants that were imaged under stationary conditions without fluid flow through the vessel lumen. The first method to estimate GCX thickness under flow conditions without fixation was described by Vink and Duling.[49] Using a 70 kDa dextran plasma tracer which was sterically excluded by the GCX, they were able to estimate the thickness of the GCX under flow conditions in live capillaries to be in the range of 0.4–0.5 μm. This estimate of the *in vivo* thickness of the GCX is two to five times greater than previous estimates derived from EM studies, which likely significantly underestimated the value owing either to the dehydration of the extracellular matrix or the cleavage of its outer matrix components that accompanies tissue fixation.

The dye-exclusion technique developed by Duling and coworkers does not provide adequate resolution in vessels larger than ~12–15 μm due to optical difficulties reviewed by Henry and Duling.[43] A new method based on high resolution, near wall, intravital fluorescent micro-particle image velocimetry (μ-PIV) to examine the velocity profile near the vessel wall in post-capillary venules of the mouse cremaster muscle was described by Smith *et al.*[50] and elaborated by Long *et al.*[51] and Damiano *et al.*[52]. Ultimately these methods led to estimates of a GCX thickness of 0.5 μm in a 20–40 μm thick mouse cremaster venule. The μ-PIV method, like the dye-exclusion technique, was applied under live (un-fixed) conditions in a physiological flow field.

Another new approach to GCX imaging, based on the use of confocal laser scanning microscopy, was used by van den Berg and colleagues[6] who imaged sections of explanted mouse carotid arteries and found a GCX thickness of about 4 μm in the common region. These results confirmed earlier findings of Megens *et al.*[53] that were obtained using yet another novel method, two-photon laser scanning microscopy, by which a 4.5 μm

GCX was found in explanted intact mouse carotid arteries. The use of confocal laser scanning microscopy to assess GCX thickness on ECs cultured *in vitro* was first described by Barker *et al.*[54] A fluorescein isothiocyanate (FITC)-linked wheat germ agglutinin was used for the detection of sialic acid on the surface of human umbilical vein endothelial cells (HUVECs) with a confocal microscope using z-section scans at intervals of 0.5 μm. The GCX thickness was deduced to be 2.5 μm on these live cells *in vitro*, imaged under stationary (no flow) conditions. When these same cells were viewed under EM after conventional fixation and staining with ruthenium red, as in Luft[4], a GCX thickness of only 100 nm was apparent. This study clearly demonstrates the marked differences in estimates of GCX thickness for live cells versus fixed cells. In subsequent related studies, conventional aldehyde fixation and EM were used by Ueda *et al.*[55] to detect a GCX layer of 20–30 nm thickness on ruthenium red stained bovine aortic endothelial cells (BAECs) *in vitro* and by Devaraj *et al.*[56] to record a GCX layer of 850 nm thickness on human aortic endothelial cells (HAECs) processed with Alcian Blue and lanthanum nitrate, whereas Stevens *et al.*[57] applied confocal laser scanning microscopy and fluorescence correlation spectroscopy on live bovine lung microvascular endothelial cells (BLMVEC) labeled with both heparan sulfate and hyaluronan and estimated GCX thickness of 2–3 μm (see Fig. 2).

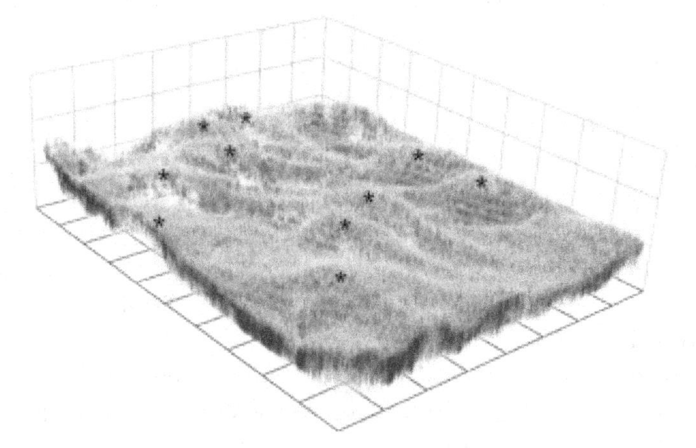

Fig. 2. Confocal image of the glycocalyx (green fluorescence) on the surface of an endothelial monolayer *in vitro*. This 3D reconstruction shows that the surfaces of 10 bovine lung capillary endothelial cells (*) are covered with a heparan sulfate layer measuring 2.8 $\pm$ 0.5 μm ($n = 10$). 1 Unit = 7.2 μm. *Adapted from Fig. 6, Stevens et al.*[57]

A few recent studies have suggested that the GCX is not a significant structure on cells cultured *in vitro.* Potter and Damiano[58] and Potter *et al.*[59] examined HUVECs and BAECs grown on collagen microchannels using the μ-PIV method and reported that the GCX thickness was not significantly different from 0 μm. They did not report any imaging results of specific GCX localization (by immunofluorescence or other means), making it difficult to reconcile their observations with the previous EM and confocal microscopy studies showing a significant GCX on cells *in vitro.*[54,55,57] Jacob *et al.*[60] and Chappell *et al.*[61] used a lanthanum/glutaraldehyde fixation method in preparation for EM to visualize the GCX on HUVECs *in vitro.* They measured a GCX thickness of 29 nm *in vitro* compared to 878 nm for *ex vivo* cells on intact umbilical veins. Again, these results are difficult to reconcile with the results of Barker *et al.*[54] and Stevens *et al.*[57] There were some anomalies in the cell culture methods reported by Chappell *et al.*[61] For example, it required 10 days for their HUVEC monolayers to reach confluency. This is abnormally long compared to standard practice[62] and suggests that the nature of the GCX *in vitro* is sensitive to culture conditions and protocols. The time to confluency was not described in Potter and Damiano.[58]

A method to estimate systemic GCX volume *in vivo* was developed by Nieuwdorp *et al.*[8] In this method the total plasma volume is estimated from the fraction of labeled erythrocytes in the blood, and the total intravascular volume is estimated from the volume occupied by the GCX permeable tracer, dextran 40. The difference in volume is attributed to the GCX. Measurements are consistent and estimate in humans a GCX volume of 1.6 liters.[63] Across various species (i.e., mouse, dog, goat, and human), the estimated GCX volume is between 15 and 20 ml/kg body weight.[63] This is a systemic value and does not account for variations across organs and vascular beds. If one applies a typical estimate for total vascular surface area of 4000 m^2[64] and the total volume estimate 1.6 liters, an average systemic GCX thickness of 0.4 μm is deduced. The exact physical significance of the GCX volume estimated in this manner is not clear. However, changes due to systemic challenges such as hyperglycemia and elevated oxidized LDL–cholesterol plasma levels that lead to reduced GCX volume can be detected and estimated differences between GCX volume in healthy and diseased states correlated.

In summary, it appears that live cell imaging under stationary (no flow) conditions both *in vitro* and *in vivo* lead to estimates of GCX thickness on the order of several microns. Cells prepared for EM by conventional fixation produce estimates of thickness that are two orders of magnitude lower. Alternative EM fixation methods designed to reduce damage to fragile GAG structures produce larger estimates of GCX thickness, but still well below the live cell imaging values. On the other hand, when the glycocalyx on live endothelial cells are analyzed under physiological flow conditions *in vitro* or *in vivo*, the estimated GCX thickness is well below that estimated for stationary conditions. One possible explanation for the lower estimates of thickness under flow conditions is that the GCX is deformed under flow (like trees bending in the wind). However, theoretical estimates suggest that the core proteins are quite stiff and would not be expected to deform significantly under physiological shear stress conditions.[65] Thus, it may be that the outer regions of the GCX that are visualized by confocal microscopy have a "loose" (more porous) structure that is penetrated by the 70 kD dextran employed by Vink and Duling[49] in their estimates of GCX thickness under flowing conditions or the micro-particles used by Smith *et al.*[50] in determining near wall velocity profiles. Further studies will be required to unravel these seeming contradictions.

3. Glycocalyx Role in Mechanotransduction

A major recent development is the growing recognition that the GCX serves a critical role in the transmission of fluid flow associated shear stress (FSS) to the actin cytoskeleton and in the initiation of intracellular signaling. While numerous studies have demonstrated that FSS stimulates intracellular biomolecular responses and vascular regulation, it was widely assumed that this signaling was initiated either at the base of the cell via focal adhesion complexes or by the direct action of FSS on proteins in the apical membrane. Theoretical models of the structural integrity of the GCX have led to a fundamental paradox since they predict that the fluid flow within the GCX is negligible and, consequently, the FSS at the level of the membrane is vanishingly small. Furthermore, recent experiments in which the structural integrity of the GCX is compromised clearly demonstrate that cytoskeletal reorganization and biochemical responses can be nearly entirely abolished if the GCX is not intact. The studies described in this section show, quite convincingly, that the GCX plays a vital role in mechanotransduction.

3.1. *Biomolecular Response to FSS*

The primary evidence that supports a central role for the GCX in mechanotransduction comes from experiments in which enzymes were used to selectively degrade specific components of the GCX, followed by a reassessment of function, or, by using perfusion solutions without plasma proteins where the GCX is collapsed, as first demonstrated by Adamson and Clough,[14] and then reexamining function. Florian *et al.*[66] used the enzyme heparinase III to selectively degrade the HS component of bovine aortic endothelial cell (BAEC) GAGs *in vitro*, and observed that the substantial production of nitric oxide (NO) induced over 3 hours by steady or oscillatory FSS (20 or $10 \pm 15\,\text{dyn/cm}^2$) could be completely inhibited by an enzyme dose that removed only 46% of the fluorescence intensity associated with a HS antibody. The enzyme did not degrade CS and displayed negligible protease activity. It was also demonstrated that receptor mediated NO induction by bradykinin and histamine were not affected by the enzymatic treatment, demonstrating that endothelial-type NO synthase (eNOS) activity was not impaired directly by the enzyme and that NO depletion was not mediated by release of reactive oxygen species (ROS) sequestered in the GCX.

In an earlier study, the enzyme neuraminidase was used to remove sialic acid (SA) residues from saline-perfused rabbit mesenteric arteries, and it was observed that flow-dependent vasodilation was abolished by a 30-minute enzymatic pretreatment.[67] Because flow-dependent vasodilation is mediated by NO release in many arteries, this study suggested that SA also contributes to FSS-induced production of NO. Similarly, Hecker *et al.*[68] showed that when intact segments of rabbit femoral arteries were pre-treated with neuraminidase, FSS-induced NO production was inhibited. They also demonstrated that the same enzyme treatment had no effect on another hallmark response of ECs, the FSS-induced production of prostacyclin (PGI_2).[69] This study illustrated the fact that there are multiple mechanisms of mechanotransduction and not a single mechanotransducer. In a more recent study, the enzyme hyaluronidase was used in isolated canine femoral arteries to degrade HA from the GCX layer, and a significant inhibition of FSS-induced NO production was demonstrated.[70] Rubio and Ceballos[71] using guinea pig hearts showed related influences of the GCX on the responses of coronary arteries to changes in coronary flow.

Another recent *in vitro* study using bovine aortic endothelial cells examined all of the basic GCX degrading enzymes: heparinase (heparin sulfate), neuraminidase (sialic acid), hyaluronidase (hyaluronic acid) and chondroitinase (chondroitin sulfate), and showed that NO induced by a steady shear stress of 13.3 dyn/cm^2 was substantially blocked by heparinase, neuraminidase and hyaluronidase, but not chondroitinase.[72] In support of the earlier work of Hecker *et al.*,[68] none of these enzymes affected the shear-induced PGI_2 production, again reinforcing the idea that there are multiple sites for mechanotransduction. The interpretation of these results relies on the biomolecular structure of the GCX as described in Fig. 1. There are several possible mechanisms relating the GCX to NO production. HS proteoglycans can be linked to both the decentralized and centralized mechanisms of mechanotransduction put forth by Davies.[73] Syndecans that contain both HS and CS have an established association with the cytoskeleton,[31] and through it can decentralize the signal by distributing it to multiple sites within the cell (i.e., nucleus, organelles, focal adhesions, intercellular junctions). Significantly, the platelet-endothelial cell adhesion molecule (PECAM-1) associates with the cytoskeleton through catenins, and has been linked to shear-induced eNOS activation.[74] In terms of central transduction, it is noteworthy that glypicans which contain HS, but not CS, are linked to caveolae where eNOS resides along with many other signaling molecules.[12] The observation of Pahakis *et al.*[72] that the depletion of HS, but not CS, inhibits shear-induced NO production, favors a glypican-caveolae-eNOS mechanism. It is also important to note that HA binds to its CD44 receptor that is localized in caveolae.[44] This provides a link between HA and shear-induced NO. The role of SA that is removed by neuraminidase is less clear, but it is known that CD44 can have oligosaccharides (that are capped by SA) attached to it.[75]

Of course all of the glycocalyx components investigated by Pahakis *et al.*[72] provide net negative charges to the surface layer that enhance hydration and extension of the multicomponent structure in aqueous media. Loss of charge through enzyme degradation could lead to partial collapse of the integrated structure and reduction of fluid shear sensing.[76] The lack of influence of chondroitinase may be associated with chondroitin sulfate's location that is closer to the plasma membrane than the other components, thus allowing the more apical drag sensing elements to remain extended in its absence (Fig. 1).

The fact that shear-induced PGI_2 production was not inhibited by any of the GCX degradation enzymes suggests that the transduction machinery for this molecule resides in a location distinct from the NO machinery. One possibility was presented in studies of shear-induced prostaglandin release from cultured osteoblasts, where it was shown that none of the three major cytoskeletal networks (actin microfilaments, microtubules, or intermediate filaments) is required, but rather, fibronectin-induced focal adhesions promote shear-induced prostaglandin release and upregulation of cyclooxygenase-2 (COX-2) protein.[77] A similar mechanism may be operative in endothelial cells.

The experiments reviewed in this section so far suggest the mechanotransduction hypothesis that is summarized in the cartoon of Fig. 3. It shows ECs in a shear field with an intact GCX (top panel)

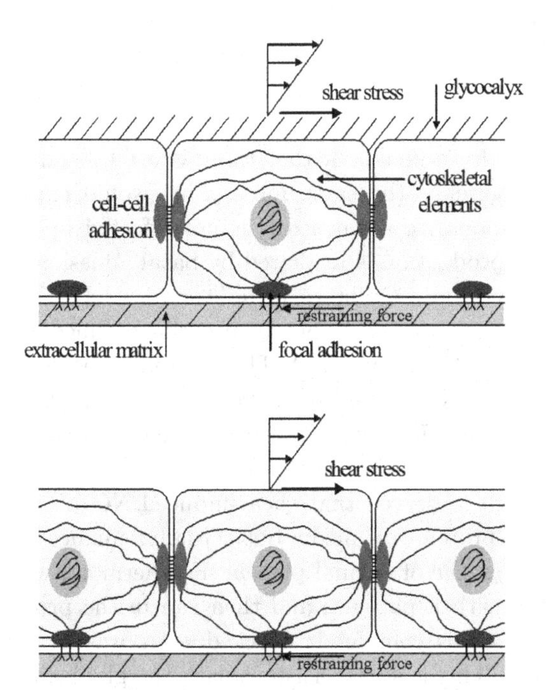

Fig. 3. Mechanotransduction hypothesis. Endothelial cells in a shear field with the GCX intact (top) or degraded (bottom). When the GCX is intact, it senses the shear force of blood flow, transmits this force, and decentralizes mechanotransduction to cellular sites that include the apical cell membrane, intercellular junctions, the basal adhesion plaques, the nucleus, and the cytoskeleton. When the GCX is degraded, the cell detects shear force directly at the apical membrane. Due to mechanical equilibrium, the basal adhesion plaques feel the same force whether or not the GCX is present.

and with a degraded GCX (bottom panel). When the GCX is intact, it senses the shear force of blood flow through the extended surface of its GAG chains, much like the leaves of a tree sense the force of wind. This force is transmitted to the cell through the core proteins (tree trunks) of the proteoglycans that decorate the cell surface. The force is further distributed throughout the cell by the structures of the cytoskeleton. Mechanotransduction may then take place at many locations in the cell, including the apical membrane (for example, the glypican-eNOS-caveolae pathway that was proposed for the production of NO), intercellular junctions, basal adhesion plaques, and the cytoskeleton itself. When the GCX is degraded by enzymes, the cell senses the shear force directly at the apical plasma membrane. In this scenario, the distribution of force to the apical aspects of the cell, including the actin cortical web and intercellular junctions, is altered. However, because the cell is in a state of mechanical equilibrium, the restraining force experienced by the basal adhesion plaques to balance the applied force on the surface will not be different whether the GCX is intact or degraded. Another way of saying this is that the basal adhesion plaques don't know whether there is a GCX on the EC surface or not—they experience the same force. This would explain why PGI_2 production in response to shear stress is not affected by GCX-degrading enzymes if PGI_2 production is mediated by basal adhesion plaques.

More recently, Lopez-Quintero *et al.*[78] exposed BAECs to the same shear stress as Pahakis *et al.*,[72] but in protein-free media that is known to induce collapse of the GCX.[14] The protein-free media was highly disruptive to the GCX as it led to a 900% increase in the EC monolayer hydraulic conductivity (Lp), whereas heparinase increased Lp by only 25%, hyaluronidase by 97% and chondroitinase by 81%. However, Lopez-Quintero *et al.*[78] surprisingly observed that shear-induced NO production was not suppressed in the protein-free media but actually enhanced above the level induced in the presence of normal protein. Furthermore, when monolayers were pre-treated with heparinase and then run in the protein-free media, shear-induced NO was completely blocked as it was in normal protein-containing media. This is still consistent with the glypican-caveolae-eNOS mechanism described above since these connections would be expected to remain intact even when the GCX has collapsed due to a lack of protein interactions.

HS may be involved in mechanotransduction through effects that are secondary to eNOS activation, but crucial to NO signaling. Nieuwdorp *et al.*[79] suggested that lack of HS on the EC surface could result in loss of extracellular superoxide dismutase (EC-SOD), an enzyme that catalyzes the reaction of superoxide to oxygen. This would result in a pro-oxidant state, damaging both the GCX and eNOS, which would lead to a decreased NO availability.[80] In a recent study using porcine femoral arteries *ex vivo*, Kumagai *et al.*[81] presented data indicating that HS and SA are not directly involved in shear-mediated NO production but only indirectly because their degradation by enzymes released reactive oxygen that reacts with NO to form peroxynitrite. On the other hand, they found that HA had a direct effect in shear-induced NO release. Their findings for HS and SA are not consistent with studies using BAECs *in vitro*,[66,72] as these studies showed that heparinase and neuraminidase did not block NO production induced by bradykinin or histamine that act through surface receptors. If heparinase or neuraminidase were releasing reactive oxygen from the GCX it would have reacted with NO induced by bradykinin (histamine) as well. This suggests the possibility that mechanisms of mechanotransduction mediated by the glycocalyx may differ among species as well as between *in vitro* conditions and intact vessels.

Along the same lines is the hypothesis that HS plays a role in the availability of arginine close to the EC surface and its transporters. The supporting evidence for this comes from several different sources. First, HS displays high affinities for polycationic molecules, such as poly-L-arginines, and the binding sites of all of their ligands involve arginine residues.[18,25,39] Thus HS proteoglycans may serve as a means of concentrating arginine close to the plasma membrane. In an older study, it was shown that HS proteoglycans adsorbed to a surface undergo a conformational change when exposed to flow, their core proteins unfolding from a random coil to an extended filament, and their HS chains elongating by 35%.[82] This was used to illustrate how sodium ions bound to HS could be delivered by the stretched GAGs to their transporter channels; an analogous hypothesis can be made for the case of L-arginine. But again, if these mechanisms were operative in the studies of Florian *et al.*[66] and Pahakis *et al.*[72] there would have been a reduction in bradykinin (histamine)-induced NO formation when GCX degrading enzymes were employed. But GCX degrading enzymes had no effect on bradykinin (histamine)-induced NO in those studies.

Another aspect of mechanotransduction that appears to be mediated by the GCX is the sensing of hypotonic stress. Oike *et al.*[86] reported that hypotonic cell swelling is sensed by heparin sulfate proteoglycans. They showed that heparinase treatment of BAECs abolished hypotonic stress induced tyrosine phosphorylation of 125 kDa focal adhesion kinase (FAK). It also affected the amplitude of the volume-regulated ion channel current and associated adenosine triphosphate (ATP) release and calcium (Ca^{2+}) transients that are induced by hypotonic stress, but did not affect the change in cell volume.

3.2. *Endothelial Cell Remodeling in Response to FSS*

A related response of endothelial cells (ECs) to FSS is their morphological and cytoskeletal remodeling. The early stages of these processes are observed within hours after the exposure of cultured EC to FSS and the culmination is observed after 24–48 hours of exposure when the distinct morphology of cells elongated and aligned in the direction of flow is observed, as reported by Remuzzi *et al.*[87] and others. This morphological response has been used as an indicator of shear stress magnitude and direction *in vivo*[88] and is considered to be one of the hallmarks of EC response to FSS. Recent work has demonstrated that this quintessential response is mediated by the glycocalyx.

Thi *et al.*[76] performed a series of experiments to explore the role of the GCX in the remodeling of the actin cytoskeleton, intercellular junctions and basal focal-adhesions in response to FSS when the GCX is either intact or compromised (by enzymatic degradation or by the absence of plasma proteins). In particular, the redistribution of F-actin, vinculin, zonula occludens-1 (ZO-1), paxillin and connexin 43 (Cx43) in confluent rat fat pad ECs were examined in response to 5 hours of FSS in four different bathing media. The four types of bathing media included Dulbecco's Modified Eagle Medium (DMEM), DMEM containing 10% fetal bovine serum (FBS), DMEM containing 1% bovine serum albumin (BSA), and DMEM containing 1% BSA and Heparinase III. DMEM alone (no protein) and DMEM with 1% BSA and Heparinase III were associated with a disruption of the GCX.

The most striking observations in these experiments were that with an intact GCX there was a severe disruption of the dense peripheral actin band (DPAB), a formation of stress fibers, and a migration of vinculin to cell borders after exposure to FSS. While this has been seen in numerous previous studies, this early remodeling was completely abolished when the integrity of the GCX was compromised. Similarly, there were disruptions of the tight junctions (indicated by ZO-1) and gap junctions (indicated by Cx43) for the intact GCX and no changes in the distribution of either of these junction-associated proteins when the GCX was compromised. In marked contrast, the distribution of paxillin, a marker for basal focal adhesions, was unaffected by the integrity of the GCX. This surprising observation (paxillin) can be understood when we remember that, for a cell in mechanical equilibrium (steady state), the applied stress at the apical surface (10 dyn/cm^2) must be balanced by an equal reaction stress at the basal surface. Therefore, a focal adhesion at the basal surface of the cell would feel the same mechanical stress regardless of whether the glycocalyx were present or not, and any remodeling events mediated by basal adhesion plaques would not be sensitive to the status of the glycocalyx (recall Fig. 3).

These remodeling results, which were obtained for a steady FSS of 10 dyn/cm^2, were substantially reduced for a FSS of 5 dyn/cm^2 applied for the same duration. This demonstrated that the GCX was central to EC remodeling in response to FSS and that there was a threshold FSS for the cytoskeletal reorganization to occur. The foregoing results are explained in Thi *et al.*[76] in terms of a 'bumper-car' conceptual model to describe the role of the GCX in activating cytoskeletal reorganization.

The early remodeling (5 hrs) described in Thi *et al.*[76] was further examined by Moon *et al.*[89] who showed, using BAECs *in vitro*, that the directional migration of ECs that is characterized by a distinct tendency to align with the applied shear direction, even at 5 hrs, is essentially abolished by pre-treatment of the BAEC monolayer with heparinase. This remodeling process culminates in cell elongation and strong alignment in the direction of shear after 24–48 hours at physiological levels of shear stress, but only when the glycocalyx is intact. Dewey's group[90] subsequently showed that disruption of the glycocalyx with heparinase completely blocks this characteristic elongation and alignment in the direction of shear after 24 hours. These studies clearly indicate the importance of the glycocalyx in remodeling of endothelial cells to FSS.

3.3. *Theoretical Models of Mechanotransduction*

One simple conceptual model of fluid flow mechanotransduction envisions the extended GAGs as drag sensors that transmit force from the flow to the core proteins, which in turn transmit the force to either the plasma membrane or the cytoskeleton. This is the 'wind in the trees' model wherein wind (fluid flow) is sensed by the branches (GAGs), and the force is transmitted to the ground (membrane) through the tree trunk (core protein). Various theoretical models that treat the GCX as a porous gel layer with a characteristic hydraulic permeability (K) that can be estimated from transport experiments, predict that when the GCX is intact, the fluid shear stress imposed on the uppermost surface is completely dissipated within the layer, such that the plasma membrane itself senses essentially zero fluid shear stress.[91,92] Most of the fluid shear stress is transmitted to the solid components of the glycocalyx and these solid structures actually deliver the force to the cell. This picture is consistent with the 'wind in the trees' model mentioned above. On the other hand, if the glycocalyx is degraded by disease states,[7,79,93–99] the permeability of the layer may be increased or its thickness decreased so that a greater fraction of the external shear stress is actually transmitted closer to or even directly on the cell membrane by the fluid itself. Using a structural model of the glycocalyx derived from the observations of Squire *et al.*,[48] Weinbaum *et al.*[92] have shown that the core proteins in the bush-like structures comprising the glycocalyx are sufficiently stiff to act as transmitters of fluid shear stress without significant deflection. They propose that the fluid shear force dissipated in the outer region of the glycocalyx imposes a torque on the relatively stiff core proteins that is transmitted to the actin cortical cytoskeleton via transmembrane domains. Their calculations suggest displacements of individual actin filaments in the cortical web in the order of 10 nm for typical fluid shear stresses, and this could drive intracellular signaling.[92] Additional theoretical models of the GCX including the oncotic model of Secomb *et al.*,[100] the mechano-electrochemical model of Damiano and Stace[101] and the elastohydrodynamic model of Han *et al.*[65] are thoroughly reviewed in Weinbaum *et al.*[13]

4. Concluding Remarks

We have seen that what would seem to be the most rudimentary characteristic of the glycocalyx — its thickness — has not been completely resolved. While early estimates based on ruthenium red and conventional electron microscopy (order 20 nm) surely under estimate the *in vivo* thickness, confocal microscopy images of live cells in a static fluid environment (order several microns) may over estimate the *in vivo* thickness. Blood flow is bound to deform the GCX and in the microcirculation, blood cells interact with the GCX to alter its effective thickness. The relationship of the molecular organization of the GCX to its physical organization as revealed by microscopy is not known either. For example, do HS and HA extend throughout the GCX? Are there inner and outer regions where specific components are concentrated?

There is still controversy about the status of the GCX *in vitro*, with several studies showing an abundant and thick layer while others report a barely detectable layer. We must remember, however, that most of what we know about mechanotransduction in endothelial cells is based on *in vitro* experiments. It is therefore imperative to establish the nature of the GCX *in vitro* and its relationship to the *in vivo* state.

The GCX, when it is intact, is the sensor of FSS through its extended GAGs. The shear force is transmitted to the cell membrane and cytoskeleton through the core proteins, and transduction to a biomolecular response may occur at the apical membrane (centralized transduction) or remotely at the intercellular junctions, basal adhesion plaques, or within the cytoskeleton itself (decentralized transduction). A number of studies have examined the roles of various GAG components in mechanotransduction and remodeling using enzymes to selectively deplete GAG components, but there have been no systematic studies of the core proteins involved. Knowledge of the core proteins mediating specific responses will help to unravel the signaling networks that encode information about the fluid mechanical forces imposed on the cell.

The GCX also plays a role in mechanotransduction of transvascular flow (shear stress) across the endothelium and the sensing of osmotic stress. Preliminary evidence has been reported to suggest that the GCX also plays a role in sensing of interstitial flow shear stress by smooth muscle cells.[102] Thus it appears the GCX plays a role in sensing of mechanical stress by many cell types and that we are at the beginning of a new age of discovery concerning this most fascinating structure.

Acknowledgement

This work was supported by NIH Grant HL 57093.

References

1. Danielli, J. F. (1940) Capillary permeability and oedema in the perfused frog. *J Physiol* **98**(1), 109–129.

2. Chambers, R., and Zweifach, B. W. (1947) Intercellular cement of capillary permeability. *Physiol Rev* **27**, 436–463.
3. Copley, A. L. (1974) Hemorheological aspects of the endothelium-plasma interface. *Microvasc Res* **8**(2), 192–212.
4. Luft, J. H. (1966) Fine structures of capillary and endocapillary layer as revealed by ruthenium red. *Fed Proc* **25**(6), 1773–1783.
5. Lewis, J. C., Taylor, R. G., Jones, N. D., St Clair, R. W., and Cornhill, J. F. (1982) Endothelial surface characteristics in pigeon coronary artery atherosclerosis. I. Cellular alterations during the initial stages of dietary cholesterol challenge. *Lab Invest* **46**(2), 123–138.
6. van den Berg, B. M., Spaan, J. A., and Vink, H. (2009) Impaired glycocalyx barrier properties contribute to enhanced intimal low-density lipoprotein accumulation at the carotid artery bifurcation in mice. *Pflugers Arch* **457**(6), 1199–1206.
7. van den Berg, B. M., Spaan, J. A., Rolf, T. M., and Vink, H. (2006) Atherogenic region and diet diminish glycocalyx dimension and increase intima-to-media ratios at murine carotid artery bifurcation. *Am J Physiol Heart Circ Physiol* **290**(2), H915–920.
8. Nieuwdorp, M., van Haeften, T. W., Gouverneur, M. C., Mooij, H. L., van Lieshout, M. H., Levi, M., Meijers, J. C., Holleman, F., Hoekstra, J. B., Vink, H., Kastelein, J. J., and Stroes, E. S. (2006) Loss of endothelial glycocalyx during acute hyperglycemia coincides with endothelial dysfunction and coagulation activation *in vivo*. *Diabetes* **55**(2), 480–486.
9. van den Berg, B. M., Nieuwdorp, M., Stroes, E. S., and Vink, H. (2006) Glycocalyx and endothelial (dys) function: from mice to men. *Pharmacol Rep* **58**(Suppl), 75–80.
10. Gouverneur, M., Berg, B., Nieuwdorp, M., Stroes, E., and Vink, H. (2006) Vasculoprotective properties of the endothelial glycocalyx: effects of fluid shear stress. *J Intern Med* **259**(4), 393–400.
11. Pries, A. R., Secomb, T. W., and Gaehtgens, P. (2000) The endothelial surface layer. *Pflugers Arch* **440**(5), 653–666.
12. Tarbell, J. M., and Pahakis, M. Y. (2006) Mechanotransduction and the glycocalyx. *J Intern Med* **259**(4), 339–350.
13. Weinbaum, S., Tarbell, J. M., and Damiano, E. R. (2007) The structure and function of the endothelial glycocalyx layer. *Annu Rev Biomed Eng* **9**, 121–167.
14. Adamson, R. H., and Clough, G. (1992) Plasma proteins modify the endothelial cell glycocalyx of frog mesenteric microvessels. *J Physiol* **445**, 473–486.
15. Bernfield, M., Gotte, M., Park, P. W., Reizes, O., Fitzgerald, M. L., Lincecum, J., and Zako, M. (1999) Functions of cell surface heparan sulfate proteoglycans. *Annu Rev Biochem* **68**, 729–777.
16. Osterloh, K., Ewert, U., and Pries, A. R. (2002) Interaction of albumin with the endothelial cell surface. *Am J Physiol Heart Circ Physiol* **283**(1), H398–405.

17. Coombe, D. R., and Kett, W. C. (2005) Heparan sulfate-protein interactions: therapeutic potential through structure-function insights. *Cell Mol Life Sci* **62**(4), 410–424.
18. Hileman, R. E., Fromm, J. R., Weiler, J. M., and Linhardt, R. J. (1998) Glycosaminoglycan-protein interactions: definition of consensus sites in glycosaminoglycan binding proteins. *Bioessays* **20**(2), 156–167.
19. Kan, M., Wang, F., To, B., Gabriel, J. L., and McKeehan, W. L. (1996) Divalent cations and heparin/heparan sulfate cooperate to control assembly and activity of the fibroblast growth factor receptor complex. *J Biol Chem* **271**(42), 26143–26148.
20. Kijewska, I., and Hawlicka, E. (2005) A new radiochemical method to investigate ion binding with polyelectrolytes. *Carbohydr Res* **340**(6), 1185–1191.
21. McGee, M. P., and Liang, J. (2001) Regulation of glycosaminoglycan function by osmotic potentials. Measurement of water transfer during antithrombin activation by heparin. *J Biol Chem* **276**(52), 49275–49282.
22. Arisaka, T., Mitsumata, M., Kawasumi, M., Tohjima, T., and Hirose, S., (1995) Yoshida Y. Effects of shear stress on glycosaminoglycan synthesis in vascular endothelial cells. *Ann N Y Acad Sci* **748**, 543–554.
23. Paka, L., Kako, Y., Obunike, J. C., and Pillarisetti, S. (1999) Apolipoprotein E containing high density lipoprotein stimulates endothelial production of heparan sulfate rich in biologically active heparin-like domains. A potential mechanism for the anti-atherogenic actions of vascular apolipoprotein e. *J Biol Chem* **274**(8), 4816–4823.
24. Vijayagopal, P., Figueroa, J. E., and Levine, E. A. (1998) Altered composition and increased endothelial cell proliferative activity of proteoglycans isolated from breast carcinoma. *J Surg Oncol* **68**(4), 250–254.
25. Jackson, R. L., Busch, S. J., and Cardin, A. D. (1991) Glycosaminoglycans: molecular properties, protein interactions, and role in physiological processes. *Physiol Rev* **71**(2), 481–539.
26. Oohira, A., Wight, T. N., and Bornstein, P. (1983) Sulfated proteoglycans synthesized by vascular endothelial cells in culture. *J Biol Chem* **258**(3), 2014–2021.
27. Camejo, G., Hurt-Camejo, E., Wiklund, O., and Bondjers, G. (1998) Association of apo B lipoproteins with arterial proteoglycans: pathological significance and molecular basis. *Atherosclerosis* **139**(2), 205–222.
28. Almond, A., and Sheehan, J. K. (2000) Glycosaminoglycan conformation: do aqueous molecular dynamics simulations agree with x-ray fiber diffraction? *Glycobiology* **10**(3), 329–338.
29. Seog, J., Dean, D., Rolauffs, B., Wu, T., Genzer, J., Plaas, A. H., Grodzinsky A. J., and Ortiz, C. (2005) Nanomechanics of opposing glycosaminoglycan macromolecules. *J Biomech* **38**(9), 1789–1797.
30. van Haaren, P. M., VanBavel, E., Vink, H., and Spaan, J. A. (2005) Charge modification of the endothelial surface layer modulates the permeability

barrier of isolated rat mesenteric small arteries. *Am J Physiol Heart Circ Physiol* **289**(6), H2503–2507.
31. Tkachenko, E., Rhodes, J. M., and Simons, M. (2005) Syndecans: new kids on the signaling block. *Circ Res* **96**(5), 488–500.
32. Zimmermann, P., and David, G. (1999) The syndecans, tuners of transmembrane signaling. *FASEB J* **13**(Suppl), S91–S100.
33. Rosenberg, R. D., Shworak, N. W., Liu, J., Schwartz, J. J., and Zhang, L. (1997) Heparan sulfate proteoglycans of the cardiovascular system. Specific structures emerge but how is synthesis regulated? *J Clin Invest* **100**(11 Suppl), S67–75.
34. Halden, Y., Rek, A., Atzenhofer, W., Szilak, L., Wabnig, A., and Kungl, A. J. (2004) Interleukin-8 binds to syndecan-2 on human endothelial cells. *Biochem J* **377**(Pt 2), 533–538.
35. Kokenyesi, R., and Bernfield, M. (1994) Core protein structure and sequence determine the site and presence of heparan sulfate and chondroitin sulfate on syndecan-1. *J Biol Chem* **269**(16), 12304–12309.
36. Simons, M., and Horowitz, A. (2001) Syndecan-4-mediated signalling. *Cell Signal* **13**(12), 855–862.
37. Yoneda, A., and Couchman, J. R. (2003) Regulation of cytoskeletal organization by syndecan transmembrane proteoglycans. *Matrix Biol* **22**(1), 25–33.
38. Fransson, L. A., Belting, M., Cheng, F., Jonsson, M., Mani, K., and Sandgren, S. (2004) Novel aspects of glypican glycobiology. *Cell Mol Life Sci* **61**(9), 1016–1024.
39. Belting, M. (2003) Heparan sulfate proteoglycan as a plasma membrane carrier. *Trends Biochem Sci* **28**(3), 145–151.
40. Cheng, F., Mani, K., van den Born, J., Ding, K., Belting, M., and Fransson, L. A. (2002) Nitric oxide-dependent processing of heparan sulfate in recycling S-nitrosylated glypican-1 takes place in caveolin-1-containing endosomes. *J Biol Chem* **277**(46), 44431–44439.
41. van Deurs, B., Roepstorff, K., Hommelgaard, A. M., and Sandvig, K. (2003) Caveolae: anchored, multifunctional platforms in the lipid ocean. *Trends Cell Biol* **13**(2), 92–100.
42. Laurent, T. C., and Fraser, J. R. (1992) Hyaluronan. *FASEB J* **6**(7), 2397–2404.
43. Henry, C. B., and Duling, B. R. (1999) Permeation of the luminal capillary glycocalyx is determined by hyaluronan. *Am J Physiol* **277**(2 Pt 2), H508–514.
44. Singleton, P. A., and Bourguignon, L. Y. (2004) CD44 interaction with ankyrin and IP3 receptor in lipid rafts promotes hyaluronan-mediated Ca2+ signaling leading to nitric oxide production and endothelial cell adhesion and proliferation. *Exp Cell Res* **295**(1), 102–118.
45. Varki, A. (1997) Sialic acids as ligands in recognition phenomena. *FASEB J* **11**(4), 248–255.

46. Rostgaard, J., and Qvortrup, K. (1997) Electron microscopic demonstrations of filamentous molecular sieve plugs in capillary fenestrae. *Microvasc Res* **53**(1), 1–13.
47. van den Berg, B. M., Vink, H., and Spaan, J. A. (2003) The endothelial glycocalyx protects against myocardial edema. *Circ Res* **92**(6), 592–594.
48. Squire, J. M., Chew, M., Nneji, G., Neal, C., Barry, J., and Michel, C. (2001) Quasi-periodic substructure in the microvessel endothelial glycocalyx: a possible explanation for molecular filtering? *J Struct Biol* **136**(3), 239–255.
49. Vink, H., and Duling, B. R. (1996) Identification of distinct luminal domains for macromolecules, erythrocytes, and leukocytes within mammalian capillaries. *Circ Res* **79**(3), 581–589.
50. Smith, M. L., Long, D. S., Damiano, E. R., and Ley, K. (2003) Near-wall micro-PIV reveals a hydrodynamically relevant endothelial surface layer in venules *in vivo*. *Biophys J* **85**(1), 637–645.
51. Long, D. S., Smith, M. L., Pries, A. R., Ley, K., and Damiano, E. R. (2004) Microviscometry reveals reduced blood viscosity and altered shear rate and shear stress profiles in microvessels after hemodilution. *Proc Natl Acad Sci U S A* **101**(27), 10060–10065.
52. Damiano, E. R., Long, D. S., and Smith, M. L. (2004) Estimation of viscosity profiles using velocimetry data from parallel flows of linearly viscous fluids: application to microvascular haemodynamics. *J Fluid Mech* **512**, 1–19.
53. Megens, R. T., Reitsma, S., Schiffers, P. H., Hilgers, R. H., De Mey, J. G., Slaaf D. W., oude Egbrink, M. G., and van Zandvoort, M. A. (2007) Two-photon microscopy of vital murine elastic and muscular arteries. Combined structural and functional imaging with subcellular resolution. *J Vasc Res* **44**(2), 87–98.
54. Barker, A. L., Konopatskaya, O., Neal, C. R., Macpherson, J. V., Whatmore, J. L., Winlove, C. P., Unwin, P. R., and Shore, A. C. (2004) Observation and characterisation of the glycocalyx of viable human endothelial cells using confocal laser scanning microscopy. *Physical Chemistry Chemical Physics* **6**, 1006–1011.
55. Ueda, A., Shimomura, M., Ikeda, M., Yamaguchi, R., and Tanishita, K. (2004) Effect of glycocalyx on shear-dependent albumin uptake in endothelial cells. *Am J Physiol Heart Circ Physiol* **287**(5), H2287–2294.
56. Devaraj, S., Yun, J. M., Adamson, G., Galvez, J., and Jialal, I. (2009) C-reactive protein impairs the endothelial glycocalyx resulting in endothelial dysfunction. *Cardiovasc Res* **84**(3), 479–484.
57. Stevens, A. P., Hlady, V., and Dull, R. O. (2007) Fluorescence correlation spectroscopy can probe albumin dynamics inside lung endothelial glycocalyx. *Am J Physiol Lung Cell Mol Physiol* **293**(2), L328–335.
58. Potter, D. R., and Damiano, E. R. (2008) The hydrodynamically relevant endothelial cell glycocalyx observed *in vivo* is absent *in vitro*. *Circ Res* **102**(7), 770–776.

59. Potter, D. R., Jiang, J., and Damiano, E. R. (2009) The recovery time course of the endothelial cell glycocalyx *in vivo* and its implications *in vitro*. *Circ Res.* **104**(11), 1318–1325.
60. Jacob, M., Rehm, M., Loetsch, M., Paul, J. O., Bruegger, D., Welsch, U., Conzen, P., and Becker, B. F. (2007) The endothelial glycocalyx prefers albumin for evoking shear stress-induced, nitric oxide-mediated coronary dilatation. *J Vasc Res* **44**(6), 435–443.
61. Chappell, D., Jacob, M., Paul, O., Rehm, M., Welsch, U., Stoeckelhuber, M., Conzen, P., and Becker, B. F. (2009) The glycocalyx of the human umbilical vein endothelial cell: an impressive structure *ex vivo* but not in culture. *Circ Res* **104**(11), 1313–1317.
62. Cheung, A. L. (2007) Isolation and culture of human umbilical vein endothelial cells (HUVEC). *Curr Protoc Microbiol*; Appendix 4: Appendix 4B.
63. Nieuwdorp, M., Meuwese, M. C., Mooij, H. L., Ince, C., Broekhuizen, L. N., Kastelein, J. J., Stroes, E. S., and Vink, H. (2008) Measuring endothelial glycocalyx dimensions in humans: a potential novel tool to monitor vascular vulnerability. *J Appl Physiol* **104**(3), 845–852.
64. Aird, W. C. (2005) Spatial and temporal dynamics of the endothelium. *J Thromb Haemost* **3**(7), 1392–1406.
65. Han, Y., Weinbaum, S., Spaan, J. A., and Vink, H. (2006) Large-deformation analysis of the elastic recoil of fiber layers in a Brinkman medium with application to the endothelial glycocalyx. *J Fluid Mech* **554**, 217–235.
66. Florian, J. A., Kosky, J. R., Ainslie, K., Pang, Z., Dull, R. O., and Tarbell, J. M. (2003) Heparan sulfate proteoglycan is a mechanosensor on endothelial cells. *Circ Res* **93**(10), e136–142.
67. Pohl, U., Herlan, K., Huang, A., and Bassenge, E. (1991) EDRF-mediated shear-induced dilation opposes myogenic vasoconstriction in small rabbit arteries. *Am J Physiol* **261**(6 Pt 2), H2016–2023.
68. Hecker, M., Mulsch, A., Bassenge, E., and Busse, R. (1993) Vasoconstriction and increased flow: two principal mechanisms of shear stress-dependent endothelial autacoid release. *Am J Physiol* **265**(3 Pt 2), H828–833.
69. Frangos, J. A., Eskin, S. G., McIntire, L. V., and Ives, C. L. (1985) Flow effects on prostacyclin production by cultured human endothelial cells. *Science* **227**(4693), 1477–1479.
70. Mochizuki, S., Vink, H., Hiramatsu, O., Kajita, T., Shigeto, F., Spaan, J. A., and Kajiya, F. (2003) Role of hyaluronic acid glycosaminoglycans in shear-induced endothelium-derived nitric oxide release. *Am J Physiol Heart Circ Physiol* **285**(2), H722–726.
71. Rubio, R., and Ceballos, G. (2000) Role of the endothelial glycocalyx in dromotropic, inotropic, and arrythmogenic effects of coronary flow. *Am J Physiol Heart Circ Physiol* **278**(1), H106–116.
72. Pahakis, M. Y., Kosky, J. R., Dull, R. O., and Tarbell, J. M. (2007) The role of endothelial glycocalyx components in mechanotransduction of fluid shear stress. *Biochem Biophys Res Commun* **355**(1), 228–233.

73. Davies, P. F. (1995) Flow-mediated endothelial mechanotransduction. *Physiol Rev* **75**(3), 519–560.
74. Dusserre, N., L'Heureux, N., Bell, K. S., Stevens, H. Y., Yeh, J., Otte, L. A., Loufrani, L., and Frangos, J. A. (2004) PECAM-1 interacts with nitric oxide synthase in human endothelial cells: implication for flow-induced nitric oxide synthase activation. *Arterioscler Thromb Vasc Biol* **24**(10), 1796–1802.
75. Forster-Horvath, C., Meszaros, L., Raso, E., Dome, B., Ladanyi, A., Morini, M., Albini, A., and Timar, J. (2004). Expression of CD44v3 protein in human endothelial cells in vitro and in tumoral microvessels *in vivo*. *Microvasc Res* **68**(2), 110–118.
76. Thi, M. M., Tarbell, J. M., Weinbaum, S., and Spray, D. C. (2004) The role of the glycocalyx in reorganization of the actin cytoskeleton under fluid shear stress: a "bumper-car" model. *Proc Natl Acad Sci U S A* **101**(47), 16483–16488.
77. Norvell, S. M., Ponik, S. M., Bowen, D. K., Gerard, R., and Pavalko, F. M. (2004) Fluid shear stress induction of COX-2 protein and prostaglandin release in cultured MC3T3-E1 osteoblasts does not require intact microfilaments or microtubules. *J Appl Physiol* **96**(3), 957–966.
78. Lopez-Quintero, S. V., Amaya, R., Pahakis, M., and Tarbell, J. M. (2009) The endothelial glycocalyx mediates shear-induced changes in hydraulic conductivity. *Am J Physiol Heart Circ Physiol* **296**(5), H1451–1456.
79. Nieuwdorp, M., Meuwese, M. C., Vink, H., Hoekstra, J. B., Kastelein, J. J., and Stroes E.S. (2005) The endothelial glycocalyx: a potential barrier between health and vascular disease. *Curr Opin Lipidol* **16**(5), 507–511.
80. Faraci, F. M., and Didion, S. P. (2004) Vascular protection: superoxide dismutase isoforms in the vessel wall. *Arterioscler Thromb Vasc Biol* **24**(8), 1367–1373.
81. Kumagai, T., Osada, Y., Ohta, N., and Kanazawa, T. (2009) Peroxiredoxin-1 from Schistosoma japonicum functions as a scavenger against hydrogen peroxide but not nitric oxide. *Mol Biochem Parasitol* **164**(1), 26–31.
82. Bevan, J. A., and Siegel, G. (1991) Blood vessel wall matrix flow sensor: evidence and speculation. *Blood Vessels* **28**(6), 552–556.
83. Dull, R. O., Mecham, I., and McJames, S. (2007) Heparan sulfates mediate pressure-induced increase in lung endothelial hydraulic conductivity via nitric oxide/reactive oxygen species. *Am J Physiol Lung Cell Mol Physiol* **292**(6), L1452–1458.
84. Tarbell, J. M., Demaio, L., and Zaw, M. M. (1999) Effect of pressure on hydraulic conductivity of endothelial monolayers: role of endothelial cleft shear stress. *J Appl Physiol* **87**(1), 261–268.
85. Burns, A. R., Zheng, Z., Soubra, S. H., Chen, J., and Rumbaut, R. E. (2007) Transendothelial flow inhibits neutrophil transmigration through a nitric oxide-dependent mechanism: potential role for cleft shear stress. *Am J Physiol Heart Circ Physiol* **293**(5), H2904–2910.

86. Oike, M., Watanabe, M., and Kimura, C. (2008) Involvement of heparan sulfate proteoglycan in sensing hypotonic stress in bovine aortic endothelial cells. *Biochim Biophys Acta* **1780**(10), 1148–1155.
87. Remuzzi, A., Dewey, C. F. Jr., Davies, P. F., Gimbrone, M. A. Jr. (1984) Orientation of endothelial cells in shear fields *in vitro*. *Biorheology* **21**(4), 617–630.
88. Langille, B. L., and Adamson, S. L. (1981) Relationship between blood flow direction and endothelial cell orientation at arterial branch sites in rabbits and mice. *Circ Res* **48**(4), 481–488.
89. Moon, J. J., Matsumoto, M., Patel, S., Lee, L., Guan, J. L., and Li, S. (2005) Role of cell surface heparan sulfate proteoglycans in endothelial cell migration and mechanotransduction. *J Cell Physiol* **203**(1), 166–176.
90. Yao, Y., Rabodzey, A., and Dewey, C. F. Jr. (2007) Glycocalyx modulates the motility and proliferative response of vascular endothelium to fluid shear stress. *Am J Physiol Heart Circ Physiol* **293**(2), H1023–1030.
91. Secomb, T. W., Hsu, R., and Pries, A. R. (2001) Effect of the endothelial surface layer on transmission of fluid shear stress to endothelial cells. *Biorheology* **38**(2–3), 143–150.
92. Weinbaum, S., Zhang, X., Han, Y., Vink, H., and Cowin, S. C. (2003) Mechanotransduction and flow across the endothelial glycocalyx. *Proc Natl Acad Sci U S A* **100**(13), 7988–7995.
93. Mulivor, A. W., Lipowsky, H. H. (2004) Inflammation- and ischemia-induced shedding of venular glycocalyx. *Am J Physiol Heart Circ Physiol* **286**(5), H1672–1680.
94. Zuurbier, C. J., Demirci, C., Koeman, A., Vink, H., and Ince, C. (2005) Short-term hyperglycemia increases endothelial glycocalyx permeability and acutely decreases lineal density of capillaries with flowing red blood cells. *J Appl Physiol* **99**(4), 1471–1476.
95. Edwards, I. J., Wagner, J. D., Vogl-Willis, C. A., Litwak, K. N., and Cefalu, W. T. (2004) Arterial heparan sulfate is negatively associated with hyperglycemia and atherosclerosis in diabetic monkeys. *Cardiovasc Diabetol* **3**, 6.
96. Constantinescu, A. A., Vink, H., and Spaan, J. A. (2001) Elevated capillary tube hematocrit reflects degradation of endothelial cell glycocalyx by oxidized LDL. *Am J Physiol Heart Circ Physiol* **280**(3), H1051–1057.
97. Henry, C. B., and Duling, B. R. (2000) TNF-alpha increases entry of macromolecules into luminal endothelial cell glycocalyx. *Am J Physiol Heart Circ Physiol* **279**(6), H2815–2823.
98. Kurzelewski, M., Czarnowska, E., and Beresewicz, A. (2005) Superoxide- and nitric oxide-derived species mediate endothelial dysfunction, endothelial glycocalyx disruption, and enhanced neutrophil adhesion in the post-ischemic guinea-pig heart. *J Physiol Pharmacol* **56**(2), 163–178.

99. Ward, B. J., and Donnelly, J. L. (1993) Hypoxia induced disruption of the cardiac endothelial glycocalyx: implications for capillary permeability. *Cardiovasc Res* **27**(3), 384–389.
100. Secomb, T. W., Hsu, R., and Pries, A. R. (1998) A model for red blood cell motion in glycocalyx-lined capillaries. *Am J Physiol* **274**(3 Pt 2), H1016–1022.
101. Damiano, E. R., and Stace, T. M. (2002) A mechano-electrochemical model of radial deformation of the capillary glycocalyx. *Biophys J* **82**(3), 1153–1175.
102. Ainslie, K. M., Garanich, J. S., Dull, R. O., and Tarbell, J. M. (2005) Vascular smooth muscle cell glycocalyx influences shear stress-mediated contractile response. *J Appl Physiol* **98**(1), 242–249.

Chapter 4

ROLE OF KRÜPPEL-LIKE FACTORS IN SHEAR STRESS-MEDIATED VASOPROTECTION

DAIJI KAWANAMI, G. BRANDON ATKINS, ANNE HAMIK
and MUKESH K. JAIN*

University Hospitals Harrington-McLaughlin Heart & Vascular Institute and Case Cardiovascular Research Institute, Case Western Reserve University School of Medicine, 2103 Cornell Road, Room 4-522, Cleveland, OH, 44106, USA
**mukesh.jain2@case.edu*

Laminar shear stress protects against atherogenesis and thrombosis by inducing anti-inflammatory and anti-coagulant gene expression in endothelial cells. Krüppel-like factors (KLFs) are zinc-finger type transcription factors that play important roles in modulating cellular function in a broad range of mammalian cell types. Several KLFs have been reported to be expressed in endothelial cells. Of these, KLF2 and KLF4 have been shown to be upregulated by laminar shear stress. Interestingly, the vasoprotective functions of shear stress overlap with described functions of KLF2, and accumulating evidence demonstrates that KLF2 mediates these favorable effects. This chapter will focus on the emerging role of Krüppel-like factors in endothelial cell biology with an emphasis on their role in laminar shear stress-mediated vasoprotection.

1. Introduction

Cardiovascular disease, in particular coronary heart disease (defined as impaired blood flow to cardiac muscle leading to ischemia and ultimately heart failure), is the principal cause of mortality worldwide.[1] Atherosclerosis is the underlying disorder in the majority of patients with coronary heart disease and a better understanding of the molecular mechanisms that underlie its pathogenesis is crucial for both scientific and therapeutic reasons. Although the development of atherosclerosis is dependent upon a complex interplay between many factors and processes, accumulating evidence demonstrates that shear stress plays a central role in atherosclerosis. It has been well established that there is a non-uniform distribution of atherosclerosis within the vasculature.[2,3] Atherosclerosis occurs more frequently at branch points of the arterial tree; areas that are exposed to turbulent blood flow. In contrast, laminar shear stress is present in unbranched portions of vessels and induces anti-inflammatory and anti-coagulant genes such as endothelial nitric oxide synthase (eNOS) and thrombomodulin (TM), thereby conferring an atheroprotective phenotype to the vessel wall.

Studies from the our group and others have demonstrated a critical role for the Krüppel-like Factor (KLF) family of zinc-finger transcription factors in endothelial biology. KLF2 and KLF4 are upregulated by laminar shear stress. Moreover, KLF2 has been shown to mediate the atheroprotective effects of laminar shear stress in endothelial cells. This chapter describes our current understanding of the role of KLFs in the shear stress-mediated endothelial phenotype.

1.1. *Krüppel-Like Factors*

The Sp/KLF family of transcription factors is a subclass of the zinc-finger family of transcriptional regulators that broadly regulate cellular growth and differentiation.[4–7] KLFs exhibit homology to the *Drosophila melanogaster* segmentation gene product Krüppel. Krüppel is the German word for "cripple"; the name derives from the observation that mutation of this protein causes deletion of thoracic and anterior abdominal segments in Drosophila embryos.[8–10] The first mammalian KLF to be discovered (KLF1, also referred to as to erythroid Kruppel-like factor, EKLF) was cloned from red blood cells in 1993 by Bieker and colleagues.[11] To date 21 members have been identified, including 4 Sp factors (Sp1–4) and 17 KLF factors (KLF1–17) (Black *et al.*, 2001; van Vliet *et al.*, 2006).[12,13] Members of this family bind with varying affinities to a consensus DNA sequence (termed GC-box or CACCC element) and exert diverse transcriptional functions.[6,12] Furthermore, members of this family can modulate one another's function through a number of distinct mechanisms, such as cross-regulation of expression or through direct protein-protein interaction.[6,12,14,15]

1.2. *Krüppel-Like Factor 2*

KLF2 was isolated and cloned by Lingrel and colleagues in 1995 using the zinc finger domain of ELKF as a hybridization probe. The full-length mouse KLF2 cDNA encodes a protein of 354 amino acids (355 amino acids in human) and a molecular weight of 38 kDa. The human and mouse KLF2 homologs exhibit an 85% nucleotide identity and 90% amino acid similarity. Within the 5' proximal promoter of KLF2, a region of 75 nucleotides appears particularly important in transcriptional regulation of KLF2. Mutagenesis of this region significantly impairs the ability of the KLF2 promoter to drive reporter gene expression.[16]

KLF2 has both activating and inhibitory effects on gene transcription via both direct and indirect promoter activity. Transcriptional regulation by KLF2 is mediated by a potent transcriptional activation domain (amino acids 1–110) as well as an (auto)inhibitory domain encoded by amino acids 111–267.[17] An interesting function of the inhibitory domain of KLF2 was described by Conkwright *et al.* This domain, by binding to WW domain-containing E3 ubiquitin protein ligase 1 (WWP1), mediates polyubiquitination and proteasomal degradation of KLF2.[18]

The developmental expression of KLF2 is highly regulated with initial expression at embryonic day 7 (E7), deactivation at E11, and subsequent reactivation at E15.[19] KLF2 is expressed in multiple cell types and has been implicated in endothelial biology,[20–24] monocyte/macrophage biology,[25,26] T-cell biology,[27–30] erythropoiesis,[31] adipocyte biology,[32,33] and stem cell biology.[34] KLF2 is highly expressed in the lung and thus was initially termed lung Krüppel-like factor (LKLF).[19] In fact, KLF2 is indispensable for normal lung development as demonstrated by chimeric KLF2-null mice. These mice fail to develop normal lung tissue whereas other tissues are normally developed.[16] KLF2 knockout mice have a grossly normal vascular network, with vasculogenesis and angiogenesis seemingly intact.[35,36] However, as will be described in detail below, vessel maturation is impaired, leading to embryonic death from hemorrhage. Thus, KLF2 has been shown to have a role in multiple cell types, and a crucial function in lung and vascular development.

1.3. *Regulation of KLF2 by Laminar Shear Stress*

The susceptibility of vascular branch points and curvatures to atherosclerosis is in large part related to exposure to turbulent flow. In contrast, the portion of the arterial tree exposed to unidirectional laminar shear stress tends to be protected. In 2002, Horrevoets and colleagues used microarray analysis to identify endothelial KLF2 as induced by prolonged laminar shear stress.[37] *In situ* hybridization assays in the human aorta have revealed that KLF2 is consistently expressed in the endothelium of the aorta but its expression level is lower at branch points of the aortic arch and the abdominal aorta.[38] Shear stress-mediated KLF2 induction has also been observed during cardiovascular development in chicken embryos. Groenendijk *et al.* demonstrated the overlap of KLF2's expression pattern with the distribution of high shear levels, which occurs in the narrow regions of the cardiovascular system such as the cardiac inflow/outflow tracts, the atrioventricular canal and, in the early stages of development, in the aortic sac and the pharyngeal arch arteries.[39,40] Using a murine carotid artery collar model to focally increase flow, Dekker *et al.* demonstrated the direct involvement of high shear stress in the *in vivo* induction of KLF2 expression in the endothelium.[38] Laminar shear stress induces KLF2 expression by increasing both transcription and mRNA stability.[37,41]

Lingrel and colleagues identified a novel 62 bp shear stress responsive element in the KLF2 promoter that contains a 30 bp tripartite palindrome motif.[42,43] Furthermore, they demonstrated binding of PCAF (p300/cAMP-response element-binding protein-binding protein-associated factor) and heterogenous nuclear ribonucleoprotein D (hnRNP D) to this region as components of a shear stress-specific regulatory complex. Binding of these factors was dependent upon the activation of phosphatidylinositol 3-kinase (PI3K) pathway and correlated with histone H3 and H4 acetylation.[42] In a subsequent study, this group identified nucleolin, an abundant and ubiquitous cellular protein that plays important roles in DNA transcription, chromatin remodeling and mRNA stability,[44] as a factor which binds the shear stress-responsive site of the KLF2 promoter. The binding of nucleolin is PI3K-dependent and required for the induction of KLF2 by laminar shear stress.[45] Wang and colleagues reported that the Src signaling pathway is also involved in the shear stress-mediated regulation of KLF2. They demonstrated that Src mediates the inhibitory effect of oscillatory or disturbed flow on KLF2 expression.[46]

Additional investigation of the mechanism of flow induced KLF2 expression has demonstrated that the MEK5 (MAP/ERK kinase 5)/ERK5 (extracellular signal regulated kinase 5)/MEF2 (myocyte enhancer factor 2) signaling pathway mediates the increase of KLF2 by laminar shear stress. Kumar and colleagues showed that a single consensus MEF2 binding site in the conserved region of the KLF2 promoter regulates KLF2 promoter activity.[21] ERK5 (also referred as to Big MAPK1 (BMK1)) is highly induced by laminar shear stress, and MEF2 is a well-characterized target gene of ERK5. Winoto and colleagues found that ERK5 plays a crucial role in KLF2 expression in embryos and that MEF2 mediates ERK5-induced KLF2 expression.[47] Building on these observations, Parmar *et al.* demonstrated that dominant negative MEF2 or mutant MEK5 (an upstream activator of ERK5) abolished flow-mediated KLF2 induction in endothelial cells (Parmar *et al.*, 2006). More recently, Young *et al.* demonstrated that the shear stress regulated factor AMP-activated protein kinase (AMPK) is also able to activate the ERK5/MEF2 pathway, thereby increasing KLF2 expression.[48] Woo and colleagues demonstrated that sumoylation of ERK5 by H_2O_2 and AGEs (advanced glycation end products), major transducers of diabetic vasculopathy, inhibits shear stress-mediated KLF2 induction in endothelial cells.[49] They observed that H_2O_2 and AGEs induce endogenous sumoylation of ERK5, leading to reduction of shear stress-induced eNOS expression. Sumoylation of ERK5 downregulates MEF2 and subsequently reduces KLF2 transcriptional activity, thereby suppressing induction of eNOS and the anti-inflammatory response by shear stress.[49] It has been shown that angiopoeitin-1 (Ang-1) also upregulates KLF2 expression through the PI3K/Akt-dependent activation of MEF2.[50] Recently, the adaptor protein p66shc, known to promote cellular oxidative stress and apoptosis, has been demonstrated to inhibit KFL2 transcription by suppression of MEF2A expression.[51] These observations indicate that ERK5/MEF2 signaling pathway plays a crucial role in regulating KLF2 expression by laminar shear stress.

The identification of MEF2 as being critical in the regulation of KLF2 also has implications for the downregulation of KLF2 expression observed in the setting of cytokine stimulation. Specifically, Kumar *et al.* showed that TNF-α downregulates KLF2 expression in endothelial cells. Inhibition of NF-κB abolishes the reduction of KLF2 by TNF-α as supported by inability of TNF-α to downregulate KLF2 in p65 null cells. Mechanistic studies revealed that histone deacetylase 4/5 and p65 form a complex and binding of this complex to myocyte enhancing factor 2 (MEF2) site of the KLF2 promoter causes TNF-α-mediated KLF2 repression.[52] A schematic diagram of the regulation of KLF2 in endothelial cells is shown in Fig. 1.

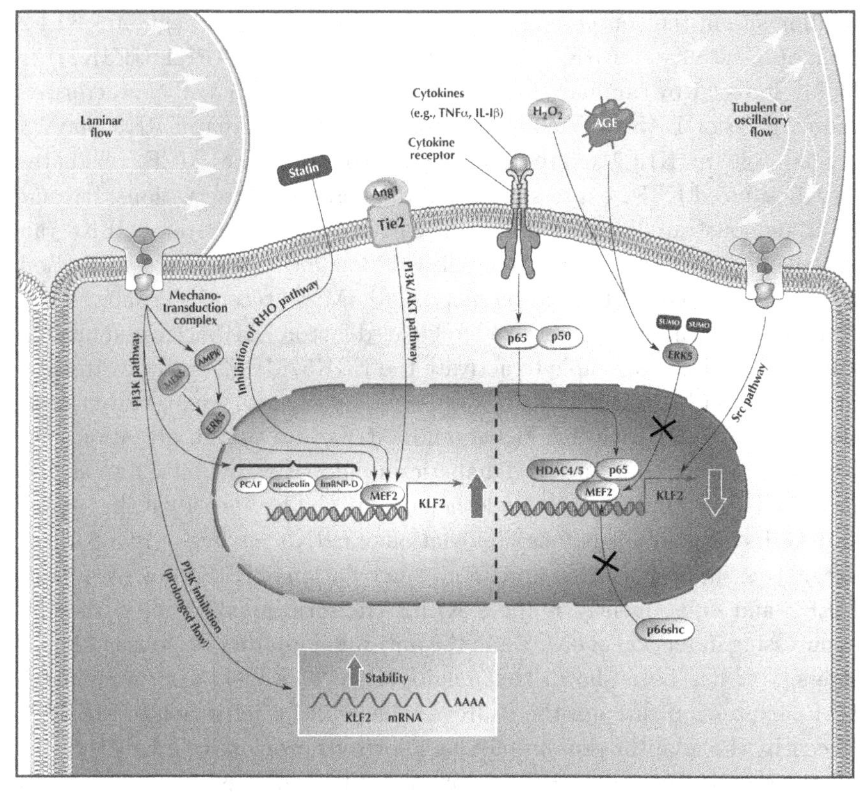

Fig. 1. Schematic diagram of the regulation of KLF2 in endothelial cells. Ang1 indicates Angiopoietin 1; AGE, advanced glycation end products.

1.4. *Targets of Shear-Stress Induced KLF2*

1.4.1. *Inflammation and atherogenesis*

Of particular importance is the ability of shear-induced KLF2 to mediate the favorable effects of shear stress. Indeed, more than 15% of all flow-regulated genes are dependent on flow-mediated KLF2 induction, and of those most highly regulated by flow, approximately 50% are KLF2-dependent.[53] The Horrevoets laboratory has suggested that three characteristics of KLF2, 1)potent up-regulation by prolonged laminar shear stress 2)lack of up-regulation by other physiological mediators, and 3)vascular expression limited to the endothelium, make it an attractive candidate as an integral mediator of laminar flow.[37] Targets of KLF2 (direct or indirect) are involved in mediating a broad range of shear-regulated systemic, cellular, and molecular events. The effect of KLF2 on regulation of the expression of two critical mediators of vascular tone, eNOS and endothelin-1 (ET-1) has been published by several laboratories.[24,38,53] As described in detail in earlier chapters, nitric oxide production in response to shear stress is a fundamental mechanism of regulation of vascular tone. KLF2 is one of the most potent inducers of eNOS expression yet described.[24] Mechanistic studies have revealed that KLF2 directly binds to the eNOS promoter. Furthermore, KLF2 recruits the co-activator CBP/p300 to the eNOS promoter.[24] KLF2 has also been shown to induce C-natriuretic peptide and arginosuccinate synthase, a limiting enzyme in eNOS substrate bioavailability.[38,54,55] Finally, KLF2 reduces expression of caveolin-1 which negatively regulates eNOS activity.[56] In contrast, KLF2 inhibits the expression of adrenomedullin, ET-1 and angiotensin-converting enzyme (ACE), all of which increase vascular tone.[38] Surprisingly, the *in vivo* phenotype of conditional embryonic loss of systemic or endothelial-specific KLF2 is lethal embryonic heart failure, thought to be secondary to low vascular tone.[57] The phenotype, demonstrated in both mice and zebrafish, is rescued by the administration of phenylephrine. A molecular mechanism for the phenotype could not be demonstrated in this study, as the expression of target genes known to affect vascular tone (including eNOS, adrenomedullin, and ET-1, as well as smooth muscle cell function) were similar in the controls and knockout mice. The authors of the study hypothesized that the phenotype is due to loss of an as yet unidentified gene or is a result of small changes in a large number of known target genes.

Endothelial homeostasis, driven by shear stress-dependent gene expression, is an important regulator of protective responses to acute and chronic inflammation.[58] Inflammation plays a central role in the development of atherosclerosis.[59] In response to inflammatory mediators, the expression of adhesion molecules such as vascular cell adhesion molecule-1 (VCAM-1) is induced on the surface of vascular endothelial cells. Adhesion molecules mediate the recruitment of leukocytes to the endothelium, and their expression is a crucial step in the formation of atherosclerotic lesions. Our group demonstrated that KLF2 functions as an anti-inflammatory factor in endothelial cells and that it inhibits cytokine-mediated VCAM-1 induction.[24] NF-κB is a well-established key regulator of cytokine-induced endothelial cell activation. We have demonstrated that

KLF2 inhibits NF-κB function by inhibiting recruitment of CBP/p300, a NF-κB co-factor critical in mediating NF-κB activity. Binding of KLF2 to CBP/p300 inhibits the interaction between p65 and CBP/p300. As a consequence, NF-κB is not optimally activated.[24]

The inflammatory effects of TNF-α on human umbilical vein endothelial cells (HUVECs) are considered a reasonable model for atherogenesis[60] and are mediated by both NF-κB and MAPK, which activates activation protein 1 (AP-1). Shear stress-induced KLF2 inhibits activating transcription factor 2 (ATF2), one of the heterodimeric components of AP-1.[61] Increased levels of phosphorylated ATF2 are seen in endothelial cells overlying early atherosclerotic plaques. Knockdown studies using siRNA against KLF2 suppressed the inhibitory effect of shear stress on ATF2. Furthermore, KLF2 excluded phosphorylated ATF2 from the nucleus,[61] thereby inhibiting ATF2's ability to activate inflammatory pathways.

TGF-β has been proposed to regulate endothelial cell activation.[62] KLF2 regulates the TGF-β-mediated proinflammatory response in endothelial cells by inducing Smad7, a potent attenuator of TGF-β signaling. This results in a reduction of the phosphorylation and nuclear accumulation of Smad2 and the Smad3/4-dependent transcriptional cascade, thereby abrogating TGFβ signaling. Furthermore, they demonstrated that KLF2 can inhibit AP-1, an important co-factor in TGF-β-mediated inflammatory activity.[63]

Consistent with these *in vitro* observations, Atkins and colleagues demonstrated that hemizygous deficiency of KLF2 promotes diet-induced atherosclerosis in apolipoprotein E deficient mice.[25] To date this is the only evidence that KLF2 functions as an athero-protective factor *in vivo*. Hemizygous deficiency of KLF2 did not, however, show significant changes in endothelial mediators of inflammation, including VCAM-1, eNOS and TM. This may be due to a compensatory effect of KLF4 (discussed below), which was increased in KLF2-deficient mice compared to control animals.[25] The mechanism of increased susceptibility to atherosclerosis may also be a result of alterations in macrophage activity; hemizygous deficiency of KLF2 enhances the expression of the key lipid binding protein adipocyte protein 2/fatty acid-binding protein 4 and increases macrophage lipid. It will be critically important to study the cell-specific mechanisms that underlie the regulation of vascular inflammation by KLF2 in this model by utilizing tissue-specific KLF2 knockout mice.

1.4.2. *Thrombosis*

Numerous studies have demonstrated the importance of cross-talk between the coagulation and inflammatory pathways.[64–66] Inflammatory stimuli induce the expression of tissue factor (TF) and plasminogen activator inhibitor 1 (PAI-1) by endothelial cells, resulting in a local imbalance of anticoagulant and procoagulant proteins, and development of clot. We have shown that KLF2 inhibits cytokine-mediated PAI-1 and TF induction in endothelial cells.[23] The relationship between shear stress and endothelial expression of coagulation proteins has been described for several of the factors regulated by KLF2. While a transient *increase* in tissue factor expression is seen in cultured endothelial cells exposed to laminar shear stress,[67] *in vivo* studies in rat carotid arteries show tissue factor expression only in vessels subjected to mechanical stenosis.[68] Analysis of human autopsy specimens demonstrate a selective lack of expression of TF and PAI-1 in regions of the carotid artery exposed to atheroprotective flow.[69] We have also demonstrated that KLF2 robustly induces TM, a potent inhibitor of blood coagulation.[23] Consistent with these observations, over-expression of KLF2 in HUVECs increases blood clotting time under flow conditions. Conversely, knockdown of KLF2 by siRNA leads to a reduced time to clot formation. Our mechanistic studies demonstrate that KLF2 binds to specific sites within the TM promoter and thereby induces transcription of the TM promoter.[23] TM expression is enhanced by fluid shear stress.[70,71] In cultured endothelial cells made deficient in KLF2 (via siRNA technology) and exposed to atheroprotective flow, upregulation of TM is significantly diminished.[53] Thrombin is a key component of the coagulation cascade and has been shown to induce inflammatory genes expression via NF-κB activation (Minami and Aird, 2001). Lin and colleagues demonstrated that KLF2 inhibits thrombin-mediated expression of pro-inflammatory and chemokine including IL-6, IL-8 and monocyte chemoattractant protein-1 (MCP-1) in endothelial cells.[22] The majority of thrombin's activity is mediated via protease-activated receptor 1 (PAR-1), a G-coupled protein receptor. Thrombin cleaves the receptor, unmasking a tethered ligand that then activates the receptor.[64,72,73] KLF2 negatively regulates PAR-1 expression and inhibits thrombin-mediated NF-κB activation.[22] Interestingly, PAR-1 expression is increased at sites of vascular injury (and thus altered flow mechanics), but down-regulated by laminar shear stress.[74] Thus, while direct evidence is incomplete, the pattern of expression of these coagulation-active factors is consistent with an antithrombotic role for KLF2 *in vivo*.

1.4.3. *Vascular Development/Maturation/Remodeling*

Shear stress appears to control key aspects of embryonic cardiovascular development[75] as well as remodeling of developing and mature arteries.[76,77] KLF2 knockout mice are embryonic lethal at E12.5-14.5 due to severe intra-embryonic and intra-amniotic hemorrhaging.[36,78] In this model, formation of the vascular network appeared normal and both vasculogenesis and arteriogenesis were intact, but the vessel morphology was abnormal. KLF2-/- mice showed umbilical vessel and aortic defects resulting from impaired smooth muscle cell recruitment and tunica media formation, causing aortic dilation and rupture.[78] Of note, significant structural vascular defects (hemorrhage, aneurysm, or abnormal smooth muscle morphology) were not observed by Lee *et al.*[57] in KLF2-/- mice, with the exception of a few late-stage embryos. These authors explain the apparent discrepancy by interpreteing the morphological defects to be a late, secondary effect of the primary physiologic event (low vascular tone). Lingrel and colleagues have subsequently demonstrated that KLF2-/- embryos have a normal development pattern of endothelial cells but a reduced number of smooth muscle cells in the aorta. Deficiency of KLF2 also inhibited smooth muscle cell migration in response to platelet-derived growth factor B (PDGF-B), resulting in a lack of vessel maturation and stability.[79] Furthermore, shear stress waveforms designed to mimic those seen in coronary collateral vessels induce KLF2 as well as genes important for endothelium-smooth muscle interactions.[80]

1.4.4. *Angiogenesis*

Angiogenesis is a complex process that involves multiple gene products expressed by different cell types and recapitulates many of the molecular events that occur during vascular development. Imbalance of this process results in malignant and ischemic disorders.[81] The effect of shear stress on angiogenesis is not well described; most of the expected effects are extrapolated from the pattern of growth factors, such as VEGF, induced by *in vitro* shear stress experiments. Studies from our laboratory demonstrate that KLF2 potently inhibits VEGF-mediated angiogenesis.[20] In the nude mouse ear model of angiogenesis, KLF2 potently inhibits permeability, tissue edema and angiogenesis. From a mechanistic stand point, KLF2 inhibits, cell proliferation, VEGF receptor 2 (VEGFR2) expression, and VEGF-induced endothelial activation (characterized by reduction of calcium influx, suppression of VCAM-1, TF and cyclooxygenase 2).[20] KLF2 has been shown to regulate VEGFR2 (also referred as to Flt1 or KDR) by cooperating with Ets during vascular development in *Xenopus* embryos.[82]

Ang-1 and -2 are Tie ligands that have critical roles in regulating angiogenesis.[83,84] Ang-1-mediated Tie2 activation is required to maintain the quiescent resting state of the endothelium. Agonistic Ang-1 functions are antagonized by Ang-2, which is believed to inhibit Ang-1/Tie2 signaling. Ang-2 destabilizes the quiescent endothelium and primes it to respond to exogenous stimuli, thereby facilitating the activities of inflammatory and angiogenic cytokines.[83] KLF2 has been shown to inhibit cytokine-mediated Ang-2 expression in endothelial cells.[53] Furthermore, KLF2 has been shown to induce Tie2 expression.[53] A fundamental aspect of sprouting angiogeneis is the migration of endothelial cells. Studies from the Horrevoetts laboratory showed that KLF2 inhibits endothelial cell migration by upregulating semaphorin-3F, a potent anti-migratory factor.[54]

As described above, KLF2 has been implicated as an anti-angiogenic factor. However, role of KLF2 in hypoxia-mediated angiogenesis has not been elucidated. Our laboratory identified KLF2 as a negative regulator of hypoxia-mediated angiogenesis. KLF2 protein expression is acutely upregulated by hypoxia. Adenoviral overexpression of KLF2 inhibited matrigel tube formation whereas primary microvascular endothelial cells from KLF2+/- mice showed enhanced tube formation in response to hypoxia. Hypoxia inducible factor 1 (HIF-1)α is a key regulator of angiogensis under hypoxic conditions (e.g. ischemic heart disease, cancer). We showed that KLF2 inhibits HIF-1α expression and function in endothelial cells.[85] Interestingly, KLF2 limits accumulation of HIF-1α protein in response to hypoxia. Loss of function studies using siRNA-mediated KLF2 knockdown and mouse KLF2-/- embryonic fibroblasts showed accelerated HIF-1α accumulation in response to hypoxia. We found that KLF2 promotes HIF-1α degradation in a von Hippel Lindau protein (VHL)-independent, p53-independent but proteasome-dependent pathway.[85] The mechanism of increased HIF-1α degradation may be explained by the ability of KLF2 to disrupt the interaction between HIF-1α and its chaperone Hsp90, suggesting that KLF2 promotes degradation of HIF-1α by affecting its folding and maturation.[85] These observations indicate that KLF2 negatively regulates hypoxia-mediated angiogenesis through inhibiting HIF-1α expression and function.

1.4.5. *Vascular Stress/Injury*

While oscillatory or absent shear stress in areas of disturbed blood flow enable oxidative stress to take full effect, laminar shear stress results in elaboration of several anti-oxidant factors.[86] Recent studies have identified novel factors that are induced by laminar shear stress in a KLF2-dependent manner. Laminar shear stress induces expression and nuclear accumulation of nuclear factor erythroid 2-related factor 2 (Nrf2), an antioxidant transcription factor that activates antioxidant response element (ARE)-dependent transcriptional programs.[87] Interestingly, expression of Nrf2 and its target genes such as NAD(P)H dehydrogenase quinon 1 (NQO1) and heme oxygenase (HO-1) were upregulated by laminar shear stress and KLF2. Knockdown of KLF2 resulted in loss of induction of NQO1 but not Nrf2 by shear stress. KLF2 does, however, enhance the nuclear localization and activation of Nrf2 and promotes its antioxidant activity.[87] Together KLF2 and Nrf2 govern approximately 70% of the shear stress-induced gene set.[63,87]

Mason and colleagues have identified CD59 as a novel factor that is induced by laminar shear stress in a KLF2-dependent fashion.[88] Complement activation occurs in vascular injury and is thought to have a capability to induce a proinflammatory response in endothelial cells. CD59 blocks the terminal pathway of complement activation. Functionally, the increase of CD59 by laminar shear stress reduces C9 deposition and complement lysis. CD59 induction is dependent upon the magnitude of shear force. This characteristic is manifested in it's differential expression pattern in murine aorta.[88] Mechanistic analysis using inhibitors of signaling pathways revealed that CD59 induction is independent of PI3K, ERK1/2 and nitric oxide (NO). Knockdown studies by use of siRNA demonstrated that the induction is ERK5 and KLF2-dependent.[88] These observations indicate that CD59 is a KLF2-dpendent anti-atherogenic factor that is induced by laminar shear stress in endothelial cells.

In sum, induction of KLF2 in regions of high shear stress and the subsequent effects of KLF2 on the entire range of shear-induced molecular, cellular, and systemic functions prove KLF2 to be one of the most important mediators of shear stress yet described (summarized in Fig. 2).

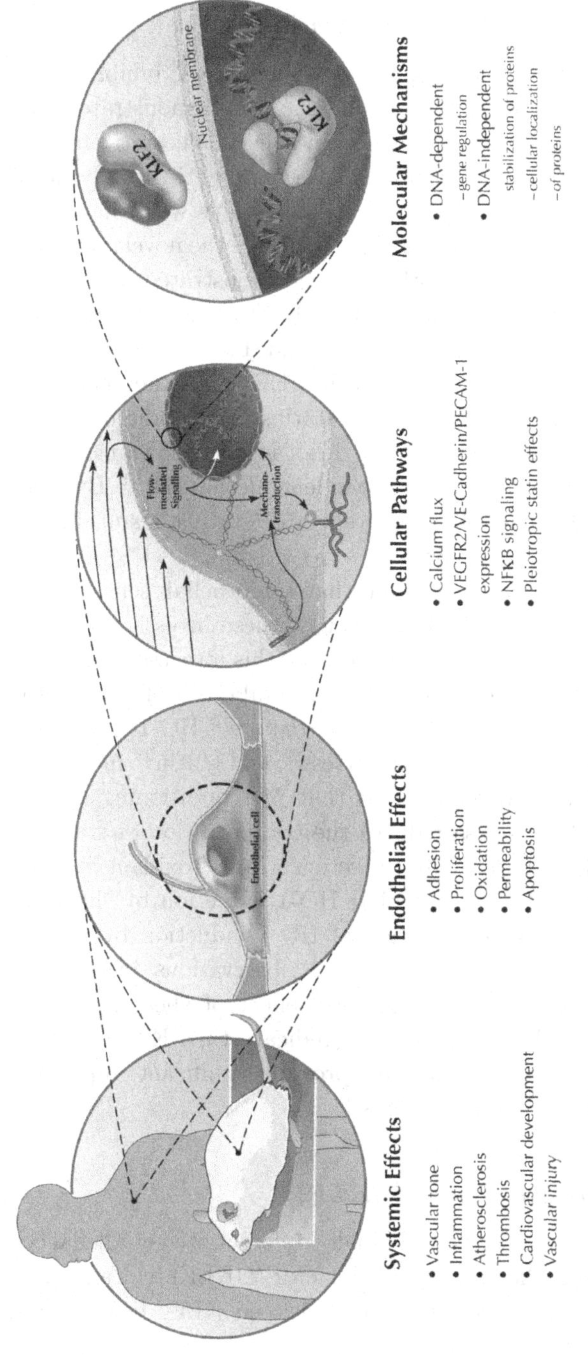

Fig. 2. Schematic overview of the role of KLF2 in shear stress-induced vasoprotection. See text for details.

1.5. *KLF2, Shear Stress, and Statins*

Statins (3-hydroxy-3-methylglutaryl coenzyme A inhibitors) are widely used in the treatment of hyperlipidemia.[1] As demonstrated by basic and clinical studies, statins also have numerous homeostatic functions in the endothelium, including anti-inflammatory and anti-thrombotic effects. The effect of statins on endothelial function overlaps with that of KLF2. This fact led us to speculate whether there might be the novel link between KLF2 and statins. Indeed, we and others have demonstrated that multiple statins robustly induce KLF2 in endothelial cells.[89,90] Importantly, knockdown of KLF2 inhibits statin-mediated eNOS and TM induction, indicating that KLF2 mediates statin effects.[89] Both MEF2 and Rho activity are critical for regulating KLF2 expression by statins. MEF2 directly transactivates the KLF2 promoter. Constitutive Rho activity downregulates KLF2 by geranylgeranyl pyrophosphate-dependent mechanism.[89] By inhibiting the conversion of HMG-CoA to mevalonate, statins result in depletion of geranylgeranyl pyrophosphate.

Ali *et al.* recently reported that endothelial sensitivity to statins depends on shear stress.[91] Interestingly, these investigators demonstrated that KLF2 plays an important role in this process. Heme oxygenase-1 (HO-1) is a rate limiting factor in the catabolism of heme into biliverdin and functions as an anti-atherogenic factor.[92] HO-1 has been shown to be upregulated by laminar shear stress[86] and statin[93] in endothelial cells. These investigators demonstrated that pre-conditioning endothelial cells with laminar shear stress reduces the concentration of statin required to enhance HO-1-mediated cytoprotection against oxidant-induced injury.[91] Knockdown of KLF2 did not alter HO-1 induction by shear stress alone, however, it resulted in inhibition of HO-1 induction by the combination of shear stress and statins.[91] These observations indicate that KLF2 mediates a synergistic vasoprotective effect of shear stress and statins. Taken together, these observations indicate that KLF2 is a mediator of pleiotropic effects of statins and provide significant implications in the treatment of cardiovascular disease.

1.6. *Krüppel-Like Factor 4 (KLF4)*

KLF4 is highly expressed in terminally differentiated epithelial cells and was cloned as gut-enriched Kruppel-like factor (GKLF) by Yang and colleagues in 1996.[94] Katz and colleagues have deleted KLF4 in gastric epithelia.[95]

These mice survive to adulthood and show increased proliferation and altered differentiation of their gastric epithelia, suggesting that KLF4 is a critical factor for normal gastric epithelial homeostasis. Furthermore, KLF4 has been implicated as a crucial factor in the development and maintenance of mouse cornea.[96,97] KLF4 plays an important role in skin barrier function.[98] Segre and colleagues showed that KLF4-/- mice die shortly after birth; death was postulated to be due to dehydration resulting from loss of skin barrier function.[98]

KLF4 is expressed in many cell types besides epithelial cells and has been shown to have significant roles in endothelial cell biology,[99] vascular smooth muscle cell biology,[100–103] monocyte/macrophage biology,[104,105] and tumor biology.[106–108] In 2006, Yamanaka and colleagues identified KLF4 as a crucial factor in generating inducible pluripotent stem cells.[109] Studies from this group and others demonstrate that introduction of Oct3/4, Sox2, c-Myc and KLF4 by retrovirus or plasmid can induce reprogram mouse fibroblasts into pluripotent stem cells.[110–112]

The first description of KLF4 in endothelial cells was provided by Yet and colleagues in 1998.[113] A subsequent study by McCormick and colleagues identified KLF4 as a shear stress-inducible gene by DNA microarray analysis of HUVECs.[114] Hamik and colleagues first revealed *in vivo* expression of endothelial cells and demonstrated that KLF4 negatively regulates endothelial inflammation.[99] Functionally, forced expression of KLF4 induced atheroprotective genes such as eNOS and TM.[99] Furthermore, KLF4 reduced cytokine-mediated VCAM-1, PAI-1 and TF induction in endothelial cells. Consistent with these observations, KLF4 inhibited cytokine-mediated monocyte adhesion on endothelial cells. The induction of KLF4 by shear stress was dependent upon the magnitude of shear force; arterial stress was more potent than venous shear stress.[99] All these characteristics are reminiscent of KLF2. Intriguingly, and in contradistinction to KLF2, inflammatory cytokines induce KLF4. This raises the question of whether KLF4 can compensate for KLF2 under inflammatory conditions. In fact, it is postulated that the lack of a pro-inflammatory expression pattern in the endothelium of the heterozygous KLF2 ApoE null mouse may be due to the compensatory increase in KLF4 expression.[25] Further studies will be critical to elucidate the mechanisms by which shear stress induces KLF4 expression and how shear-induced KLF4 effects endothelial function.

1.7. *Future Directions*

KLF2 has been proven to be a central regulator of endothelial function. It controls endothelial inflammation, thrombosis, and vascular tone, serving as a "molecular switch" in regulating endothelial quiescence. In addition, a significant body of evidence demonstrates that KLF2 is a transducer of the vasoprotective effects of laminar shear stress. Furthermore, the findings that KLF2 mediates the non-lipid-lowering effects of statins suggest that expression of endothelial KLF2 has significant clinical implications. Substantial progress has been made in this field but important questions remain to be addressed.

To date, the PI3K, AMPK, and MEK5/ERK5/MEF2 pathways have been implicated in laminar shear stress mediated induction of KLF2. The likelihood that other shear stress activated signaling pathways are involved in regulating KLF2 warrants further investigation. Furthermore, identification of novel flow-inducible factors that upregulate or interact with KLF2 would be intriguing. Sumoylation of ERK5 results in the reduction of KLF2 promoter activity. It would be of interest to study the effects of protein modification of other factors upstream of KLF2, such as MEK5 or MEF2, on KLF2 expression. In addition, post-translational modification of KLF2 itself needs to be examined. For example, does shear stress result in post-translational modification of KLF2 and subsequently alter KLF2's cellular localization and/or function?

Further elucidation of KLF2's *in vivo* endothelial functions is of considerable interest. The role of KLF2 in cardiovascular development has been studied in systemic and endothelial specific KLF2 knockout mice. Beyond developmental studies, it is extremely important to understand the role of KLF2 in endothelial cells in adult animals. Our laboratory has shown that hemizygous deficiency of KLF2 promotes atherosclerosis. Interestingly, no obvious endothelial phenotype was identified but we demonstrated that the macrophages from these mice play a substantial role in the development of disease. To investigate more precisely the *in vivo* role of KLF2 in regulating endothelial function, it is important to develop an inducible endothelial cell specific KLF2 knockout mouse and assess models of vascular inflammation, atherosclerosis and angiogenesis. Furthermore, maintaining barrier function is one of the canonical endothelial functions, and shear stress has been implicated as playing a role.[115] Given KLF2's function as a vasoprotective agent, it is likely that KLF2 has some role in regulating endothelial permeability.

In addition to the knock-out experiments described above, *in vivo* endothelial cell KLF2 overexpresion studies would be of interest to be considered. Besides genetic approaches, further investigation is warranted to identify compounds that regulate or interact with KLF2. Screening compounds that increase KLF2 levels, similar to statins, may provide new clinical implications for the treatment of disease.

The role of KLF4 in endothelial cell biology remains largely unknown. Although KLF4 has been shown to be induced by laminar shear stress, the mechanisms underlying this observation remain unclear and should be a subject of future investigation. Furthermore, it is critically important to understand whether KLF4 has the same shear stress-induced vasoprotective effects demonstrated by KLF2. In addition, the mechanism by which KLF4 regulates inflammation in endothelial cells should be elucidated (e.g. examination of NF-κB signaling pathway). Just as with KLF2, it is very important to establish tissue/cell-specific gain or loss of function approaches to understand the precise role of KLF4 in regulating endothelial function.

Finally, overlapping and distinct functions between KLF2 and KLF4 in endothelial cells should be further investigated. Both KLF2 and KLF4 have anti-inflammatory and anti-thrombotic effects in endothelial cells. Consistent with *in vitro* observations, KLF2 has been shown to serve as an anti-atherogenic factor *in vivo*. However, the role of KLF4 in atherosclerosis *in vivo* has not been elucidated and its role in angiogenesis is unknown. In addition to functional analysis, simultaneous regulation of KLF2 and KLF4 should be studied. For example, it has been shown that shear stress induces both KLF2 and KLF4, but is the induction of both factors mediated by a common signaling pathway or are there distinct mechanisms? Do KLF2 and KLF4 regulate, compensate, or antagonize each other in physiological and/or disease conditions? These questions should be addressed in future studies. In summary, KLF2 and KLF4 are laminar shear stress induced factors with important functions in endothelial biology. Therefore, they are attractive as targets for the development of novel therapeutic strategies for cardiovascular disease.

Acknowledgements

This work was supported by NIH grants HL72952, HL75427, HL76754, HL086548, HL084154, and P01 HL48743 (to M.K.J.); and HL088740 (to

G.B.A.); and HL083090 (to A.H.); an Alliance for Cancer Gene Therapy grant (to M.K.J.); a Robert Wood Johnson/Harold Amos Medical Faculty Development grant (to G.B.A.); a Dominic Visconsi Scholar Award (to G.B.A., A.H.); and American Heart Association Postdoctoral Fellowship 0725297B (to D.K.); and a Kanae Foundation for the Promotion of Medical Science grant (to D.K.).

References

1. Jain, M. K., Ridker, P. M. (2005) Anti-inflammatory effects of statins: clinical evidence and basic mechanisms. *Nat Rev Drug Discov* **4**(12), 977–987.
2. Glagov, S. (1973) Mechanical stresses on vessels and the non-uniform distribution of atherosclerosis. *Med Clin North Am* **57**(1), 63–77.
3. Weinberg, P. D. (Jan-Feb 2004) Rate-limiting steps in the development of atherosclerosis: the response-to-influx theory. *J Vasc Res* **41**(1), 1–17.
4. Atkins, G. B., Jain, M. K. (Jun 22 2007) Role of Kruppel-like transcription factors in endothelial biology. *Circ Res* **100**(12), 1686–1695.
5. Feinberg, M. W., Lin, Z., Fisch, S., Jain, M. K. (Aug 2004) An emerging role for kruppel-like factors in vascular biology. *Trends Cardiovasc Med* **14**(6), 241–246.
6. Haldar, S. M., Ibrahim, O. A., Jain, M. K. (Jul 2007) Kruppel-like Factors (KLFs) in muscle biology. *J Mol Cell Cardiol* **43**(1), 1–10.
7. Hamik, A., Wang, B., Jain, M. K. (Sep 2006) Transcriptional regulators of angiogenesis. *Arterioscler Thromb Vasc Biol* **26**(9), 1936–1947.
8. Jackle, H., Rosenberg, U. B., Preiss, A., *et al.* (1985) Molecular analysis of Kruppel, a segmentation gene of Drosophila melanogaster. *Cold Spring Harb Symp Quant Biol* **50**, 465–473.
9. Preiss, A., Rosenberg, U. B., Kienlin, A., Seifert, E., Jackle, H. (Jan 3–9 1985) Molecular genetics of Kruppel, a gene required for segmentation of the Drosophila embryo. *Nature* **313**(5997), 27–32.
10. Rosenberg, U. B., Preiss, A., Seifert, E., Jackle, H., Knipple, D. C. (Feb 21–27 1985) Production of phenocopies by Kruppel antisense RNA injection into Drosophila embryos. *Nature* **313**(6004), 703–706.
11. Miller, I. J., Bieker, J. J. (1993) A novel, erythroid cell-specific murine transcription factor that binds to the CACCC element and is related to the Kruppel family of nuclear proteins. *Molecular & Cellular Biology* **13**(5), 2776–2786.
12. Black, A. R., Black, J. D. (Aug 2001) Azizkhan-Clifford J. Sp1 and kruppel-like factor family of transcription factors in cell growth regulation and cancer. *J Cell Physiol* **188**(2), 143–160.
13. van Vliet, J., Crofts, L. A., Quinlan, K. G., Czolij, R., Perkins, A. C. (Apr 2006) Crossley M. Human KLF17 is a new member of the Sp/KLF family of transcription factors. *Genomics* **87**(4), 474–482.

14. Dang, D. T., Zhao, W., Mahatan, C. S., Geiman, D. E., Yang, V. W. (Jul 1 2002) Opposing effects of Kruppel-like factor 4 (gut-enriched Kruppel-like factor) and Kruppel-like factor 5 (intestinal-enriched Kruppel-like factor) on the promoter of the Kruppel-like factor 4 gene. *Nucleic Acids Res* **30**(13), 2736–2741.
15. Zhang, W., Shields, J. M., Sogawa, K., Fujii-Kuriyama, Y., Yang, V. W. (1998) The gut-enriched Kruppel-like factor suppresses the activity of the CYP1A1 promoter in an Sp1-dependent fashion. *Journal of Biological Chemistry* **273**(28), 17917–17925.
16. Wani, M. A., Wert, S. E., Lingrel, J. B. (Jul 23 1999) Lung Kruppel-like factor, a zinc finger transcription factor, is essential for normal lung development. *J Biol Chem* **274**(30), 21180–21185.
17. Conkright, M. D., Wani, M. A., Lingrel, J. B. (2001) Lung Kruppel-like factor contains an autoinhibitory domain that regulates its transcriptional activation by binding WWP1, an E3 ubiquitin ligase. *Journal of Biological Chemistry* **276**(31), 29299–29306.
18. Zhang, X., Srinivasan, S. V., Lingrel, J. B. (Mar 26 2004) WWP1-dependent ubiquitination and degradation of the lung Kruppel-like factor, KLF2. *Biochem Biophys Res Commun* **316**(1), 139–148.
19. Anderson, K. P., Kern, C. B., Crable, S. C., Lingrel, J. B. (Nov 1995) Isolation of a gene encoding a functional zinc finger protein homologous to erythroid Kruppel-like factor: identification of a new multigene family. *Mol Cell Biol* **15**(11), 5957–5965.
20. Bhattacharya, R., Senbanerjee, S., Lin, Z., *et al.* (Aug 12 2005) Inhibition of vascular permeability factor/vascular endothelial growth factor-mediated angiogenesis by the Kruppel-like factor KLF2. *J Biol Chem* **280**(32), 28848–28851.
21. Kumar, A., Lin, Z., Senbanerjee, S., Jain, M. K. (Jul 2005) Tumor Necrosis Factor Alpha-Mediated Reduction of KLF2 Is Due to Inhibition of MEF2 by NF-{kappa}B and Histone Deacetylases. *Mol Cell Biol* **25**(14), 5893–5903.
22. Lin, Z., Hamik, A., Jain, R., Kumar, A., Jain, M. K. (May 2006) Kruppel-like factor 2 inhibits protease activated receptor-1 expression and thrombin-mediated endothelial activation. *Arterioscler Thromb Vasc Biol* **26**(5), 1185–1189.
23. Lin, Z., Kumar, A., Senbanerjee, S., *et al.* (Feb 17 2005) Kruppel-Like Factor 2 (KLF2) Regulates Endothelial Thrombotic Function. *Circ Res.*
24. SenBanerjee, S., Lin, Z., Atkins, G. B. *et al.* (May 17 2004) KLF2 Is a novel transcriptional regulator of endothelial proinflammatory activation. *J Exp Med* **199**(10), 1305–1315.
25. Atkins, G. B., Wang, Y., Mahabeleshwar, G. H., *et al.* (Sep 26 2008) Hemizygous deficiency of Kruppel-like factor 2 augments experimental atherosclerosis. *Circ Res* **103**(7), 690–693.
26. Das, H., Kumar, A., Lin, Z., *et al.* (Apr 25 2006) Kruppel-like factor 2 (KLF2) regulates proinflammatory activation of monocytes. *Proc Natl Acad Sci U S A.* **103**(17), 6653–6658.

27. Wu, J., Lingrel, J. B. (Sep 1 2005) Kruppel-like factor 2, a novel immediate-early transcriptional factor, regulates IL-2 expression in T lymphocyte activation. *J Immunol* **175**(5), 3060–3066.
28. Carlson, C. M., Endrizzi, B. T., Wu, J., *et al.* (Jul 20 2006) Kruppel-like factor 2 regulates thymocyte and T-cell migration. *Nature* **442**(7100), 299–302.
29. Kuo, C. T., Veselits, M. L., Leiden, J. M. (Sep 26 1997) LKLF: A transcriptional regulator of single-positive T cell quiescence and survival. *Science* **277**(5334), 1986–1990.
30. Sebzda, E., Zou, Z., Lee, J. S., Wang, T., Kahn, M. L. (Mar 2008) Transcription factor KLF2 regulates the migration of naive T cells by restricting chemokine receptor expression patterns. *Nat Immunol* **9**(3), 292–300.
31. Basu, P., Morris, P. E., Haar, J. L., *et al.* (Oct 1 2005) KLF2 is essential for primitive erythropoiesis and regulates the human and murine embryonic beta-like globin genes *in vivo*. *Blood* 106(7), 2566–2571.
32. Banerjee, S. S., Feinberg, M. W., Watanabe, M., *et al.* (2003) The Kruppel-like factor KLF2 inhibits peroxisome proliferator-activated receptor-gamma expression and adipogenesis. *Journal of Biological Chemistry* **278**(4), 2581–2584.
33. Wu, J., Srinivasan, S. V., Neumann, J. C., Lingrel, J. B. (Aug 23 2005) The KLF2 transcription factor does not affect the formation of preadipocytes but inhibits their differentiation into adipocytes. *Biochemistry* **44**(33), 11098–11105.
34. Jiang, J., Chan, Y. S., Loh, Y. H., *et al.* (Mar 2008) A core Klf circuitry regulates self-renewal of embryonic stem cells. *Nat Cell Biol* **10**(3), 353–360.
35. Kuo, C. T., Veselits, M. L., Barton, K. P., Lu, M. M., Clendenin, C., Leiden, J. M. (1997) The LKLF transcription factor is required for normal tunica media formation and blood vessel stabilization during murine embryogenesis. *Genes & Development* **11**(22), 2996–3006.
36. Wani, M. A., Means, R. T., Jr., Lingrel, J. B. (Jul 1998) Loss of LKLF function results in embryonic lethality in mice. *Transgenic Res* **7**(4), 229–238.
37. Dekker, R. J., van Soest, S., Fontijn, R. D., *et al.* (Sep 1 2002) Prolonged fluid shear stress induces a distinct set of endothelial cell genes, most specifically lung Kruppel-like factor (KLF2). *Blood* **100**(5), 1689–1698.
38. Dekker, R. J., van Thienen, J. V., Rohlena, J., *et al.* (Aug 2005) Endothelial KLF2 links local arterial shear stress levels to the expression of vascular tone-regulating genes. *Am J Pathol* **167**(2), 609–618.
39. Groenendijk, B. C., Hierck, B. P., Vrolijk, J., *et al.* (Jun 24 2005) Changes in shear stress-related gene expression after experimentally altered venous return in the chicken embryo. *Circ Res* **96**(12), 1291–1298.
40. Groenendijk, B. C., Van der Heiden, K., Hierck, B. P., Poelmann, R. E. (Dec 2007) The role of shear stress on ET-1, KLF2, and NOS-3 expression in the

developing cardiovascular system of chicken embryos in a venous ligation model. *Physiology (Bethesda)* **22**, 380–389.
41. van Thienen, J. V., Fledderus, J. O., Dekker, R. J., *et al.* (Nov 1 2006) Shear stress sustains atheroprotective endothelial KLF2 expression more potently than statins through mRNA stabilization. *Cardiovasc Res* **72**(2), 231–240.
42. Huddleson, J. P., Ahmad, N., Srinivasan, S., Lingrel, J. B. (Jun 17 2005) Induction of KLF2 by fluid shear stress requires a novel promoter element activated by a phosphatidylinositol 3-kinase-dependent chromatin-remodeling pathway. *J Biol Chem* **280**(24), 23371–23379.
43. Huddleson, J. P., Srinivasan, S., Ahmad, N., Lingrel, J. B. (Sep 2004) Fluid shear stress induces endothelial KLF2 gene expression through a defined promoter region. *Biol Chem* **385**(8), 723–729.
44. Storck, S., Shukla, M., Dimitrov, S., Bouvet, P. (2007) Functions of the histone chaperone nucleolin in diseases. *Subcell Biochem* **41**, 125–144.
45. Huddleson, J. P., Ahmad, N., Lingrel, J. B. (Jun 2 2006) Up-regulation of the KLF2 transcription factor by fluid shear stress requires nucleolin. *J Biol Chem* **281**(22), 15121–15128.
46. Wang, N., Miao, H., Li, Y. S., *et al.* (Mar 24 2006) Shear stress regulation of Kruppel-like factor 2 expression is flow pattern-specific. *Biochem Biophys Res Commun* **341**(4), 1244–1251.
47. Sohn, S. J., Li, D., Lee, L. K., Winoto, A. (Oct 2005) Transcriptional regulation of tissue-specific genes by the ERK5 mitogen-activated protein kinase. *Mol Cell Biol* **25**(19), 8553–8566.
48. Young, A., Wu, W., Sun, W., *et al.* (Aug 20 2009) Flow Activation of AMP-Activated Protein Kinase in Vascular Endothelium Leads to Kruppel-Like Factor 2 Expression. *Arterioscler Thromb Vasc Biol*
49. Woo, C. H., Shishido, T., McClain, C. *et al.* (Mar 14 2008) Extracellular signal-regulated kinase 5 SUMOylation antagonizes shear stress-induced antiinflammatory response and endothelial nitric oxide synthase expression in endothelial cells. *Circ Res* **102**(5), 538–545.
50. Sako, K., Fukuhara, S., Minami, T. *et al.* (Feb 27 2009) Angiopoietin-1 induces Kruppel-like factor 2 expression through a phosphoinositide 3-kinase/AKT-dependent activation of myocyte enhancer factor 2. *J Biol Chem* **284**(9), 5592–5601.
51. Kumar, A., Hoffman, T. A., Dericco, J., Naqvi, A., Jain, M. K., Irani, K. (Aug 24 2009) Transcriptional repression of Kruppel like factor-2 by the adaptor protein p66shc. FASEB J.
52. Kumar, A., Lin, Z., SenBanerjee, S., Jain, M. K. (Jul 2005) Tumor necrosis factor alpha-mediated reduction of KLF2 is due to inhibition of MEF2 by NF-kappaB and histone deacetylases. *Mol Cell Biol* **25**(14), 5893–5903.
53. Parmar, K. M., Larman, H. B., Dai G., *et al.* (Jan 4 2006) Integration of flow-dependent endothelial phenotypes by Kruppel-like factor 2. *J Clin Invest* **116**(1), 49–58.
54. Dekker, R. J., Boon, R. A., Rondaij, M. G., *et al.* (Jun 1 2006) KLF2 provokes a gene expression pattern that establishes functional quiescent differentiation of the endothelium. *Blood* **107**(11), 4354–4363.

55. Goodwin, B. L., Solomonson, L. P., Eichler, D. C. (Apr 30 2004) Argininosuccinate synthase expression is required to maintain nitric oxide production and cell viability in aortic endothelial cells. *J Biol Chem* **279**(18), 18353–18360.
56. Razani, B., Zhang, X. L., Bitzer, M., von Gersdorff, G., Bottinger, E. P., Lisanti, M. P. (Mar 2 2001) Caveolin-1 regulates transforming growth factor (TGF)-beta/SMAD signaling through an interaction with the TGF-beta type I receptor. *J Biol Chem* **276**(9), 6727–6738.
57. Lee, J. S., Yu, Q., Shin, J. T., *et al.* (Dec 2006) Klf2 is an essential regulator of vascular hemodynamic forces *in vivo*. *Dev Cell* **11**(6), 845–857.
58. Hwa, C., Sebastian, A., Aird, W. C. (May-Jun 2005) Endothelial biomedicine: its status as an interdisciplinary field, its progress as a basic science, and its translational bench-to-bedside gap. *Endothelium* **12**(3), 139–151.
59. Ross, R. (Nov 1999) Atherosclerosis is an inflammatory disease. *Am Heart J* **138**(5 Pt 2), S419–420.
60. Horrevoets, A. J., Fontijn, R. D., van Zonneveld, A. J., de Vries C. J., ten Cate, J. W., Pannekoek, H. (May 15 1999) Vascular endothelial genes that are responsive to tumor necrosis factor-alpha *in vitro* are expressed in atherosclerotic lesions, including inhibitor of apoptosis protein-1, stannin, and two novel genes. *Blood* **93**(10), 3418–3431.
61. Fledderus, J. O., van Thienen, J. V., Boon, R. A., *et al.* (May 15 2007) Prolonged shear stress and KLF2 suppress constitutive proinflammatory transcription through inhibition of ATF2. *Blood* **109**(10), 4249–4257.
62. Goumans, M. J., Liu, Z., ten Dijke, P. (Jan 2009) TGF-beta signaling in vascular biology and dysfunction. *Cell Res* **19**(1), 116–127.
63. Boon, R. A., Fledderus, J. O., Volger, O. L., *et al.* (Mar 2007) KLF2 suppresses TGF-beta signaling in endothelium through induction of Smad7 and inhibition of AP-1. *Arterioscler Thromb Vasc Biol* **27**(3), 532–539.
64. Coughlin, S. R. (Sep 14 2000) Thrombin signalling and protease-activated receptors. *Nature* **407**(6801), 258–264.
65. Jialal, I., Devaraj, S., Venugopal, S. K. (Jul 2004) C-reactive protein: risk marker or mediator in atherothrombosis? *Hypertension* **44**(1), 6–11.
66. Minami, T., Sugiyama, A., Wu, S. Q., Abid, R., Kodama, T., Aird, W. C. (Jan 2004) Thrombin and phenotypic modulation of the endothelium. *Arterioscler Thromb Vasc Biol* **24**(1), 41–53.
67. Lin, M. C., Almus-Jacobs, F., Chen, H. H., *et al.* (Feb 15 1997) Shear stress induction of the tissue factor gene. *J Clin Invest* **99**(4), 737–744.
68. Houston, P., Dickson, M. C., Ludbrook, V., *et al.* (Feb 1999) Fluid shear stress induction of the tissue factor promoter *in vitro* and *in vivo* is mediated by Egr-1. *Arterioscler Thromb Vasc Biol* **19**(2), 281–289.
69. Tohgi, H., Utsugisawa, K., Yoshimura, M., Nagane, Y., Ukitsu, M. (Aug 1999) Local variation in expression of pro- and antithrombotic factors in vascular endothelium of human autopsy brain. *Acta Neuropathol* **98**(2), 111–118.

70. Malek, A. M., Jackman, R., Rosenberg, R. D., Izumo, S. (May 1994) Endothelial expression of thrombomodulin is reversibly regulated by fluid shear stress. *Circ Res* **74**(5), 852–860.
71. Takada, Y., Shinkai, F., Kondo, S. *et al.* (Dec 15 1994) Fluid shear stress increases the expression of thrombomodulin by cultured human endothelial cells. *Biochem Biophys Res Commun* **205**(2), 1345–1352.
72. Gerszten, R. E., Chen, J., Ishii, M., *et al.* (Apr 14 1994) Specificity of the thrombin receptor for agonist peptide is defined by its extracellular surface. *Nature* **368**(6472), 648–651.
73. Vu, T. K., Hung, D. T., Wheaton, V. I., Coughlin, S. R. (Mar 22 1991) Molecular cloning of a functional thrombin receptor reveals a novel proteolytic mechanism of receptor activation. *Cell* **64**(6), 1057–1068.
74. Nguyen, K. T., Eskin, S. G., Patterson, C., Runge, M. S., McIntire, L. V. (Feb 2001) Shear stress reduces protease activated receptor-1 expression in human endothelial cells. *Ann Biomed Eng* **29**(2), 145–152.
75. Lucitti, J. L., Jones, E. A., Huang, C, Chen, J., Fraser, S. E., Dickinson, M. E. (Sep 2007) Vascular remodeling of the mouse yolk sac requires hemodynamic force. *Development* **134**(18), 3317–3326.
76. Zarins, C. K., Bomberger, R. A., Glagov, S. (Aug 1981) Local effects of stenoses: increased flow velocity inhibits atherogenesis. *Circulation* **64**(2 Pt 2), II221–227.
77. Langille, B. L. (1993) Remodeling of developing and mature arteries: endothelium, smooth muscle, and matrix. *J Cardiovasc Pharmacol* **21** Suppl 1, S11–17.
78. Kuo, C. T., Veselits, M. L., Barton, K. P., Lu, M. M., Clendenin, C., Leiden, J. M. (Nov 15 1997) The LKLF transcription factor is required for normal tunica media formation and blood vessel stabilization during murine embryogenesis. *Genes Dev* **11**(22), 2996–3006.
79. Wu, J., Bohanan, C. S., Neumann, J. C., Lingrel, J. B. (Feb 15 2008) KLF2 transcription factor modulates blood vessel maturation through smooth muscle cell migration. *J Biol Chem* **283**(7), 3942–3950.
80. Mack, P. J., Zhang, Y., Chung, S., Vickerman, V., Kamm, R. D., Garcia-Cardena, G. (Mar 27 2009) Biomechanical Regulation of Endothelium-dependent Events Critical for Adaptive Remodeling. *J Biol Chem* **284**(13), 8412–8420.
81. Carmeliet, P. (Dec 15 2005) Angiogenesis in life, disease and medicine. *Nature* **438**(7070), 932–936.
82. Meadows, S. M., Salanga, M. C., Krieg, P. A. (Apr 2009) Kruppel-like factor 2 cooperates with the ETS family protein ERG to activate Flk1 expression during vascular development. *Development* **136**(7), 1115–1125.
83. Fiedler, U., Augustin, H. G. (Dec 2006) Angiopoietins: a link between angiogenesis and inflammation. *Trends Immunol* **27**(12), 552–558.
84. Fiedler, U., Reiss, Y., Scharpfenecker, M., *et al.* (Feb 2006) Angiopoietin-2 sensitizes endothelial cells to TNF-alpha and has a crucial role in the induction of inflammation. *Nat Med* **12**(2), 235–239.

85. Kawanami, D., Mahabeleshwar, G. H., Lin, Z., *et al.* (Jun 1 2009) Kruppel-like factor 2 inhibits Hypoxia-Inducible-Factor-1alpha expression and function in the endothelium. *J Biol Chem.*
86. Chen, X. L., Varner, S. E., Rao, A. S., *et al.* (Jan 10 2003) Laminar flow induction of antioxidant response element-mediated genes in endothelial cells. A novel anti-inflammatory mechanism. *J Biol Chem* **278**(2), 703–711.
87. Fledderus, J. O., Boon, R. A., Volger, O. L., *et al.* (Jul 2008) KLF2 primes the antioxidant transcription factor Nrf2 for activation in endothelial cells. *Arterioscler Thromb Vasc Biol* **28**(7), 1339–1346.
88. Kinderlerer, A. R., Ali, F., Johns, M., *et al.* (May 23 2008) KLF2-dependent, shear stress-induced expression of CD59: a novel cytoprotective mechanism against complement-mediated injury in the vasculature. *J Biol Chem* **283**(21), 14636–14644.
89. Sen-Banerjee, S., Mir, S., Lin, Z., *et al.* (Jul 25 2005) Kruppel-Like Factor 2 as a Novel Mediator of Statin Effects in Endothelial Cells. *Circulation.*
90. Parmar, K. M., Nambudiri, V., Dai, G., Larman, H. B., Gimbrone, M. A., Jr., Garcia-Cardena, G. (May 4 2005) Statins exert endothelial atheroprotective effects via the KLF2 transcription factor. *J Biol Chem.*
91. Ali, F., Zakkar, M., Karu, K., *et al.* (May 19 2009) Induction of the cytoprotective enzyme heme oxygenase-1 by statins is enhanced in vascular endothelium exposed to laminar shear stress and impaired by disturbed flow. *J Biol Chem.*
92. Morita, T. (Sep 2005) Heme oxygenase and atherosclerosis. *Arterioscler Thromb Vasc Biol* **25**(9), 1786–1795.
93. Lee, T. S., Chang, C. C., Zhu, Y., Shyy, J. Y. (Sep 7 2004) Simvastatin induces heme oxygenase-1: a novel mechanism of vessel protection. *Circulation* **110**(10), 1296–1302.
94. Shields, J. M., Christy, R. J., Yang, V. W. (1996) Identification and characterization of a gene encoding a gut-enriched Kruppel-like factor expressed during growth arrest. *Journal of Biological Chemistry* **271**(33), 20009–20017.
95. Katz, J. P., Perreault, N., Goldstein, B. G., *et al.* (Apr 2005) Loss of Klf4 in mice causes altered proliferation and differentiation and precancerous changes in the adult stomach. *Gastroenterology* **128**(4), 935–945.
96. Swamynathan, S. K., Davis, J., Piatigorsky, J. (Aug 2008) Identification of candidate Klf4 target genes reveals the molecular basis of the diverse regulatory roles of Klf4 in the mouse cornea. *Invest Ophthalmol Vis Sci* **49**(8), 3360–3370.
97. Swamynathan, S. K., Katz, J. P., Kaestner, K. H., Ashery-Padan, R., Crawford, M. A., Piatigorsky, J. (Jan 2007) Conditional deletion of the mouse Klf4 gene results in corneal epithelial fragility, stromal edema, and loss of conjunctival goblet cells. *Mol Cell Biol* **27**(1), 182–194.
98. Segre, J. A., Bauer, C., Fuchs, E. (Aug 1999) Klf4 is a transcription factor required for establishing the barrier function of the skin. *Nat Genet* **22**(4), 356–360.

99. Hamik, A., Lin, Z., Kumar, A., *et al.* (May 4 2007) Kruppel-like factor 4 regulates endothelial inflammation. *J Biol Chem* **282**(18), 13769–13779.
100. Yoshida, T., Gan, Q., Owens, G. K. (Nov 2008) Kruppel-like factor 4, Elk-1, and histone deacetylases cooperatively suppress smooth muscle cell differentiation markers in response to oxidized phospholipids. *Am J Physiol Cell Physiol* **295**(5), C1175–1182.
101. Yoshida, T., Kaestner, K. H., Owens, G. K. (Jun 20 2008) Conditional deletion of Kruppel-like factor 4 delays downregulation of smooth muscle cell differentiation markers but accelerates neointimal formation following vascular injury. *Circ Res* **102**(12), 1548–1557.
102. Liu, Y., Sinha, S., McDonald, O. G., Shang, Y., Hoofnagle, M. H., Owens, G. K. (Mar 11 2005) Kruppel-like factor 4 abrogates myocardin-induced activation of smooth muscle gene expression. *J Biol Chem* **280**(10), 9719–9727.
103. Adam, P. J., Regan, C. P., Hautmann, M. B., Owens, G. K. (2000) Positive- and negative-acting Kruppel-like transcription factors bind a transforming growth factor beta control element required for expression of the smooth muscle cell differentiation marker SM22alpha *in vivo*. *Journal of Biological Chemistry* **275**(48), 37798–37806.
104. Feinberg, M. W., Cao, Z., Wara, A. K., Lebedeva, M. A., Senbanerjee, S., Jain, M. K. (Nov 18 2005) Kruppel-like factor 4 is a mediator of proinflammatory signaling in macrophages. *J Biol Chem* **280**(46), 38247–38258.
105. Feinberg, M. W., Wara, A. K., Cao, Z., *et al.* (Sep 19 2007) The Kruppel-like factor KLF4 is a critical regulator of monocyte differentiation. *Embo J* **26**(18), 4138–4148.
106. Zhang, G., Zhu, H., Wang, Y., *et al.* (May-Jun 2009) Kruppel-like factor 4 represses transcription of the survivin gene in esophageal cancer cell lines. *Biol Chem* **390**(5–6), 463–469.
107. Zhang, W., Chen, X., Kato, Y., *et al.* (Mar 2006) Novel cross talk of Kruppel-like factor 4 and beta-catenin regulates normal intestinal homeostasis and tumor repression. *Mol Cell Biol* **26**(6), 2055–2064.
108. Ghaleb, A. M., McConnell, B. B., Nandan, M. O., Katz, J. P., Kaestner, K. H., Yang, V. W. (Aug 1 2007) Haploinsufficiency of Kruppel-like factor 4 promotes adenomatous polyposis coli dependent intestinal tumorigenesis. *Cancer Res* **67**(15), 7147–7154.
109. Takahashi, K., Yamanaka, S. (Aug 25 2006) Induction of pluripotent stem cells from mouse embryonic and adult fibroblast cultures by defined factors. *Cell* **126**(4), 663–676.
110. Okita, K., Ichisaka, T., Yamanaka, S. (Jul 19 2007) Generation of germline-competent induced pluripotent stem cells. *Nature* **448**(7151), 313–317.
111. Maherali, N., Sridharan, R., Xie, W., *et al.* (Jun 7 2007) Directly reprogrammed fibroblasts show global epigenetic remodeling and widespread tissue contribution. *Cell Stem Cell* **1**(1), 55–70.

112. Wernig, M., Meissner, A., Foreman, R., *et al.* (Jul 19 2007) *In vitro* reprogramming of fibroblasts into a pluripotent ES-cell-like state. *Nature* **448**(7151), 318–324.
113. Yet, S. F., McA'Nulty, M. M., Folta, S. C., *et al.* (Jan 9 1998) Human EZF, a Kruppel-like zinc finger protein, is expressed in vascular endothelial cells and contains transcriptional activation and repression domains. *J Biol Chem* **273**(2), 1026–1031.
114. McCormick, S. M., Eskin, S. G., McIntire, L. V., *et al.* (Jul 31 2001) DNA microarray reveals changes in gene expression of shear stressed human umbilical vein endothelial cells. *Proc Natl Acad Sci U S A* **98**(16), 8955–8960.
115. Li, Y. S., Haga, J. H., Chien, S. (Oct 2005) Molecular basis of the effects of shear stress on vascular endothelial cells. *J Biomech* **38**(10), 1949–1971.

Chapter 5

RHO FAMILY SMALL GTPASES IN SHEAR STRESS SIGNALING

DANIEL T. SWEET and ELLIE TZIMA
Department of Cell and Molecular Physiology,
University of North Carolina at Chapel Hill
eleni_tzima@med.unc.edu

Fluid shear stress is a major determinant of endothelial cell shape, function, and gene transcription. Shear stress activates several signaling cascades in endothelial cells including the following: opening of K^+ and CA^{+2} channels,[1–3] activation of heterotrimeric G proteins,[4] production of Nitric Oxide,[5] tyrosine phosphorylation of proteins such as Shc, c-src, and focal adhesion kinase (FAK),[6,7] activation of MAP kinase pathway, protein kinase C (PKC) and jun C-terminal kinase (JNK),[8–10] release of reactive oxygen species (ROS),[11] and activation of important transcription factors such as c-fos, c-jun, c-myc and NF-kB.[12] The hallmark of the endothelial cell responses to fluid shear stress is the rearrangement of cytoskeleton and the elongation of microfilaments and microtubules in the direction of flow.[13–15] Shear stress can also modulate endothelial monolayer permeability of macromolecules[16] and leukocytes from the blood into the underlying tissue, which is an early characteristic of atherosclerotic lesion development.[17]

A remarkable number of events stimulated by shear are downstream of small GTPases, and in particular Rho family GTPases. There are at least 150 small GTPases encoded by the human genome. The various subclasses of this superfamily, including Ras, Rho, Arf, Rab and Ran GTPases, have been implicated in almost all aspects on cell biology including proliferation, differentiation, cytoskeletal organization, vesicle trafficking, nucleocytoplasmic transport and gene expression.[18,19] All of the small GTPases function as binary 'molecular switches' that are active when bound to GTP and inactive when bound to GDP. The regulation of these states is tightly controlled by Guanine nucleotide Exchange Factors (GEFs) which activate the protein by exchanging a GDP for a GTP, and GTPase Activating Proteins (GAPs) which catalyze the hydrolysis of GTP to GDP to inactivate the protein.

The Rho family of small GTPases has been found to be critical in endothelial signaling pathways activated by shear stress, and the Rho subclass of GTPases will be the focus in this chapter. Three GTPases; namely, RhoA, Rac1 and Cdc42, are known to be crucial in regulating cell shape changes through the rearrangements of the cytoskeleton,[20] but they also have roles in endothelial adhesion, permeability and gene expression which are equally significant. This chapter will describe the well known roles for Rho family small GTPases in morphological and cytoskeletal rearrangements, and then discuss what is known about their roles in permeability and gene transcription in response to shear stress.

1. Cytoskeletal Rearrangement in Response to Shear Stress

Shear stress induces tightly controlled regulation of RhoA, Rac1 and Cdc42, which activate signaling cascades to initiate rearrangements of the cytoskeleton and cell polarity. Because each of the three GTPases controls a distinct aspect of cytoskeletal rearrangement, this section will be divided into three sections for the individual GTPase.

1.1. *Role of RhoA in Shear-Induced Cytoskeletal Alignment*

Rho GTPase regulates the assembly of actin stress fibers and focal adhesions in response to growth factors.[21] Fluid shear stress induces the rearrangement of both of these cytoskeletal structures and their alignment in the direction of flow. Not surprisingly, Rho is instrumental in stress fiber and focal adhesion reorganization in endothelial cells in response to shear stress. Fluid shear stress induces Rho translocation to the cell membrane for its activation.[22] Expression of dominant negative mutants of Rho, and its downstream effector Rho-kinase/ROCK, inhibited shear-induced stress fiber formation and cell alignment in bovine aortic endothelial cells (BAECs), supporting the importance of Rho in shear-induced endothelial signaling.[22]

Shear stress induces a transient inactivation of Rho at 5–15 minutes after onset of shear, followed by Rho activation that peaks at 60 minutes.[23] This pattern of Rho regulation is similar to what is seen when suspended endothelial cells adhere to extracellular matrix (ECM) proteins.[24] Corresponding staining of actin microfilaments in cells subjected to shear revealed an early breakdown in stress fibers, overlapping with low Rho activity at 5 minutes. At 60 minutes, when Rho activity is high, there is an increase in stress fibers and cellular alignment in the direction of flow, although maximal alignment requires longer exposure to laminar flow.[15] At longer flow times of about 2 hours, Rho activity decreases again while stress fibers and alignment remain. This could indicate that Rho activity is required for assembly of new stress fibers, while maintenance of existing stress fibers requires low Rho activity and/or other proteins.

Tight regulation of Rho is important for proper stress fiber formation and alignment in the direction of flow. The cell needs to be able to break down existing, randomly oriented stress fibers before it can re-assemble new ones in the proper orientation. Constitutively active mutants of RhoA inhibit shear stress-induced alignment of endothelial cells, indicating the importance of the initial Rho deactivation in facilitating alignment.[23] A second study of shear-induced directionality and polarization in subconfluent cells showed that Rho is required for initial polarization and retraction, and later elongation in the flow direction, but had no affect on migration rate.[25]

1.2. *Role of Rac1 in Shear-Induced Cytoskeletal Alignment*

Rac is required for actin polymerization and formation of membrane ruffles/lamellipodia in cells treated with growth factors.[26] Lamellipodia formation in the direction of flow is an early morphological response to shear stress, and it was discovered that Rac is required for endothelial cell alignment and migration in the direction of flow.[27–29] Biochemical pulldown assays and immunofluorescence studies have shown that Rac is transiently activated by shear stress. The maximal activation of Rac is within 30 minutes in response to the onset of flow, a timepoint where actin stress fibers are re-assembling in the direction of flow.[30] Similar to Rho regulation, Rac activity decreases to baseline at longer time points of shear and Rac activity may not be important in maintaining alignment. Interestingly, Rac activation has been shown to be polarized, which is thought to facilitate polarization of the cytoskeleton and alignment in the direction of flow. Importantly, Fluorescence Activation Indicator for Rho proteins (FLAIR) technique[31] has been used in cells subjected to flow to show that the Fluorescence Resonance Energy Transfer (FRET) signal is localized preferentially to the downstream edges of cells relative to the direction of flow.[30] Interestingly, expression of the Rac GEF Vav activates Rac1, but the FRET signal is not polarized, indicating that directionality of the force stimulus is important.

Akin to Rho, regulation of Rac is required for alignment in the direction of flow. Endothelial cells expressing dominant negative Rac (N17Rac) show the characteristic initial decrease in F-actin, followed by assembly of new stress fibers. However, these stress fibers are randomly oriented, even after a prolonged exposure to shear.[30,32] Similarly, cells expressing dominant active Rac (V12Rac) have high levels of active Rac-GTP; however, this active Rac is not polarized to the downstream edge and the cells are unable to align in the direction of flow.

In a separate but similar study, Rac was activated within 5–30 minutes in response to shear stress and precise regulation of Rac was required for cell re-spreading and alignment in the direction of flow using both dominant negative and dominant active mutant expression.[25] Surprisingly, PI3K, which acts upstream of Rac activation in response to growth factors,[33] is not required for cell alignment or stress fiber formation in response to shear stress.[25] Rac was also shown to be important in shear-induced orientation of cell migration and migration speed.

1.3. *Role of Cdc42 in Shear-Induced Cytoskeletal Alignment*

Cdc42 was first found in non-endothelial cells to promote formation of actin-rich finger-like membrane extensions called filopodia.[34,35] Cdc42 also controls cellular polarity during establishment of cellular asymmetry, morphogenesis and migration.[36]

Shear stress induces Cdc42 translocation to the membrane and activation of transcription factor AP-1.[22] Cdc42 activation is maximal between 5–60 minutes after onset of flow, and then returns to baseline by 60–120 minutes.[25,37] A FRET assay used to visualize Cdc42 activation in live cells showed that Cdc42 activation is polarized to the downstream edge of sheared cells, similar to Rac activation. Importantly, while Rho and Rac control shear induced polarity and alignment primarily through actin microfilaments, Cdc42 is important in regulating the flow-induced polarization of the two other cytoskeletal structures; namely, microtubules and intermediate filaments.

1.3.1. *Cdc42 Effects on the Microtubule Cytoskeleton*

Expression of dominant negative Cdc42 (N17Cdc42) in endothelial cells does not inhibit shear stress-induced alignment or stress fiber formation.[22,25] However, Cdc42 has an important role in regulating the microtubule cytoskeleton and in particular, polarization of the microtubule organizing center (MTOC) in migrating astrocytes[38] and fibroblasts,[39] and in endothelial cells exposed to shear stress.[37] Importantly, correctly polarized activation of Cdc42 is essential for localization of the MTOC on the downstream side of the nucleus in confluent sheared cells.[40] The role of Cdc42 in migrating cells under flow is unclear, as one report states that MTOC polarization is mediated by Cdc42 in 3T3 fibroblasts under flow[40] while another report using human umbilical vein endothelial cells (HUVECs) showed that dominant negative Cdc42 did not affect directionality of endothelial cell migration under flow.[25]

1.3.2. *Cdc42 Effects on Intermediate Filaments*

The importance of the intermediate filament (IF) cytoskeleton in response to flow is less well understood, but two IF proteins, in particular, vimentin and keratin have been studied recently. Activation of Rho family GTPases induces collapse of the vimentin IF network in fibroblasts.[41,42] Also, Cdc42 induces vimentin reorganization through p21 Activated Kinase (PAK)[43] and p70 S6K.[44] A series of spatial analyses of vimentin reorganization in response to flow in living endothelial cells revealed rapid regional IF displacement in response to flow.[45–47] These experiments suggested an integrated mechanism of mechanotransduction by the cytoskeleton in which spatial organization of multiple structural networks regulates cellular response to changes in shear stress. *In vivo*, vimentin knockout mice[48] exhibited attenuated flow induced vasodilation compared to controls,[49] as well as an altered balance of endothelin-1 and nitric oxide.[50] Further experiments in these vimentin knockout mice revealed a role for vimentin in arterial remodeling in response to alteration in flow,[51] and in regulating focal contact size and endothelial cell adhesion to EC.[52]

Another IF protein that has been shown to be responsive to shear stress is keratin. Shear stress induced disassembly of keratin IFs in lung epithelial cells through protein kinase C delta-mediated phosphorylation of keratin 8.[53] Also, protein kinase C zeta mediates the shear induced structural reorganization of the keratin IF network.[54] While quite a bit is being elucidated about the response of the IF cytoskeleton to shear stress, the role of Rho GTPases in reorganization of IFs, while likely, is currently not well understood.

2. The Role of Rho GTPases in Endothelial Permeability and Intercellular Adhesion

2.1. *Permeability*

Shear stress-induced small GTPase activation, which leads to cytoskeletal remodeling, has been shown to enhance the barrier protective function of the endothelium, as reflected by increased transendothelial resistance in response to shear stress.[55,56] Changes in endothelial wall permeability are associated with cytoskeletal remodeling in response to growth factors, cytokines and shear stress.[57,58] Because intercellular adhesion and permeability depend heavily on the cytoskeleton and actomyosin-based cell contractility, Rho and Rac have emerged as regulators of barrier function. Rho has been shown to increase actomyosin contractility, which facilitates breakdown of intercellular junctions and increases permeability. Conversely, Rac stabilizes endothelial junctions and antagonizes Rho to decrease permeability.[25] Furthermore, both Rho and Rac have been shown to regulate permeability independent of the effects on contractility. For instance, angiopoitin-1 promotes activation of the Rho effector mDia through Rho, resulting in stabilization of intercellular contacts and decrease in permeability in response to VEGF.[59] In addition, Rac activation has been shown to promote PAK-dependent phosphorylation of VE-cadherin, which leads to its internalization and disassembly of intercellular junctions.[60]

Shear stress was found to mediate barrier enhancement in human pulmonary endothelial cells through the activation of Rac.[58] However, activated Rac also has been shown to promote cell scattering, which involves the breakdown of cell-cell junctions. While these two opposing effects of Rac on endothelial permeability seem incompatible, it is better understood when considering the downstream effectors that are activated by Rac, which carry out signaling cascades to either strengthen endothelial junctions or break them down and scatter. Indeed, two effectors with opposing roles in regulating permeability are known to be activated downstream of Rac. IQGAP, an actin binding protein, has been implicated in stabilizing adherens junctions downstream of Rac and Cdc42.[61] Also, IQGAP has been shown to strengthen adherens junctions by Rac-mediated release of β-catenin from IQGAP and association of β-catenin with E-cadherin.[62] Alternatively, PAK can be activated through Rac and lead to increased endothelial permeability.[63] Thus, cellular conditions and co-factors that favor Rac interaction with PAK would cause junctional stabilization while conditions that favor IQGAP would lead to junctional stabilization. Future studies should investigate the conditions and mechanisms whereby Rac activates certain effectors while keeping others inactive.

2.2. *Intercellular Adhesion/Leukocyte Transmigration*

Small GTPases Rho and Rac are critical in regulation of the contractile apparatus which controls permeability, paracellular pore formation and leukocyte transendothelial migration (reviewed in Refs. 64, 65). Leukocyte transendothelial migration is an involved and quite remarkable process that has many steps and players, the details of which go beyond the scope of this chapter. In short, adhesion molecules must be expressed on the surface of both the endothelium and the leukocyte. Once a leukocyte has bound to the endothelium, endothelial cell-cell junctions must open to allow space for the leukocyte to pass through. Rho and Rac are involved in both of these processes. Many agents that promote inflammation and leukocyte transendothelial migration have been shown to activate Rho in endothelial cells, thereby stimulating endothelial cell contraction and junctional opening.[64] When RhoA is inhibited, monocyte adhesion and spreading on the endothelium are decreased, indicating that Rho is important in these processes. How exactly Rho becomes activated during adhesion of leukocytes to the endothelium is unclear, but it may involve Thy-1 (CD90). Thy-1, expressed on endothelial cells, binds Mac-1 on leukocytes, and blocking this interaction prevents leukocyte adhesion and transmigration.[66] Interestingly, Thy-1 can activate Rho by decreasing activity of p190RhoGAP[67] or through integrin β3 clustering.[68] Also, engagement of the leukocyte binding receptor, intercellular adhesion molecule (ICAM)-1, activates Rho and may help open intercellular gaps during leukocyte extravasation.[69–71]

3. Rho-, Rac- and Cdc42-Dependent Signaling Pathways Activated by Flow

Although for the most part, signaling pathways have not been thoroughly mapped out, we will attempt to shed some light into the proteins involved in regulating the Rho family GTPases upstream, as well as downstream signaling activated by the Rho family proteins.

3.1. *Upstream Signaling Pathways for GTPase Regulation*

3.1.1. *Players Upstream of Rho Activity Regulation*

The pathway upstream of Rho inactivation in response to shear stress involves conformational activation of integrins and their increased binding to ECM.[23] Similarly, new interactions between integrins and ECM are required for integrin association with Shc and JNK, a hallmark of activation of signaling from integrins.[72] These observations therefore suggest that integrin-ECM adhesion is clearly important for regulation of signaling events upstream of Rho.

The molecular signaling events responsible for the initial Rho inactivation and then re-activation downstream of shear stress and integrins are currently unknown. However, we can look at the more widely studied process of cell adhesion to ECM for clues, because the pattern of Rho regulation is the same during adhesion and shear stress, and both require integrins. Fibroblasts from FAK-null mice failed to transiently inhibit Rho activity when plated on fibronectin. This defect was rescued when FAK was re-expressed, indicating a role for FAK in Rho downregulation.[73] Another report focused on the role of integrin signaling through c-Src to decrease Rho activity by tyrosine phosphorylation of p190RhoGAP.[74] The same investigators also showed that a protein tyrosine phosphatase called Shp-2 acts upstream of RhoA.[75] Paxillin phosphorylation has also been shown to be important in Rho de-activation. The mutation of two tyrosine residues in paxillin, Y31 and Y118, abolished normal Rho inhibition and these cells showed premature formation of stress fibers.[76] The phosphorylation of these two tyrosines, which is induced by integrin mediated adhesion to ECM, creates a binding site for p120RasGAP, which displaces it from its previous binding partner, p190RhoGAP. This report stated that p190RhoGAP, when freed from p120RasGAP, was able to catalyze the hydrolysis of Rho-GTP into inactive Rho-GDP. Finally, vascular endothelial (VE-) cadherin, a major component of endothelial adherens junctions, has been shown to signal through RhoA and the actin cytoskeleton to cross talk with sites of cell-ECM adhesion.[77] Currently, little is known about signaling that triggers the re-activation of Rho, an important step in stress fiber formation and alignment. One recent report showed that Rho re-activation after adhesion to fibronectin required two Rho GEFs: Lsc/p115 RhoGEF and LARG, but not other exchange factors such as Ect2 and Dbl. Knockdown of both of these GEFs decreased RhoA activation and formation of stress fibers in response to adhesion.[78] While this paper has shed some light on the subject, the re-activation of Rho and the players involved in shear stress induced Rho de-activation and re-activation should greatly enhance our understanding of cytoskeletal reorganization.

Another important protein in Rho regulation is Rho-GDP dissociation inhibitor (Rho-GDI). Rho-GDI blocks Rho and Rac activation by preventing nucleotide exchange, so the proteins are locked in the inactive state (see Ref. 79 for review). Rho-GDI has been found to be shear stress responsive, and in *ex vivo* rat aortas exposed to laminar shear stress, Rho-GDI expression was decreased.[80]

3.1.2. *Upstream Players in Rac Activation*

Akin to Rho, Rac activation by shear stress has been shown to be downstream of integrin activation and ligand binding.[30] The signaling mediators between integrins and Rac activation are unknown, but the proteins involved in adhesion-induced Rac activation are likely to be important. Integrin mediated adhesion to ECM activates Rac[81] and this requires intact β integrins.[82,83] FAK, localized to integrins and focal adhesions, associates with p130cas and paxillin, both of which been found to be important for Rac activation. Tyrosine phosphorylation of p130cas promotes the formation of a complex between Crk, ELMO and DOCK180,[84,85] which is a Rac guanine nucleotide exchange factor (GEF).[86] Another complex of PKL (GIT) and Pak-interacting exchange factor (PIX), another Rac GEF, has been found to associate with paxillin.[87] Furthermore, integrin mediated activation of Rac also involves targeting of the activated, GTP-bound form of Rac to sites of adhesion, allowing it to interact with effectors.[88] While this pathway seems fairly well worked out, it remains to be seen if the same proteins play a role in activating Rac in response to shear stress. Recently, it was shown that shear-induced PKA-dependent alpha4 integrin phosphorylation at the downstream edge of endothelial cells promotes localized Rac1 activation, which in turn directs cytoskeletal alignment in response to shear stress.[89]

3.1.3. *Upstream Players in Cdc42 Activation*

Similar to its family members Rho and Rac, new ligand binding by integrins is also required for shear-induced Cdc42 activation.[37] The signaling proteins going from integrins and leading to Cdc42 activation/deactivation are unknown, and future work needs to be done to shed some light on the subject.

3.2. *Downstream Signaling Activated by Rho GTPases*

Signaling downstream from Rho GTPases is very complex (for a detailed review, see Ref. 90); this section will briefly review what is currently known (mostly in response to growth factors or adhesion), and then focus on gene expression changes mediated by Rho GTPases in response to shear stress.

3.2.1. *Rho Effectors and Gene Expression*

The signaling pathways downstream of activated Rho have been mostly studied in response to adhesion or growth factors, but it is likely that these pathways are also activated by shear stress. There are two main effector proteins acting directly downstream of Rho; namely, Rho kinase (ROCK) and mammalian homolog of diaphanous (mDia). ROCK activates myosin contractility by increasing phosphorylation of myosin light chain (MLC)[91,92] and by inhibiting the MLC phosphatase.[93] ROCK can also induce stress fibers through activation of LIM kinase which phosphorylates and deactivates cofilin, an actin de-polymerizing protein. Recently, a study using a new technique called ballistic intracellular nanorheology revealed that ROCK mediates a dramatic flow-induced increase in cytoplasmic viscosity.[94] mDia is a Rho effector that is also instrumental in stress fiber formation. mDia can bind Rho and polymerize actin,[95] and expression of activated mDia induces stress fiber formation.[96,97] Interestingly, mechanical force applied to single cells could stimulate stress fiber and focal adhesion formation. This study found that stress fiber formation was abolished when Rho was inhibited, but was rescued by expression of active mDia. Interestingly, myosin and ROCK are not required for stress fiber formation in response to mechanical stimulation.[98]

Rho also regulates other signal transduction pathways in addition to those linked to the actin cytoskeleton. For example, Rho mediates shear-induced activation of the transcription factor AP-1 through JNK kinase.[22] Also, Rho mediates activation of another transcription factor, *c-fos*, in response to shear stress.[99] *c-fos,* when complexed with *c-jun,* makes up the AP-1 transcription factor, which controls expression of many shear-inducible genes.[100,101] The Rho-mediated shear –induction of *c-fos* is dependant on intracellular calcium, but not on the Rho effector p160ROCK or actin filaments. In this study, the inhibition of p160ROCK and the actin cytoskeleton decreased the basal activity of *c-fos* in static cells, but did not affect the shear induced *c-fos* activation. The calcium chelator BAPTA-AM inhibits shear induction of *c-fos* activity.[99] Rho can also modulate the activity of sterol regulatory element binding proteins (SREBPs) in endothelial cells.[101] SREBPs are key regulators of cellular sterol and lipid homeostasis.[102] Shear stress activates the Rho-ROCK-LIMK-cofilin pathway which enhances the cytoskeleton and facilitates the transport of SREBPs into the nucleus where they can activate gene transcription. Disturbed shear stress also upregulates expression of connective tissue growth factor in a RhoA-dependent manner.[103]

3.2.2. *Rac Effectors and Gene Expression*

Signaling from active Rac is mediated by at least two important effectors: Arp2/3 and PAK. Arp2/3 is an actin related protein that has the ability to nucleate actin polymerization. Rac can activate Arp2/3 through activation of the WAVE/Scar protein that belongs to the WASP family.[104,105] The other main Rac effector involved in cytoskeletal rearrangement is PAK. The observations about how PAK regulates lamellipodia and actin is complex and in many cases, cell type specific (see Ref. 106 for review). PAK expression has been shown to promote formation of lamellipodia.[107] Active Rac can bind to PAK, a kinase that then signals to the actin cytoskeleton through the actin binding protein filamin, or through LIM kinase and cofilin.

The major non-cytoskeletal role of Rac in endothelial cells stimulated by flow is activation of the transcription factor nuclear factor kappa-light-chain-enhancer of activated B cells (NF-κB). NF-κB is a heterodimer complex of subunits from the Rel/NF-κB family, with the p50/p65 dimer being the predominant form. In unstimulated cells, NF-κB dimers are sequestered in the cytoplasm by binding to IκB inhibitor proteins. Upon activation by a wide array of stimuli, IκB is phosphorylated and degraded, exposing a nuclear localization sequence and freeing NF-κB to translocate to the nucleus, where it binds DNA and activates transcription of several genes.[108] Activated NF-κB was identified in endothelial cells, smooth muscle cells and macrophages in human atherosclerotic tissue samples,[109] as well as in humans with unstable angina pectoris,[110] suggesting a pathophysiological role for NF-κB in atherosclerosis.[111] Rac1 activation leads to production of reactive oxygen species (ROS) in response to shear stress.[112] Rac has been shown to mediate a cytokine-stimulated, redox dependent pathway necessary for NF-κB activation.[113] Also, Rac, Rho and Cdc42 induce transcriptional activity of NF-κB by phosphorylation of IκB,[114] and Rac activation has been shown to induce NF-κB DNA binding and transcriptional activity, and enhance NF-κB-dependant expression of cyclin D1.[115] Toll-like receptor 2-mediated NF-κB activation and integrin signaling to NF-κB are both mediated by Rac.[116,117]

NF-κB is activated by shear stress[118–120] and an NF-κB consensus sequence was identified as the shear stress response element (SSRE) within the PDGF gene that allowed PDGF expression by flow.[12,121] Cells transfected with dominant negative N17Rac failed to induce NF-κB translocation to the nucleus and showed minimal transcriptional activation of an NF-κB promoter in response to shear stress.[30] Rac1-dependent NF-κB activation is required for flow-induced cell surface expression of Intercellular Cell Adhesion molecule (ICAM)-1, a protein involved in the recruitment of leukocytes to the endothelium in atherosclerotic plaques.[122,123] Recent work has highlighted the role of the subendothelial ECM in modulating NF-κB activation by flow. Endothelial cells growing on fibronectin or fibrinogen can activate NF-κB in response to flow, whereas cells on collagen or laminin cannot.[124] Interestingly, fibronectin deposition is associated with atherosclerotic plaques, so it is possible that NF-κB is only activated at plaques and not in a normal healthy vessel. Furthermore, PAK, a downstream effector of Rac, displays the same flow induced activation on fibronectin but not collagen[125] and was later shown to mediate NF-κB activation by flow.[126] Future work aimed at determining how the ECM differentially regulates NF-κB activation by flow will be interesting in understanding Rac signaling and the development of atherosclerosis.

3.2.3. *Cdc42 Effectors and Gene Expression*

Cdc42 induces changes in the cytoskeleton through three main downstream effectors. Cdc42 can directly bind WASP and N-WASP,[127,128] inducing a conformational change that allows stimulation of Arp2/3 to nucleate actin polymerization.[129] In addition, Cdc42 is capable of activating MLC through MRCK,[130] leading to myosin contractility in a mechanism similar to Rho. Finally, Cdc42 is a potent activator of PAK,[131] which activates LIMK-cofilin and filamin to activate actin polymerization. Cdc42 also has major roles in microtubule and MTOC polarity. Par6-protein kinase C ζ (PKC) complex is the Cdc42 effector that controls cell polarity.[38–40] PAR proteins were identified as key regulators of cell polarity in C. elegans development.[132] Under flow, the activity of Par6 and PKC directs the reorganization of the MTOC[37] as well as directional migration of endothelial cells.[133]

The effects of Cdc42 in regulating gene transcription in response to shear stress are still under investigation. Like Rho, Cdc42 regulates the transcriptional activation of the serum response element (SRE) in the c-fos promoter through serum response factor.[134] Cdc42 is also required and sufficient in the shear stress-induced activation of JNK that leads to increased AP-1/TRE activity. Through this transcription factor, Cdc42 controls expression of several shear stress-inducible genes.[22]

4. Rho GTPases in Development and *in vivo*

This section will give a brief overview of the function of Rho GTPases in cardiovascular development, focusing on the three main GTPases that have been discussed in this chapter.

4.1. *RhoA*

Surprisingly, a RhoA knockout mouse has not been reported, although highly homologous isoforms RhoB and RhoC have been knocked out and yield viable, fertile and developmentally normal mice.[135,136] Two RhoA effectors, ROCK and mDia have been knocked out in the mouse, and both lines of mice are viable and anatomically normal. The viability of the homozygous ROCK knockout mouse is dependent on the strain of the mouse genetic background. The first ROCK knockout mouse was made in the C57BL/6N background and were born at expected Mendelian ratios, but most died shortly after birth. The mice exhibited defects in eyelid closure and closure of the ventral body wall due to disorganization of actin fibers.[137] Next, heterozygous ROCK knockout mice were generated, which were haploinsufficient, fully viable and developmentally normal. Basal blood pressure, heart rate, and cardiac dimension and function in ROCK1$^{+/-}$ mice were similar to those in wild-type (WT) littermates. Infusion of angiotensin II or treatment with NG-nitro-L-arginine methyl ester caused similar increases in systolic blood pressure, left ventricular wall thickness, left ventricular mass, ratio of heart weight to tibia length, and cardiomyocyte size in ROCK1$^{+/-}$ mice and WT littermates. In contrast, perivascular fibrosis in hearts was increased to a lesser extent in ROCK1$^{+/-}$ mice compared with WT littermates. This was associated with decreased expression of transforming growth factor-beta, connective tissue growth factor, and type III collagen. In addition, perivascular fibrosis induced by transaortic constriction or myocardial infarction was decreased in ROCK1$^{+/-}$ mice compared with WT littermates.[138] These results indicate that ROCK is critical in development of cardiac fibrosis, but not hypertrophy. In a separate study, these researchers performed carotid artery ligation on adult males and found reduced neointima formation in ROCK1$^{+/-}$ mice compared with that of WT mice. This correlated with decreased vascular smooth muscle cell proliferation and survival, decreased levels proinflammatory adhesion molecule expression, and reduced leukocyte infiltration.[139] These data indicate that ROCK plays an important role in vascular remodeling. A ROCK1 knockout mouse was recently made in the FVB background, and the homozygous null animals were viable and developmentally normal. However, these mice exhibited systemic insulin resistance by impaired insulin signaling compared to WT littermates, indicating an unexpected role for ROCK in glucose homeostasis.[140] A role for ROCK in atherosclerosis was reported when bone marrow from ROCK1$^{-/-}$ null mice was transplanted into atherosclerosis prone LDLR null mice. Compared to LDLR$^{-/-}$ mice, lipid accumulation and atherosclerotic lesions were reduced in LDLR$^{-/-}$ mice whose bone marrow had been replaced with bone marrow derived from ROCK1$^{-/-}$ mice[141] Also, in ApoE null mice, another hypercholesterolemic mouse model of atherosclerosis, blockade of ROCK by fasudil significantly reduced atherosclerotic lesion size compared to controls.[142] This indicates that RhoA signaling through ROCK may be important in endothelial transmigration and development of atherosclerotic lesions. Additionally, the RhoA pathway is also required for vessel remodeling during arteriogenesis, as the ROCK inhibitor fasudil inhibited arteriogenesis in response to femoral artery occlusion.[143] Another Rho effector, mDia1, has recently been knocked out, and the resulting mice were developmentally normal, but developed myeloproliferative defects later in life.[144] No cardiovascular defect was reported.

4.2. *Rac1*

Rac1 knockout mice are embryonic lethal, and the mice die so early that the three germ layers do not form during gastrulation.[145] Thus, many tissue-specific conditional knockout mice have been made to study the role of Rac function in a given tissue. Rac1 has been knocked out specifically in myeloid cells,[146] B-cells,[147] hematopoietic cells,[148] epidermal cells,[149,150] cardiomyocytes,[151] Schwann cells,[152] forebrain,[153] and endothelial cells.[154] All of these tissue-specific knockout mice were viable except for the forebrain knockout, which was lethal after E18.5, just before birth, and the endothelial cell specific knockout which died at E9.5, indicating the Rac is most important in endothelial cells during development. This endothelial-specific Rac1 knockout exhibited defective development of major vessels and complete lack of small branched vessels in embryos and their yolk sacs. These findings provide direct evidence that the activity of Rac1 in endothelial cells is essential for vascular development.[154] Confirming *in vitro* data, Rac1 null endothelial cellss were defective in lamellipodia formation.[154] Similarly, lamellipodia formation is inhibited in WAVE-null mouse embryonic fibroblasts (MEFs), indicating that WAVE is an important Rac effector *in vivo* as well as *in vitro*.[155] Rac1 null MEFs also have reduced spreading and increased apoptosis.[156]

Vav2, a GEF for Rac and Rho, has been knocked out in mice, and these mice are viable and have tachycardia, hypertension and heart defects.[157] Similarly, in a transgenic mouse that expresses constitutively active Rac in vascular smooth muscle cells, the vessels had excessive amounts of superoxide and reduced nitric oxide (NO) levels, causing moderate hypertension.[158] An endothelial cell-specific heterozygous knockout of Rac (Rac1 +/−) was viable, and had a defect in expression and activity of endothelial nitric oxide synthase and mild hypertension.[159] While these results are confusing because both upregulation and downregulation of Rac caused reduced NO, these studies indicate that tight Rac regulation is important in cardiovascular disease and vessel homeostasis.

4.3. *Cdc42*

Cdc42 global knockout mice are early embryonic lethal at day E7.5. The embryonic stem cells of these mice had aberrant actin cytoskeletal organization and reduced filopodia even though proliferation rate and MAP Kinase activation was normal.[160] While many conditional knockout mice have been generated to study Cdc42 *in vivo*, no vascular or heart tissue-specific Cdc42 null mouse has been made to date. Cdc42 null MEFs completely lack filopodia while MEFs from Cdc42GAP-null mice, with increased Cdc42 activity, have high levels of spontaneous filopodia.[161] This confirms *in vitro* data that Cdc42 is required for formation of filopodia. Cdc42-null MEFs and hematopoietic stem cells support a role for Cdc42 in chemotaxis.[161,162] Loss of Cdc42 is thought to affect Rac polarity and activation at the leading edge.[163] Cdc42-null embryoid bodies exhibited defects in cell polarity and cell-cell junctions, as well as decreased Rac activity and aPKC phosphorylation.[164]

5. A Model for Rho GTPases in Mechanotransduction

It has become increasingly clear that exogenous force transmission due to blood flow via filamentous elements linked to membrane surfaces and organelles provide exquisite sensitivity to allow appropriate cellular responses. Although each Rho GTPase mediates distinct signaling networks that are spatially organized, the overall signaling response of the endothelium to flow is integrated. Thus, a unifying model of endothelial mechanotransduction can be proposed based on the relationship between cell adhesions, Rac, Rho and Cdc42 and actin stress fibers and microtubules during shear stress-induced directional reorganization of the cytoskeleton. To this end, Civelekoglu-Scholey and colleagues formulated a mathematical model[165] based on the assumption that the cytoskeleton transfers the shear force to the adhesion sites, which allow integrins to be activated. Activated and ligated integrins signal and transiently de-activate Rho, causing disassembly of stress fibers. Ligated integrins also signal and activate Rac, which enhances focal complex assembly. When Rho activity recovers, stress fibers reappear and promote maturation of focal complexes into focal contacts. The elevated level of Rac activity at the downstream edge of the cell is translated into an alignment of the newly formed stress fibers in the direction of flow. While Rac and Rho control the actin cytoskeleton, polarized activation of Cdc42 mediates reorganization of the MTOC. In addition, all three GTPases control gene expression and regulate a complex molecular signaling network that modulates endothelial barrier permeability and intercellular communication. Recent *in vivo* data in transgenic mice confirm the *in vitro* functions of the Rho GTPases demonstrated in cell culture experiments. Also, these mouse studies clearly show that all three Rho GTPases are critical in embryonic development and atherosclerosis, and future studies should be aimed at further exploring the signaling mechanisms that control these GTPases to decide whether they could be targets for treatments of cardiovascular disease.

References

1. Olesen, S. P., Clapham, D. E., and Davies, P. F. (1988) Haemodynamic shear stress activates a K+ current in vascular endothelial cells. *Nature* **331**, 168–70.
2. Naruse, K., and Sokabe, M. (1993) Involvement of stretch-activated ion channels in Ca2+ mobilization to mechanical stretch in endothelial cells. *Am J Physiol* **264**, C1037–44.
3. Yoshikawa, N., Ariyoshi, H., Ikeda, M., Sakon, M., Kawasaki, T., and Monden, M. (1997) Shear-stress causes polarized change in cytoplasmic calcium concentration in human umbilical vein endothelial cells (HUVECs). *Cell Calcium* **22**, 189–94.

4. Gudi, S., Nolan, J. P., and Frangos, J. A. (1998) Modulation of GTPase activity of G proteins by fluid shear stress and phospholipid composition. *Proc Natl Acad Sci U S A* **95**, 2515–9.
5. Busse, R., and Fleming, I. (1998) Regulation of NO synthesis in endothelial cells. *Kidney Blood Press Res* **21**, 264–6.
6. Liu, Y., Sweet, D. T., Irani-Tehrani, M., Maeda, N., and Tzima, E. (2008) Shc coordinates signals from intercellular junctions and integrins to regulate flow-induced inflammation. *The Journal of Cell Biology* **182**, 185–196.
7. Li, S., Kim, M., Hu, Y. L., Jalali, S., Schlaepfer, D. D., Hunter, T., Chien, S., and Shyy, J. Y. (1997) Fluid shear stress activation of focal adhesion kinase. linking to mitogen-activated protein kinases. *J Biol Chem* **272**, 30455–62.
8. Li, Y. S., Shyy, J. Y., Li, S., Lee, J., Su, B., Karin, M., and Chien, S. (1996) The ras-JNK pathway is involved in shear-induced gene expression. *Mol Cell Biol* **16**, 5947–54.
9. Tseng, H., Peterson, T. E., and Berk, B. C. (1995) Fluid shear stress stimulates mitogen-activated protein kinase in endothelial cells. *Circ Res* **77**, 869–78.
10. Traub, O., and Berk, B. C. (1998) Laminar shear stress: Mechanisms by which endothelial cells transduce an atheroprotective force. *Arterioscler Thromb Vasc Biol* **18**, 677–85.
11. Hsieh, H. J., Cheng, C. C., Wu, S. T., Chiu, J. J., Wung, B. S., and Wang, D. L. (1998) Increase of reactive oxygen species (ROS) in endothelial cells by shear flow and involvement of ROS in shear-induced c-fos expression. *J Cell Physiol* **175**, 156–62.
12. Khachigian, L. M., Resnick, N., A., G. M., Jr., and Collins, T. (1995) Nuclear factor-kappa B interacts functionally with the platelet-derived growth factor B-chain shear-stress response element in vascular endothelial cells exposed to fluid shear stress. *J Clin Invest* **96**, 1169–75.
13. Girard, P. R., and Nerem, R. M. (1995) Shear stress modulates endothelial cell morphology and F-actin organization through the regulation of focal adhesion-associated proteins. *J Cell Physiol* **163**, 179–93.
14. Malek, A. M., and Izumo, S. (1996) Mechanism of endothelial cell shape change and cytoskeletal remodeling in response to fluid shear stress. *J Cell Sci* **109**, 713–26.
15. Levesque, M. J., and Nerem, R. M. (1985) The elongation and orientation of cultured endothelial cells in response to shear stress. *J Biomech Eng* **107**, 341–7.
16. Ogunrinade, O., Kameya, G. T., and Truskey, G. A. (2002) Effect of fluid shear stress on the permeability of the arterial endothelium. *Annals of Biomedical Engineering* **30**, 430–446.
17. Ross, R. (1993) The pathogenesis of atherosclerosis: A perspective for the 1990s. *Nature* **362**, 801–9.
18. Wennerberg, K., Rossman, K. L., and Der, C. J. (2005) The ras superfamily at a glance. *J Cell Sci* **118**, 843–6.

19. Takai, Y., Sasaki, T., and Matozaki, T. (2001) Small GTP-binding proteins. *Physiol Rev* **81**, 153–208.
20. Hall, A., and Nobes, C. D. (2000) Rho GTPases: Molecular switches that control the organization and dynamics of the actin cytoskeleton. *Philos Trans R Soc Lond B Biol Sci* **355**, 965–70.
21. Ridley, A. J., and Hall, A. (1992) The small GTP-binding protein rho regulates the assembly of focal adhesions and actin stress fibers in response to growth factors. *Cell* **70**, 389–99.
22. Li, S., Chen, B. P., Azuma, N., Hu, Y. L., Wu, S. Z., Sumpio, B. E., Shyy, J. Y., and Chien, S. (1999) Distinct roles for the small GTPases Cdc42 and rho in endothelial responses to shear stress. *J Clin Invest* **103**, 1141–50.
23. Tzima, E., del Pozo, M. A., Shattil, S. J., Chien, S., and Schwartz, M. A. (2001) Activation of integrins in endothelial cells by fluid shear stress mediates rho-dependent cytoskeletal alignment. *EMBO J* **20**, 4639–47.
24. Ren, X. D., Kiosses, W. B., and Schwartz, M. A. (1999) Regulation of the small GTP-binding protein rho by cell adhesion and the cytoskeleton. *Embo J* **18**, 578–85.
25. Wojciak-Stothard, B., and Ridley, A. J. (2003) Shear stress-induced endothelial cell polarization is mediated by rho and rac but not Cdc42 or PI 3-kinases. *Journal of Cell Biology* **161**, 429–39.
26. Ridley, A. J., Paterson, H. F., Johnston, C. L., Diekmann, D., and Hall, A. (1992) The small GTP-binding protein rac regulates growth factor-induced membrane ruffling. *Cell* **70**, 401–10.
27. Masuda, M., and Fujiwara, K. (1993) Morphological responses of single endothelial cells exposed to physiological levels of fluid shear stress. *Front Med Biol Eng* **5**, 79–87.
28. Masuda, M., and Fujiwara, K. (1993) The biased lamellipodium development and microtubule organizing center position in vascular endothelial cells migrating under the influence of fluid flow. *Biol Cell* **77**, 237–45.
29. Hu, Y. L., Li, S., Miao, H., Tsou, T. C., del Pozo, M. A., and Chien, S. (2002) Roles of microtubule dynamics and small GTPase rac in endothelial cell migration and lamellipodium formation under flow. *Journal of Vascular Research* **39**, 465–76.
30. Tzima, E., Del Pozo, M. A., Kiosses, W. B., Mohamed, S. A., Li, S., Chien, S., and Schwartz, M. A. (2002). Activation of Rac1 by shear stress in endothelial cells mediates both cytoskeletal reorganization and effects on gene expression. *Embo J* **21**, 6791–800.
31. Kraynov, V. S., Chamberlain, C., Bokoch, G. M., Schwartz, M. A., Slabaugh, S., and Hahn, K. M. (2000) Localized rac activation dynamics visualized in living cells. *Science* **290**, 333–7.
32. Birukov, K. G., Birukova, A. A., Dudek, S. M., Verin, A. D., Crow, M. T., Zhan, X., DePaola, N., and Garcia, J. G. (2002) Shear stress-mediated cytoskeletal remodeling and cortactin translocation in pulmonary endothelial cells. *American Journal of Respiratory Cell & Molecular Biology* **26**, 453–64.

33. Ridley, A. J. (2001) Rho proteins, PI 3-kinases, and monocyte/macrophage motility. *FEBS Letters* **498**, 168–71.
34. Nobes, C. D., and Hall, A. (1995) Rho, rac, and cdc42 GTPases regulate the assembly of multimolecular focal complexes associated with actin stress fibers, lamellipodia, and filopodia. *Cell* **81**, 53–62.
35. Kozma, R., Ahmed, S., Best, A., and Lim, L. (1995) The ras-related protein Cdc42Hs and bradykinin promote formation of peripheral actin microspikes and filopodia in swiss 3T3 fibroblasts. *Molecular & Cellular Biology* **15**, 1942–52.
36. Etienne-Manneville, S., and Hall, A. (2002) Rho GTPases in cell biology. *Nature* **420**, 629–35.
37. Tzima, E., Kiosses, W. B., del Pozo, M. A., and Schwartz, M. A. (2003) Localized cdc42 activation, detected using a novel assay, mediates microtubule organizing center positioning in endothelial cells in response to fluid shear stress. *Journal of Biological Chemistry* **278**, 31020–3.
38. Etienne-Manneville, S., and Hall, A. (2001) Integrin-mediated activation of Cdc42 controls cell polarity in migrating astrocytes through PKCzeta. *Cell* **106**, 489–98.
39. Palazzo, A. F., Joseph, H. L., Chen, Y. J., Dujardin, D. L., Alberts, A. S., Pfister, K. K., Vallee, R. B., and Gundersen, G. G. (2001) Cdc42, dynein, and dynactin regulate MTOC reorientation independent of rho-regulated microtubule stabilization. *Current Biology* **11**, 1536–41.
40. Lee, J. S., Chang, M. I., Tseng, Y., and Wirtz, D. (2005) Cdc42 mediates nucleus movement and MTOC polarization in swiss 3T3 fibroblasts under mechanical shear stress. *Molecular Biology of the Cell* **16**, 871–80.
41. Sin, W. C., Chen, X. Q., Leung, T., and Lim, L. (1998) RhoA-binding kinase alpha translocation is facilitated by the collapse of the vimentin intermediate filament network. *Molecular & Cellular Biology* **18**, 6325–39.
42. Meriane, M., Mary, S., Comunale, F., Vignal, E., Fort, P., and Gauthier-Rouviere, C. (2000) Cdc42Hs and Rac1 GTPases induce the collapse of the vimentin intermediate filament network. *Journal of Biological Chemistry* **275**, 33046–52.
43. Goto, H., Tanabe, K., Manser, E., Lim, L., Yasui, Y., and Inagaki, M. (2002) Phosphorylation and reorganization of vimentin by p21-activated kinase (PAK). *Genes to Cells* **7**, 91–7.
44. Chan, W., Kozma, R., Yasui, Y., Inagaki, M., Leung, T., Manser, E., and Lim, L. (2002) Vimentin intermediate filament reorganization by Cdc42: Involvement of PAK and p70 S6 kinase. *European Journal of Cell Biology* **81**, 692–701.
45. Helmke, B. P., Rosen, A. B., and Davies, P. F. (2003) Mapping mechanical strain of an endogenous cytoskeletal network in living endothelial cells. *Biophysical Journal* **84**, 2691–9.
46. Helmke, B. P., Thakker, D. B., Goldman, R. D., and Davies, P. F. (2001) Spatiotemporal analysis of flow-induced intermediate filament displacement in living endothelial cells. *Biophysical Journal* **80**, 184–94.

47. Helmke, B. P., Goldman, R. D., and Davies, P. F. (2000) Rapid displacement of vimentin intermediate filaments in living endothelial cells exposed to flow. *Circ Res* **86**, 745–52.
48. Colucci-Guyon, E., Portier, M. M., Dunia, I., Paulin, D., Pournin, S., and Babinet, C. (1994) Mice lacking vimentin develop and reproduce without an obvious phenotype. *Cell* **79**, 679–94.
49. Henrion, D., Terzi, F., Matrougui, K., Duriez, M., Boulanger, C. M., Colucci-Guyon, E., Babinet, C., Briand, P., Friedlander, G., Poitevin, P., and Levy, B. I. (1997) Impaired flow-induced dilation in mesenteric resistance arteries from mice lacking vimentin. *J Clin Invest* **100**, 2909–14.
50. Terzi, F., Henrion, D., Colucci-Guyon, E., Federici, P., Babinet, C., Levy, B. I., Briand, P., and Friedlander, G. (1997) Reduction of renal mass is lethal in mice lacking vimentin. role of endothelin-nitric oxide imbalance. *Journal of Clinical Investigation* **100**, 1520–8.
51. Schiffers, P. M., Henrion, D., Boulanger, C. M., Colucci-Guyon, E., Langa-Vuves, F., van Essen, H., Fazzi, G. E., Levy, B. I., and De Mey, J. G. (2000) Altered flow-induced arterial remodeling in vimentin-deficient mice. *Arterioscler Thromb Vasc Biol* **20**, 611–6.
52. Tsuruta, D., and Jones, J. C. (2003) The vimentin cytoskeleton regulates focal contact size and adhesion of endothelial cells subjected to shear stress. *Journal of Cell Science* **116**, 4977–84.
53. Ridge, K. M., Linz, L., Flitney, F. W., Kuczmarski, E. R., Chou, Y. H., Omary, M. B., Sznajder, J. I., and Goldman, R. D. (2005) Keratin 8 phosphorylation by protein kinase C delta regulates shear stress-mediated disassembly of keratin intermediate filaments in alveolar epithelial cells. *The Journal of Biological Chemistry* **280**, 30400–30405.
54. Sivaramakrishnan, S., Schneider, J. L., Sitikov, A., Goldman, R. D., and Ridge, K. M. (2009) Shear stress induced reorganization of the keratin intermediate filament network requires phosphorylation by protein kinase C zeta. *Molecular Biology of the Cell* **20**, 2755–2765.
55. DePaola, N., Phelps, J. E., Florez, L., Keese, C. R., Minnear, F. L., Giaever, I., and Vincent, P. (2001) Electrical impedance of cultured endothelium under fluid flow. *Annals of Biomedical Engineering* **29**, 648–56.
56. Seebach, J., Dieterich, P., Luo, F., Schillers, H., Vestweber, D., Oberleithner, H., Galla, H. J., and Schnittler, H. J. (2000) Endothelial barrier function under laminar fluid shear stress. *Laboratory Investigation* **80**, 1819–31.
57. Birukova, A. A., Smurova, K., Birukov, K. G., Kaibuchi, K., Garcia, J. G., and Verin, A. D. (2004) Role of rho GTPases in thrombin-induced lung vascular endothelial cells barrier dysfunction. *Microvascular Research* **67**, 64–77.
58. Shikata, Y., Rios, A., Kawkitinarong, K., DePaola, N., Garcia, J. G., and Birukov, K. G. (2005) Differential effects of shear stress and cyclic stretch on focal adhesion remodeling, site-specific FAK phosphorylation, and small GTPases in human lung endothelial cells. *Experimental Cell Research* **304**, 40–9.

59. Gavard, J., Patel, V., and Gutkind, J. S. (2008) Angiopoietin-1 prevents VEGF-induced endothelial permeability by sequestering src through mDia. *Developmental Cell* **14**, 25–36.
60. Gavard, J., and Gutkind, J. S. (2006) VEGF controls endothelial-cell permeability by promoting the beta-arrestin-dependent endocytosis of VE-cadherin. *Nature Cell Biology* **8**, 1223–1234.
61. Noritake, J., Fukata, M., Sato, K., Nakagawa, M., Watanabe, T., Izumi, N., Wang, S., Fukata, Y., and Kaibuchi, K. (2004) Positive role of IQGAP1, an effector of Rac1, in actin-meshwork formation at sites of cell-cell contact. *Molecular Biology of the Cell* **15**, 1065–76.
62. Kuroda, S., Fukata, M., Nakagawa, M., Fujii, K., Nakamura, T., Ookubo, T., Izawa, I., Nagase, T., Nomura, N., Tani, H., Shoji, I., Matsuura, Y., Yonehara, S., and Kaibuchi, K. (1998) Role of IQGAP1, a target of the small GTPases Cdc42 and Rac1, in regulation of E-cadherin- mediated cell-cell adhesion. *Science (New York, N.Y.)* **281**, 832–835.
63. Stockton, R. A., Schaefer, E., and Schwartz, M. A. (2004) p21-activated kinase regulates endothelial permeability through modulation of contractility. *Journal of Biological Chemistry* **279**, 46621–30.
64. Dudek, S. M., and Garcia, J. G. (2001) Cytoskeletal regulation of pulmonary vascular permeability. *Journal of Applied Physiology* **91**, 1487–500.
65. Wittchen, E. S., van Buul, J. D., Burridge, K., and Worthylake, R. A. (2005) Trading spaces: Rap, rac, and rho as architects of transendothelial migration. *Current Opinion in Hematology* **12**, 14–21.
66. Wetzel, A., Chavakis, T., Preissner, K. T., Sticherling, M., Haustein, U. F., Anderegg, U., and Saalbach, A. (2004) Human thy-1 (CD90) on activated endothelial cells is a counterreceptor for the leukocyte integrin mac-1 (CD11b/CD18). *Journal of Immunology* **172**, 3850–9.
67. Barker, T. H., Grenett, H. E., MacEwen, M. W., Tilden, S. G., Fuller, G. M., Settleman, J., Woods, A., Murphy-Ullrich, J., and Hagood, J. S. (2004) Thy-1 regulates fibroblast focal adhesions, cytoskeletal organization and migration through modulation of p190 RhoGAP and rho GTPase activity. *Experimental Cell Research* **295**, 488–96.
68. Avalos, A. M., Arthur, W. T., Schneider, P., Quest, A. F., Burridge, K., and Leyton, L. (2004) Aggregation of integrins and RhoA activation are required for thy-1-induced morphological changes in astrocytes. *Journal of Biological Chemistry* **279**, 39139–45.
69. Thompson, P. W., Randi, A. M., and Ridley, A. J. (2002) Intercellular adhesion molecule (ICAM)-1, but not ICAM-2, activates RhoA and stimulates c-fos and rhoA transcription in endothelial cells. *Journal of Immunology (Baltimore, Md.: 1950)* **169**, 1007–1013.
70. Etienne-Manneville, S., Manneville, J. B., Adamson, P., Wilbourn, B., Greenwood, J., and Couraud, P. O. (2000) ICAM-1-coupled cytoskeletal rearrangements and transendothelial lymphocyte migration involve intracellular calcium signaling in brain endothelial cell lines. *Journal of Immunology (Baltimore, Md.: 1950)* **165**, 3375–3383.

71. Adamson, P., Etienne, S., Couraud, P. O., Calder, V., and Greenwood, J. (1999) Lymphocyte migration through brain endothelial cell monolayers involves signaling through endothelial ICAM-1 via a rho-dependent pathway. *Journal of Immunology (Baltimore, Md.: 1950)* **162**, 2964–2973.
72. Jalali, S., del Pozo, M., Chen, K. D., Miao, H., Li, Y. S., Schwartz, M. A., Shyy, J. Y., and Chien, S. (2001) Integrin-mediated mechanotransduction requires its dynamic interaction with specific extracellular matrix (ECM) ligands. *Proc Natl Acad Sci U S A* **98**, 1042–1046.
73. Ren, X., Kiosses, W. B., Sieg, D. J., Otey, C. A., Schlaepfer, D. D., and Schwartz, M. A. (2000) Focal adhesion kinase suppresses rho activity to promote focal adhesion turnover. *J Cell Sci* **113**, 3673–8.
74. Arthur, W. T., Petch, L. A., and Burridge, K. (2000) Integrin engagement suppresses RhoA activity via a c-src-dependent mechanism. *Curr Biol* **10**, 719–22.
75. Schoenwaelder, S. M., Petch, L. A., Williamson, D., Shen, R., Feng, G., and Burridge, K. (2000) The protein tyrosine phosphatase shp-2 regulates RhoA activity [in process citation]. *Curr Biol* **10**, 1523–6.
76. Tsubouchi, A., Sakakura, J., Yagi, R., Mazaki, Y., Schaefer, E., Yano, H., and Sabe, H. (2002) Localized suppression of RhoA activity by Tyr31/118-phosphorylated paxillin in cell adhesion and migration. *Journal of Cell Biology* **159**, 673–83.
77. Nelson, C. M., Pirone, D. M., Tan, J. L., and Chen, C. S. (2004) Vascular endothelial-cadherin regulates cytoskeletal tension, cell spreading, and focal adhesions by stimulating RhoA. *Molecular Biology of the Cell* **15**, 2943–53.
78. Dubash, A. D., Wennerberg, K., Garcia-Mata, R., Menold, M. M., Arthur, W. T., and Burridge, K. (2007) A novel role for Lsc/p115 RhoGEF and LARG in regulating RhoA activity downstream of adhesion to fibronectin. *Journal of Cell Science* **120**, 3989–3998.
79. Dovas, A., and Couchman, J. R. (2005) RhoGDI: Multiple functions in the regulation of rho family GTPase activities. *The Biochemical Journal* **390**, 1–9.
80. Qi, Y. X., Qu, M. J., Long, D. K., Liu, B., Yao, Q. P., Chien, S., and Jiang, Z. L. (2008) Rho-GDP dissociation inhibitor alpha downregulated by low shear stress promotes vascular smooth muscle cell migration and apoptosis: A proteomic analysis. *Cardiovascular Research* **80**, 114–122.
81. Price, L. S., Leng, J., Schwartz, M. A., and Bokoch, G. M. (1998) Activation of rac and Cdc42 by integrins mediates cell spreading. *Mol Biol Cell* **9**, 1863–71.
82. Berrier, A. L., Martinez, R., Bokoch, G. M., and LaFlamme, S. E. (2002) The integrin beta tail is required and sufficient to regulate adhesion signaling to Rac1. *Journal of Cell Science* **115**, 4285–91.
83. Hirsch, E., Barberis, L., Brancaccio, M., Azzolino, O., Xu, D., Kyriakis, J. M., Silengo, L., Giancotti, F. G., Tarone, G., Fassler, R., and Altruda, F. (2002) Defective rac-mediated proliferation and survival after targeted mutation of the beta1 integrin cytodomain. *Journal of Cell Biology* **157**, 481–92.

84. Vuori, K., Hirai, H., Aizawa, S., and Ruoslahti, E. (1996) Introduction of p130cas signaling complex formation upon integrin- mediated cell adhesion: A role for src family kinases. *Mol Cell Biol* **16**, 2606–13.
85. Brugnera, E., Haney, L., Grimsley, C., Lu, M., Walk, S. F., Tosello-Trampont, A. C., Macara, I. G., Madhani, H., Fink, G. R., and Ravichandran, K. S. (2002) Unconventional rac-GEF activity is mediated through the Dock180-ELMO complex.[see comment]. *Nature Cell Biology* **4**, 574–82.
86. Cote, J. F., and Vuori, K. (2002) Identification of an evolutionarily conserved superfamily of DOCK180-related proteins with guanine nucleotide exchange activity. *Journal of Cell Science* **115**, 4901–13.
87. Turner, C. E. (2000) Paxillin interactions. *Journal of Cell Science* **113** Pt 23, 4139–40.
88. Del Pozo, M. A., Kiosses, W. B., Alderson, N. B., Meller, N., Hahn, K. M., and Schwartz, M. A. (2002) Integrins regulate GTP-rac localized effector interactions through dissociation of rho-GDI. *Nat Cell Biol* **4**, 232–9.
89. Goldfinger, L. E., Tzima, E., Stockton, R., Kiosses, W. B., Kinbara, K., Tkachenko, E., Gutierrez, E., Groisman, A., Nguyen, P., Chien, S., and Ginsberg, M. H. (2008) Localized alpha4 integrin phosphorylation directs shear stress-induced endothelial cell alignment. *Circulation Research* **103**, 177–185.
90. Burridge, K., and Wennerberg, K. (2004) Rho and rac take center stage. *Cell* **116**, 167–179.
91. Chrzanowska-Wodnicka, M., and Burridge, K. (1996) Rho-stimulated contractility drives the formation of stress fibers and focal adhesions. *J Cell Biol* **133**, 1403–15.
92. Amano, M., Ito, M., Kimura, K., Fukata, Y., Chihara, K., Nakano, T., Matsuura, Y., and Kaibuchi, K. (1996) Phosphorylation and activation of myosin by rho-associated kinase (rho-kinase). *The Journal of Biological Chemistry* **271**, 20246–20249.
93. Kimura, K., Ito, M., Amano, M., Chihara, K., Fukata, Y., Nakafuku, M., Yamamori, B., Feng, J., Nakano, T., Okawa, K., Iwamatsu, A., and Kaibuchi, K. (1996) Regulation of myosin phosphatase by rho and rho-associated kinase (rho-kinase)[see comment]. *Science* 273, 245–8.
94. Lee, J. S., Panorchan, P., Hale, C. M., Khatau, S. B., Kole, T. P., Tseng, Y., and Wirtz, D. (2006) Ballistic intracellular nanorheology reveals ROCK-hard cytoplasmic stiffening response to fluid flow. *Journal of Cell Science* **119**, 1760–1768.
95. Li, F., and Higgs, H. N. (2003) The mouse formin mDial is a potent actin nucleation factor regulated by autoinhibition. *Current Biology : CB* **13**, 1335–1340.
96. Watanabe, N., Kato, T., Fujita, A., Ishizaki, T., and Narumiya, S. (1999) Cooperation between mDial and ROCK in rho-induced actin reorganization. *Nature Cell Biology* **1**, 136–143.
97. Watanabe, N., Madaule, P., Reid, T., Ishizaki, T., Watanabe, G., Kakizuka, A., Saito, Y., Nakao, K., Jockusch, B. M., and Narumiya, S.

(1997) p140mDia, a mammalian homolog of drosophila diaphanous, is a target protein for rho small GTPase and is a ligand for profilin. *Embo J* **16**, 3044–56.

98. Riveline, D., Zamir, E., Balaban, N. Q., Schwarz, U. S., Ishizaki, T., Narumiya, S., Kam, Z., Geiger, B., and Bershadsky, A. D. (2001) Focal contacts as mechanosensors: Externally applied local mechanical force induces growth of focal contacts by an mDial-dependent and ROCK-independent mechanism. *The Journal of Cell Biology* **153**, 1175–1186.
99. Shiu, Y. T., Li, S., Yuan, S., Wang, Y., Nguyen, P., and Chien, S. (2003) Shear stress-induced c-fos activation is mediated by rho in a calcium-dependent manner. *Biochemical & Biophysical Research Communications* **303**, 548–55.
100. Hsieh, H. J., Li, N. Q., and Frangos, J. A. (1993) Pulsatile and steady flow induces c-fos expression in human endothelial cells. *J Cell Physiol* **154**, 143–51.
101. Lin, T., Zeng, L., Liu, Y., DeFea, K., Schwartz, M. A., Chien, S., and Shyy, J. Y. (2003) Rho-ROCK-LIMK-cofilin pathway regulates shear stress activation of sterol regulatory element binding proteins. *Circulation Research* **92**, 1296–304.
102. Brown, M. S., and Goldstein, J. L. (1997) The SREBP pathway: Regulation of cholesterol metabolism by proteolysis of a membrane-bound transcription factor. *Cell* **89**, 331–40.
103. Cicha, I., Beronov, K., Ramirez, E. L., Osterode, K., Goppelt-Struebe, M., Raaz, D., Yilmaz, A., Daniel, W. G., and Garlichs, C. D. (2009) Shear stress preconditioning modulates endothelial susceptibility to circulating TNF-alpha and monocytic cell recruitment in a simplified model of arterial bifurcations. *Atherosclerosis.*
104. Machesky, L. M., and Insall, R. H. (1998) Scar1 and the related wiskott-aldrich syndrome protein, WASP, regulate the actin cytoskeleton through the Arp2/3 complex. *Current Biology: CB* **8**, 1347–1356.
105. Miki, H., Suetsugu, S., and Takenawa, T. (1998) WAVE, a novel WASP-family protein involved in actin reorganization induced by rac. *The EMBO Journal* **17**, 6932–6941.
106. Bokoch, G. M. (2003) Biology of the p21-activated kinases. *Annual Review of Biochemistry* **72**, 743–781.
107. Sells, M. A., Knaus, U. G., Bagrodia, S., Ambrose, D. M., Bokoch, G. M., and Chernoff, J. (1997) Human p21-activated kinase (Pak1) regulates actin organization in mammalian cells. *Current Biology: CB* **7**, 202–210.
108. Verma, I. M., Stevenson, J. K., Schwarz, E. M., Van Antwerp, D., and Miyamoto, S. (1995) Rel/NF-kappa B/I kappa B family: Intimate tales of association and dissociation. *Genes Dev* **9**, 2723–35.
109. Brand, K., Page, S., Rogler, G., Bartsch, A., Brandl, R., Knuechel, R., Page, M., Kaltschmidt, C., Baeuerle, P. A., and Neumeier, D. (1996) Activated transcription factor nuclear factor-kappa B is present in the atherosclerotic lesion. *J Clin Invest* **97**, 1715–22.

110. Ritchie, M. E. (1998) Nuclear factor-kappaB is selectively and markedly activated in humans with unstable angina pectoris. *Circulation* **98**, 1707–13.
111. Brand, K., Page, S., Walli, A. K., Neumeier, D., and Baeuerle, P. A. (1997) Role of nuclear factor-kappa B in atherogenesis. *Exp Physiol* **82**, 297–304.
112. Yeh, L. H., Park, Y. J., Hansalia, R. J., Ahmed, I. S., Deshpande, S. S., Goldschmidt-Clermont, P. J., Irani, K., and Alevriadou, B. R. (1999) Shear-induced tyrosine phosphorylation in endothelial cells requires Rac1-dependent production of ROS. *Am J Physiol* **276**, C838–47.
113. Sulciner, D. J., Irani, K., Yu, Z. X., Ferrans, V. J., Goldschmidt-Clermont, P., and Finkel, T. (1996) rac1 regulates a cytokine-stimulated, redox-dependent pathway necessary for NF-kappaB activation. *Mol Cell Biol* **16**, 7115–21.
114. Perona, R., Montaner, S., Saniger, L., Sanchez-Perez, I., Bravo, R., and Lacal, J. C. (1997) Activation of the nuclear factor-kappaB by rho, CDC42, and rac-1 proteins. *Genes Dev* **11**, 463–75.
115. Joyce, D., Bouzahzah, B., Fu, M., Albanese, C., D'Amico, M., Steer, J., Klein, J. U., Lee, R. J., Segall, J. E., Westwick, J. K., Der, C. J., and Pestell, R. G. (1999) Integration of rac-dependent regulation of cyclin D1 transcription through a nuclear factor-kappaB-dependent pathway. *J Biol Chem* **274**, 25245–9.
116. Arbibe, L., Mira, J. P., Teusch, N., Kline, L., Guha, M., Mackman, N., Godowski, P. J., Ulevitch, R. J., and Knaus, U. G. (2000) Toll-like receptor 2-mediated NF-kappaB activation requires a Rac1- dependent pathway. *Nat Immunol* **1**, 533–40.
117. Reyes-Reyes, M., Mora, N., Zentella, A., and Rosales, C. (2001) Phosphatidylinositol 3-kinase mediates integrin-dependent NF-kappaB and MAPK activation through separate signaling pathways. *J Cell Sci* **114**, 1579–89.
118. Lan, Q., Mercurius, K. O., and Davies, P. F. (1994) Stimulation of transcription factors NF kappa B and AP1 in endothelial cells subjected to shear stress. *Biochemical and Biophysical Research Communications* **201**, 950–956.
119. Bhullar, I. S., Li, Y. S., Miao, H., Zandi, E., Kim, M., Shyy, J. Y., and Chien, S. (1998) Fluid shear stress activation of IkappaB kinase is integrin-dependent. *J Biol Chem* **273**, 30544–9.
120. Nagel, T., Resnick, N., F., D. C., Jr, and A., G. M., Jr. (1999) Vascular endothelial cells respond to spatial gradients in fluid shear stress by enhanced activation of transcription factors. *Arterioscler Thromb Vasc Biol* **19**, 1825–34.
121. Resnick, N., and A., G. M., Jr. (1995) Hemodynamic forces are complex regulators of endothelial gene expression. *Faseb J* **9**, 874–82.
122. Collins, T. (1993) Endothelial nuclear factor-kappa B and the initiation of the atherosclerotic lesion. *Lab Invest* **68**, 499–508.
123. Carlos, T. M., and Harlan, J. M. (1994) Leukocyte-endothelial adhesion molecules. *Blood* **84**, 2068–101.

124. Orr, A. W., Sanders, J. M., Bevard, M., Coleman, E., Sarembock, I. J., and Schwartz, M. A. (2005) The subendothelial extracellular matrix modulates NF-kappaB activation by flow: A potential role in atherosclerosis. *Journal of Cell Biology* **169**, 191–202.
125. Orr, A. W., Stockton, R., Simmers, M. B., Sanders, J. M., Sarembock, I. J., Blackman, B. R., and Schwartz, M. A. (2007) Matrix-specific p21-activated kinase activation regulates vascular permeability in atherogenesis. *J Cell Biol* **176**, 719–27.
126. Orr, A. W., Hahn, C., Blackman, B. R., and Schwartz, M. A. (2008) p21-activated kinase signaling regulates oxidant-dependent NF-kappa B activation by flow. *Circulation Research* **103**, 671–679.
127. Miki, H., Miura, K., and Takenawa, T. (1996) N-WASP, a novel actin-depolymerizing protein, regulates the cortical cytoskeletal rearrangement in a PIP2-dependent manner downstream of tyrosine kinases. *The EMBO Journal* **15**, 5326–5335.
128. Kolluri, R., Tolias, K. F., Carpenter, C. L., Rosen, F. S., and Kirchhausen, T. (1996) Direct interaction of the wiskott-aldrich syndrome protein with the GTPase Cdc42. *Proceedings of the National Academy of Sciences of the United States of America* **93**, 5615–5618.
129. Welch, M. D. (1999) The world according to arp: Regulation of actin nucleation by the Arp2/3 complex. *Trends in Cell Biology* **9**, 423–427.
130. Dong, J. M., Leung, T., Manser, E., and Lim, L. (2002) Cdc42 antagonizes inductive action of cAMP on cell shape, via effects of the myotonic dystrophy kinase-related Cdc42-binding kinase (MRCK) on myosin light chain phosphorylation. *European Journal of Cell Biology* **81**, 231–242.
131. Manser, E., Chong, C., Zhao, Z. S., Leung, T., Michael, G., Hall, C., and Lim, L. (1995) Molecular cloning of a new member of the p21-Cdc42/Rac-activated kinase (PAK) family. *The Journal of Biological Chemistry* **270**, 25070–25078.
132. Kemphues, K. J., Priess, J. R., Morton, D. G., and Cheng, N. S. (1988) Identification of genes required for cytoplasmic localization in early C. elegans embryos. *Cell* **52**, 311–20.
133. Simmers, M. B., Pryor, A. W., and Blackman, B. R. (2007) Arterial shear stress regulates endothelial cell-directed migration, polarity, and morphology in confluent monolayers. *American Journal of Physiology. Heart and Circulatory Physiology* **293**, H1937–46.
134. Hill, C. S., Wynne, J., and Treisman, R. (1995) The rho family GTPases RhoA, Rac1, and CDC42Hs regulate transcriptional activation by SRF. *Cell* **81**, 1159–70.
135. Liu, A. X., Rane, N., Liu, J. P., and Prendergast, G. C. (2001) RhoB is dispensable for mouse development, but it modifies susceptibility to tumor formation as well as cell adhesion and growth factor signaling in transformed cells. *Molecular and Cellular Biology* **21**, 6906–6912.
136. Hakem, A., Sanchez-Sweatman, O., You-Ten, A., Duncan, G., Wakeham, A., Khokha, R., and Mak, T. W. (2005) RhoC is dispensable for embryogenesis

and tumor initiation but essential for metastasis. *Genes & Development* **19**, 1974–1979.

137. Shimizu, Y., Thumkeo, D., Keel, J., Ishizaki, T., Oshima, H., Oshima, M., Noda, Y., Matsumura, F., Taketo, M. M., and Narumiya, S. (2005) ROCK-I regulates closure of the eyelids and ventral body wall by inducing assembly of actomyosin bundles. *The Journal of Cell Biology* **168**, 941–953.
138. Rikitake, Y., Oyama, N., Wang, C. Y., Noma, K., Satoh, M., Kim, H. H., and Liao, J. K. (2005) Decreased perivascular fibrosis but not cardiac hypertrophy in ROCK1+/− haploinsufficient mice. *Circulation* **112**, 2959–2965.
139. Noma, K., Rikitake, Y., Oyama, N., Yan, G., Alcaide, P., Liu, P. Y., Wang, H., Ahl, D., Sawada, N., Okamoto, R., Hiroi, Y., Shimizu, K., Luscinskas, F. W., Sun, J., and Liao, J. K. (2008) ROCK1 mediates leukocyte recruitment and neointima formation following vascular injury. *The Journal of Clinical Investigation* **118**, 1632–1644.
140. Lee, D. H., Shi, J., Jeoung, N. H., Kim, M. S., Zabolotny, J. M., Lee, S. W., White, M. F., Wei, L., and Kim, Y. B. (2009) Targeted disruption of ROCK1 causes insulin resistance in vivo. *The Journal of Biological Chemistry* **284**, 11776–11780.
141. Wang, H. W., Liu, P. Y., Oyama, N., Rikitake, Y., Kitamoto, S., Gitlin, J., Liao, J. K., and Boisvert, W. A. (2008) Deficiency of ROCK1 in bone marrow-derived cells protects against atherosclerosis in LDLR-/- mice. *The FASEB Journal: Official Publication of the Federation of American Societies for Experimental Biology* **22**, 3561–3570.
142. Wu, D. J., Xu, J. Z., Wu, Y. J., Jean-Charles, L., Xiao, B., Gao, P. J., and Zhu, D. L. (2009) Effects of fasudil on early atherosclerotic plaque formation and established lesion progression in apolipoprotein E-knockout mice. *Atherosclerosis.*
143. Eitenmuller, I., Volger, O., Kluge, A., Troidl, K., Barancik, M., Cai, W. J., Heil, M., Pipp, F., Fischer, S., Horrevoets, A. J., Schmitz-Rixen, T., and Schaper, W. (2006) The range of adaptation by collateral vessels after femoral artery occlusion. *Circulation Research* **99**, 656–662.
144. Peng, J., Kitchen, S. M., West, R. A., Sigler, R., Eisenmann, K. M., and Alberts, A. S. (2007) Myeloproliferative defects following targeting of the Drf1 gene encoding the mammalian diaphanous related formin mDia1. *Cancer Research* **67**, 7565–7571.
145. Sugihara, K., Nakatsuji, N., Nakamura, K., Nakao, K., Hashimoto, R., Otani, H., Sakagami, H., Kondo, H., Nozawa, S., Aiba, A., and Katsuki, M. (1998) Rac1 is required for the formation of three germ layers during gastrulation. *Oncogene* **17**, 3427–3433.
146. Glogauer, M., Marchal, C. C., Zhu, F., Worku, A., Clausen, B. E., Foerster, I., Marks, P., Downey, G. P., Dinauer, M., and Kwiatkowski, D. J. (2003) Rac1 deletion in mouse neutrophils has selective effects on neutrophil functions. *Journal of Immunology (Baltimore, Md.: 1950)* **170**, 5652–5657.
147. Walmsley, M. J., Ooi, S. K., Reynolds, L. F., Smith, S. H., Ruf, S., Mathiot, A., Vanes, L., Williams, D. A., Cancro, M. P., and Tybulewicz, V. L.

(2003) Critical roles for Rac1 and Rac2 GTPases in B cell development and signaling. *Science (New York, N.Y.)* **302**, 459–462.
148. Gu, Y., Filippi, M. D., Cancelas, J. A., Siefring, J. E., Williams, E. P., Jasti, A. C., Harris, C. E., Lee, A. W., Prabhakar, R., Atkinson, S. J., Kwiatkowski, D. J., and Williams, D. A. (2003) Hematopoietic cell regulation by Rac1 and Rac2 guanosine triphosphatases. *Science (New York, N.Y.)* **302**, 445–449.
149. Benitah, S. A., Frye, M., Glogauer, M., and Watt, F. M. (2005) Stem cell depletion through epidermal deletion of Rac1. *Science (New York, N.Y.)* **309**, 933–935.
150. Chrostek, A., Wu, X., Quondamatteo, F., Hu, R., Sanecka, A., Niemann, C., Langbein, L., Haase, I., and Brakebusch, C. (2006) Rac1 is crucial for hair follicle integrity but is not essential for maintenance of the epidermis. *Molecular and Cellular Biology* **26**, 6957–6970.
151. Satoh, M., Ogita, H., Takeshita, K., Mukai, Y., Kwiatkowski, D. J., and Liao, J. K. (2006) Requirement of Rac1 in the development of cardiac hypertrophy. *Proceedings of the National Academy of Sciences of the United States of America* **103**, 7432–7437.
152. Benninger, Y., Thurnherr, T., Pereira, J. A., Krause, S., Wu, X., Chrostek-Grashoff, A., Herzog, D., Nave, K. A., Franklin, R. J., Meijer, D., Brakebusch, C., Suter, U., and Relvas, J. B. (2007) Essential and distinct roles for cdc42 and rac1 in the regulation of schwann cell biology during peripheral nervous system development. *The Journal of Cell Biology* **177**, 1051–1061.
153. Chen, L., Liao, G., Waclaw, R. R., Burns, K. A., Linquist, D., Campbell, K., Zheng, Y., and Kuan, C. Y. (2007) Rac1 controls the formation of midline commissures and the competency of tangential migration in ventral telencephalic neurons. *The Journal of Neuroscience: The Official Journal of the Society for Neuroscience* **27**, 3884–3893.
154. Tan, W., Palmby, T. R., Gavard, J., Amornphimoltham, P., Zheng, Y., and Gutkind, J. S. (2008) An essential role for Rac1 in endothelial cell function and vascular development. *The FASEB Journal: Official Publication of the Federation of American Societies for Experimental Biology* **22**, 1829–1838.
155. Yamazaki, D., Fujiwara, T., Suetsugu, S., and Takenawa, T. (2005) A novel function of WAVE in lamellipodia: WAVE1 is required for stabilization of lamellipodial protrusions during cell spreading. *Genes to Cells: Devoted to Molecular & Cellular Mechanisms* **10**, 381–392.
156. Guo, F., Debidda, M., Yang, L., Williams, D. A., and Zheng, Y. (2006) Genetic deletion of Rac1 GTPase reveals its critical role in actin stress fiber formation and focal adhesion complex assembly. *The Journal of Biological Chemistry* **281**, 18652–18659.
157. Sauzeau, V., Jerkic, M., Lopez-Novoa, J. M., and Bustelo, X. R. (2007) Loss of Vav2 proto-oncogene causes tachycardia and cardiovascular disease in mice. *Molecular Biology of the Cell* **18**, 943–952.
158. Hassanain, H. H., Gregg, D., Marcelo, M. L., Zweier, J. L., Souza, H. P., Selvakumar, B., Ma, Q., Moustafa-Bayoumi, M., Binkley, P. F., Flavahan,

N. A., Morris, M., Dong, C., and Goldschmidt-Clermont, P. J. (2007) Hypertension caused by transgenic overexpression of Rac1. *Antioxidants & Redox Signaling* **9**, 91–100.

159. Sawada, N., Salomone, S., Kim, H. H., Kwiatkowski, D. J., and Liao, J. K. (2008) Regulation of endothelial nitric oxide synthase and postnatal angiogenesis by Rac1. *Circulation Research* **103**, 360–368.
160. Chen, F., Ma, L., Parrini, M. C., Mao, X., Lopez, M., Wu, C., Marks, P. W., Davidson, L., Kwiatkowski, D. J., Kirchhausen, T., Orkin, S. H., Rosen, F. S., Mayer, B. J., Kirschner, M. W., and Alt, F. W. (2000) Cdc42 is required for PIP(2)-induced actin polymerization and early development but not for cell viability. *Current Biology: CB* **10**, 758–765.
161. Yang, L., Wang, L., and Zheng, Y. (2006) Gene targeting of Cdc42 and Cdc42GAP affirms the critical involvement of Cdc42 in filopodia induction, directed migration, and proliferation in primary mouse embryonic fibroblasts. *Molecular Biology of the Cell* **17**, 4675–4685.
162. Yang, L., Wang, L., Geiger, H., Cancelas, J. A., Mo, J., and Zheng, Y. (2007) Rho GTPase Cdc42 coordinates hematopoietic stem cell quiescence and niche interaction in the bone marrow. *Proceedings of the National Academy of Sciences of the United States of America* **104**, 5091–5096.
163. Srinivasan, S., Wang, F., Glavas, S., Ott, A., Hofmann, F., Aktories, K., Kalman, D., and Bourne, H. R. (2003) Rac and Cdc42 play distinct roles in regulating PI(3,4,5)P3 and polarity during neutrophil chemotaxis. *The Journal of Cell Biology* **160**, 375–385.
164. Wu, X., Li, S., Chrostek-Grashoff, A., Czuchra, A., Meyer, H., Yurchenco, P. D., and Brakebusch, C. (2007) Cdc42 is crucial for the establishment of epithelial polarity during early mammalian development. *Developmental Dynamics: An Official Publication of the American Association of Anatomists* **236**, 2767–2778.
165. Civelekoglu-Scholey, G., Orr, A. W., Novak, I., Meister, J. J., Schwartz, M. A., and Mogilner, A. (2005) Model of coupled transient changes of rac, rho, adhesions and stress fibers alignment in endothelial cells responding to shear stress. *Journal of Theoretical Biology* **232**, 569–585.

Chapter 6

NITRIC OXIDE AND ENDOTHELIAL MITOCHONDRIAL FUNCTION: IMPLICATIONS FOR ISCHEMIA/REPERFUSION

B. R. ALEVRIADOU*, C. I. JONES 3rd and R. J. GIEDT
Davis Heart and Lung Research Institute,
Departments of Biomedical Engineering & Internal Medicine (Cardiology),
The Ohio State University, Columbus, OH 43210
**alevriadou.1@osu.edu*

The greatest source of nitric oxide (NO) in the normal heart is the endothelial nitric oxide synthase (eNOS), which is localized in vascular endothelial cells (ECs). Endogenously synthesized NO has a variety of physiological functions. Its primary role is thought to be the control of vascular tone via its effect on the soluble guanylate cyclase enzyme of overlying smooth muscle cells. Cytochrome c oxidase (CcO or complex IV), the terminal enzyme in the mitochondrial electron transport chain (ETC) is also a NO target. NO, via its effect on the mitochondrial ETC, can regulate cellular oxygen (O_2) consumption, superoxide radical ($O_2^{\cdot -}$) production, and redox signaling. However, loss of the NO control over respiration can lead to increased formation of reactive O_2 and nitrogen species (ROS/RNS) and mitochondrial damage. Our group is particularly interested on the consequences of the NO interactions with endothelial mitochondria, because ECs under shear stress produce high levels of NO, and endothelial mitochondrial dysfunction is the hallmark of ischemia/reperfusion (I/RP) injury and is common in almost all vascular diseases. In this review, we discuss (1) the NO actions on mitochondria in general, and on mitochondria of cultured ECs exposed to shear stress in particular, and (2) the role of NO on the mitochondrial (dys)function of ECs and cardiomyocytes following I/RP. Using either *ex vivo* hearts or isolated mitochondria, it has been difficult to understand the relationship between NO, mitochondria and EC function. Cultured EC exposure to conditions of shear stress and O_2 tension (P_{O2}) that simulate the *in vivo* I/RP may provide additional insights.

1. The Mitochondrial ETC is a Source of ROS

Mammalian mitochondria consume nearly 90% of a cell's O_2 to support oxidative phosphorylation by harnessing oxidized fuel (expressed as respiration or O_2 consumption) to the synthesis of adenosine triphosphate

(ATP). The oxidative phosphorylation machinery is contained at the inner mitochondrial membrane and consists of 2 proton (H^+)-pumping systems, the ETC (also called respiratory chain) and the ATP synthase. The ETC is an assembly of 4 polypeptide complexes, nicotinamide-adenine dinucleotide (reduced) (NADH)-ubiquinone reductase (NQR; complex I), succinate-ubiquinone reductase (SQR; complex II), ubiquinol-cytochrome c reductase (QCR; complex III) and cytochrome c oxidase (CcO; complex IV), and 2 electron (e^-) carriers, ubiquinone (Q) and cytochrome c (cyt c) (Fig. 1). Electrons from the e^- donors NADH and reduced flavin-adenine dinucleotide ($FADH_2$) enter the ETC at complexes I and II, respectively. The energy released by the flow of e^- through the ETC is used to pump H^+ out of the inner membrane through complexes I, III and IV. This creates a proton gradient (pH gradient) across the inner membrane. The proton gradient generates the mitochondrial membrane potential ($\Delta\Psi_m$), which arises from the net movement of positive charge across the membrane. The potential energy stored is coupled to ATP synthesis by the ATP synthase. O_2 is the ultimate e^- acceptor and is reduced to H_2O (Wallace, 2005).

However, e^- leakage to O_2 through complexes I, II and III generates $O_2^{\cdot-}$ (Fig. 1) (Lenaz, 1998; Turrens and Boveris, 1980). The rate of $O_2^{\cdot-}$ production increases when e^- carriers harbor excess e^-, either from inhibition of oxidative phosphorylation or from excessive calorie

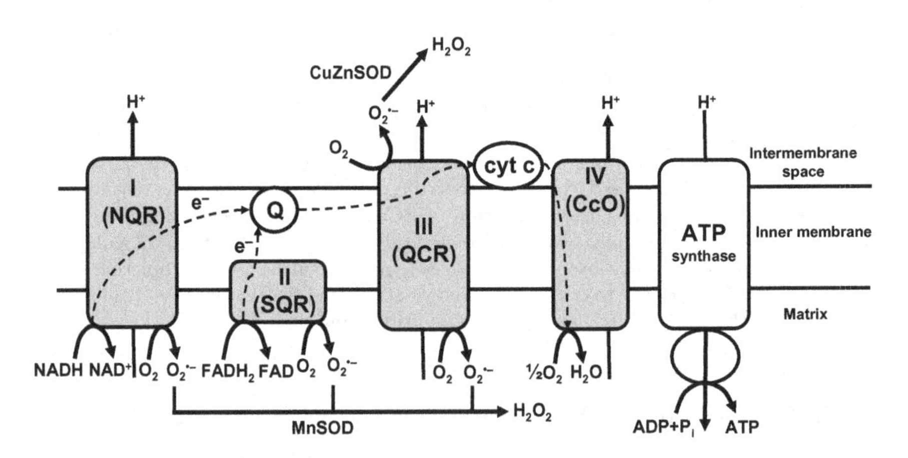

Fig. 1. Overview of the ETC and ATP synthesis on the mitochondrial inner membrane. Also shown is the mitochondrial $O_2^{\cdot-}$ production and its conversion to H_2O_2 by SOD enzymes.

consumption. The location of $O_2^{\cdot -}$ generation is important because $O_2^{\cdot -}$ does not diffuse across membranes. It is known that complexes I and II release $O_2^{\cdot -}$ into the matrix, whereas complex III releases $O_2^{\cdot -}$ both into the matrix and the intermembrane space (Muller *et al.*, 2004). $O_2^{\cdot -}$ is converted to hydrogen peroxide (H_2O_2) by manganese superoxide dismutase (MnSOD) in the matrix or by copper zinc SOD (CuZnSOD) in the intermembrane space (Fig. 1) (Gutteridge and Halliwell, 2000). The mitochondria are recognized as a major cellular source of H_2O_2, which originates from $O_2^{\cdot -}$ produced by the ETC (Boveris and Cadenas, 2000).

2. NO is a Key Mitochondrial Regulator

In cells exposed to NO donors, NO-producing cells, isolated tissues or whole animals, NO is known to modulate mitochondrial respiration as indicated by O_2 consumption measurements (Clementi *et al.*, 1999; Loke *et al.*, 1999; Shen *et al.*, 1995). At physiological concentrations (10 nM-1 μM), NO rapidly and reversibly inhibits complexes III and IV without affecting cell viability (Fig. 2) (Cleeter *et al.*, 1994; Poderoso *et al.*, 1996). Inhibition of complex III leads to autooxidation of the free radical ubisemiquinone that is generated during the oxidation of ubiquinol (QH_2) to Q. Inhibition of complex IV occurs through reversible binding to its heme a_3-copper atom Cu_B complex, and is competitive with O_2. Either inhibition results in generation of $O_2^{\cdot -}$, and subsequently H_2O_2.

At higher concentrations (>1 μM), NO promotes QH_2 oxidation with the concomitant production of $O_2^{\cdot -}$ which then reacts with NO, in a diffusion-limited reaction, to form the RNS peroxynitrite ($ONOO^-$) (Fig. 2) (Poderoso *et al.*, 1999). $ONOO^-$, as a strong oxidant, has the potential to cause persistent inhibition of complex I (due to oxidation/nitration), which greatly increases the $O_2^{\cdot -}$ production from the ETC, as well as inhibition of complex II (due to iron removal from its iron Fe^{2+}-sulfur clusters) and complex IV, the ATP synthase, MnSOD and other proteins, and to promote cell death (Fig. 2) (Brown and Borutaite, 2002; Brown and Borutaite, 2004; Cadenas, 2004; Cassina and Radi, 1996; Riobo *et al.*, 2001).

Mitochondria undergo oxidative damage when the ROS production exceeds their antioxidant capacity. H_2O_2 is decomposed by either catalase or glutathione peroxidase (GPx) to produce H_2O (Fig. 2). GPx oxidizes reduced glutathione (GSH) to its oxidized form (GSSG). GSSG is reduced to GSH by glutathione reductase (GR). GSH is synthesized

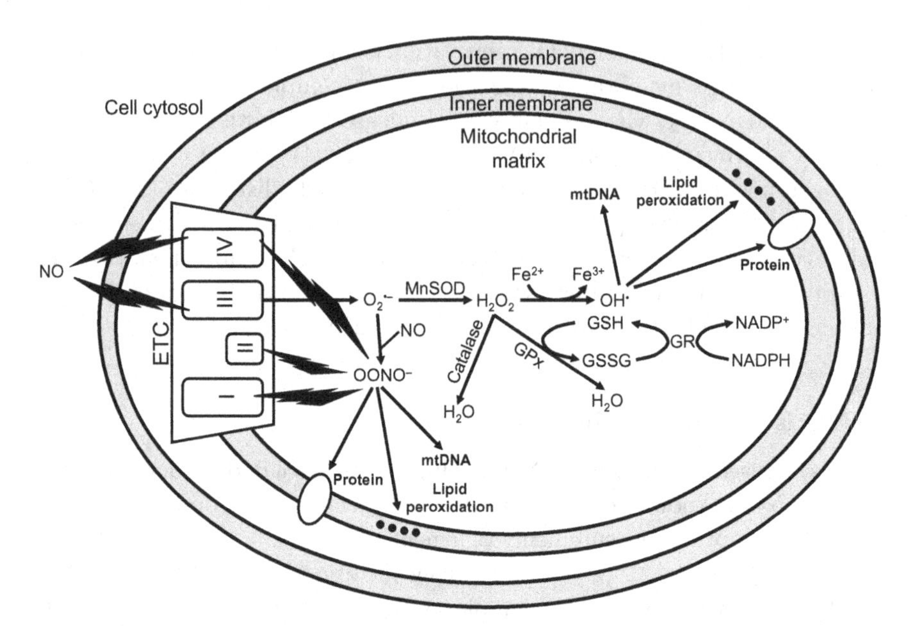

Fig. 2. Schematic representation of inhibition of respiration by NO and $ONOO^-$. NO reversibly inhibits complexes III and IV; $ONOO^-$ irreversibly inhibits complexes I, II and IV. $ONOO^-$, a potent oxidant, can cause damage to proteins, lipids and nucleic aids. H_2O_2, which originates from $O_2^{\cdot-}$ formed by the ETC, is detoxified by either catalase or the GSH-dependent pathway. $O_2^{\cdot-}$ liberates Fe^{2+} from ETC proteins, and, in the presence of Fe^{2+}, H_2O_2 is converted to $OH^{\cdot}$, another potent oxidant that can cause intramitochondrial damage.

from amino acids in the cytosol and is imported into the mitochondria. Glutathione-S-transferase then utilizes GSH as a cofactor to detoxify cytotoxic lipid peroxidation products. H_2O_2 can be converted to hydroxyl radical ($OH^{\cdot}$), a potent oxidant, via the Fe^{2+}-catalyzed (Fenton) reaction (Fig. 2). In addition to GSH, mitochondria have 2 thiol-disulfide oxidoreductases, thioredoxin and glutaredoxin, and several low molecular weight antioxidants. H_2O_2 that escapes detoxification diffuses into the cytosol where it affects the concentration of cytosolic H_2O_2 and, hence, the cell signal transduction, proliferation and apoptosis (Boveris and Cadenas, 2000; Cadenas, 2004; Lenaz, 1998). In summary, NO at medium levels is thought to increase the mitochondrial H_2O_2 production by promoting $O_2^{\cdot-}$ generation from the ETC, whereas, at high levels, it is thought to inhibit H_2O_2 production by scavenging $O_2^{\cdot-}$ and forming $ONOO^-$.

3. Cultured EC Exposure to Shear Stress Affects Mitochondrial Function: Role of NO

Moncada's group showed that endogenous NO produced by ECs under basal and stimulated conditions inhibits respiration in competition with O_2. Treatment with the neuropeptide bradykinin, which activates eNOS, generated higher NO concentrations that inhibited respiration, whereas treatment with an eNOS inhibitor caused an increase in respiration, collectively suggesting that NO interacts with complex IV and modulates the cell O_2 consumption (Clementi *et al.*, 1999).

Since cultured EC exposure to steady laminar flow, and resultant wall shear stress (using a parallel-plate flow chamber and media recirculation system), is known to produce NO by activating eNOS and, at longer times, via eNOS induction (Huddleson *et al.*, 2005; Jin *et al.*, 2003; Kuchan and Frangos, 1994), we hypothesized that the endogenous NO, by itself and possibly via formation of $ONOO^-$, would modulate the enzymatic activities of the ETC complexes and, hence, O_2 consumption. Our study (Han *et al.*, 2007) showed that cultured human umbilical vein EC (HUVEC) exposure to steady laminar shear stress (low arterial level) results in gradual inhibition of each of the respiratory complexes I, II/III and IV starting as early as 5 minutes from the flow onset and lasting throughout the shear exposure. The inhibitory effect on each of the complexes I, II/III and IV was either significantly decreased or abolished when ECs were sheared in the presence of either the eNOS inhibitor N^G-nitro-L-arginine methyl ester (L-NAME) or the $ONOO^-$ scavenger uric acid (UA). Inhibition of mitochondrial complexes occurred within minutes from the flow onset, affected all ETC complexes (not only those affected by NO), was accompanied by nitrotyrosine staining (a footprint of $ONOO^-$ formation), and was inhibited by UA suggesting that intramitochondrial $ONOO^-$ is, at least in part, responsible for the shear-induced inhibition of the ETC.

NO produced by eNOS is expected to diffuse into the mitochondria. A Ca^{2+}/calmodulin-dependent mitochondrial NOS has been reported, but questions remain regarding its precise molecular structure (Brookes, 2004). Since, in *in vitro* studies, no hemoglobin is present to scavenge NO (Azarov *et al.*, 2005) and NO is more soluble in lipid bilayers, it is possible that, within cell membranes and specifically mitochondrial membranes, the shear-induced NO reaches pathophysiological levels and reacts with the $O_2^{\cdot -}$ produced by the ETC to form $ONOO^-$.

Since it is known that the $O_2^{\cdot -}$ formation rate by the ETC increases linearly with P_{O2} (Lenaz, 1998; Turrens *et al.*, 1982), we designed experiments to test whether the relative 'hyperoxic state' of 21% O_2 of the *in vitro* flow studies is, at least in part, responsible for raising the O_2 concentration in the EC mitochondria and enhancing the formation of $O_2^{\cdot -}$, which, via its reaction with the shear-induced NO, increases the $ONOO^-$ levels and potentiates the inhibition of respiration. Since either NO or $ONOO^-$ suppresses respiration, and $ONOO^-$ suppresses respiration more than NO (Xie and Wolin, 1996), we hypothesized that the O_2 consumption rate would be lower for sheared vs. static ECs and would be modulated by the P_{O2}. A literature search confirmed that all flow studies with cultured ECs, and the reoxygenation (RO) phase of hypoxia (H)/RO studies, including our work (Han *et al.*, 2007; Jones *et al.*, 2007; Martin *et al.*, 2005; Ng *et al.*, 2002; Yeh *et al.*, 2001; Yeh *et al.*, 1999), had been carried out at the atmospheric O_2 concentration (21% O_2), which gives rise to a partial pressure of O_2 (P_{O2}) of ~160 mmHg, above the levels in arterial blood (75–100 mmHg; 10–13% O_2; 12.5% O_2 on average) and well above the levels in venous blood (35 mmHg; 5% O_2) or the levels to which ECs are exposed in tissue capillaries (mean capillary blood P_{O2} in the heart is ~20 mmHg; 2.6% O_2) (Tsai *et al.*, 2003).

To test the above hypotheses, we exposed cultured bovine aortic ECs (BAECs) to a low arterial level of shear stress under either 5%, 10% (close to the average arterial P_{O2}) or 21% O_2 in the parallel-plate flow chamber, harvested them, centrifuged and measured respiration in cell suspensions using electron paramagnetic resonance (EPR) oximetry with lithium phthalocyanine as the probe, a technique capable of measuring O_2 consumption rates from a relatively small number of cells (Ilangovan *et al.*, 2004). Our study (Jones *et al.*, 2008) showed that flow exposure inhibits EC respiration, and the shear inhibitory effect is increased when ECs are sheared at higher P_{O2}. Flow in the presence of either L-NAME or UA abolished the inhibitory effect suggesting that NO, via formation of $ONOO^-$ in the mitochondria, is responsible for the decrease in the rate of O_2 consumption by sheared ECs ((Jones *et al.*, 2008); Fig. 3A shows the effect of L-NAME on the respiration of sheared ECs). Transfection with an adenovirus that expresses MnSOD (Ad.MnSOD) in the mitochondria, and not a control virus, prior to flow exposure also blocked the shear-induced inhibitory effect providing additional evidence that the suppression of respiration is due to mitochondrial $ONOO^-$ formation (Jones *et al.*, 2008). Although $O_2^{\cdot -}$ reacts with NO faster ($k_1 = 1.9 \times 10^{10}\,M^{-1}\,s^{-1}$

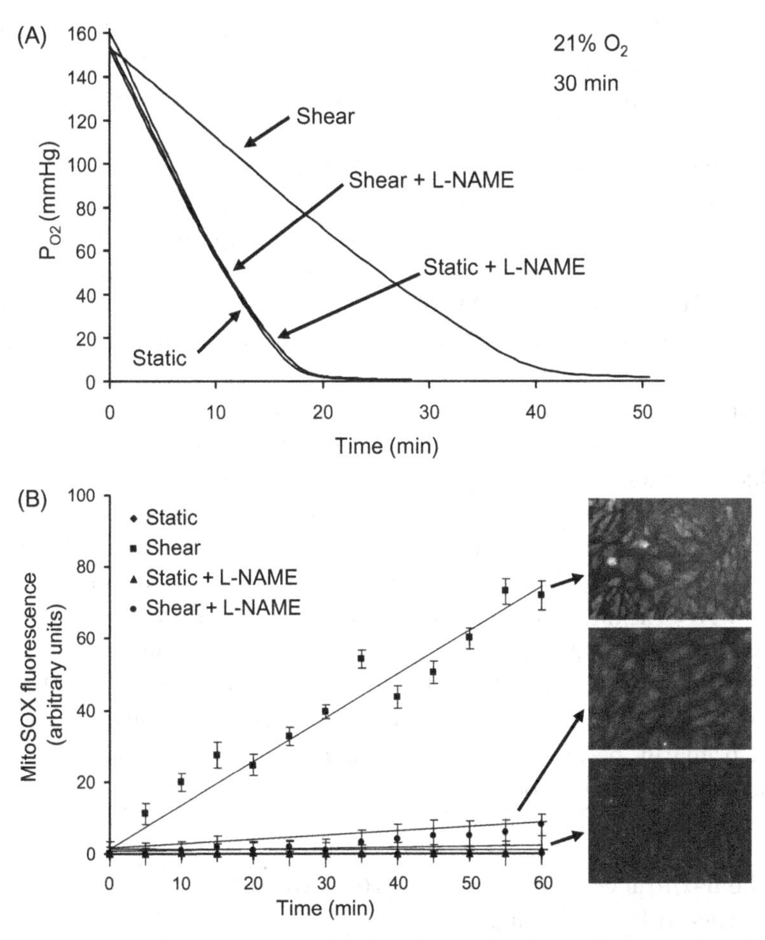

Fig. 3. Regulation of EC respiration (A) and mitochondrial $O_2^{\cdot-}$ production (B) by shear-induced NO. (A) BAECs were either sheared (10 dynes/cm^2, 30 min, 21% O_2) or left static in the incubator. Some EC monolayers were preincubated and either sheared or left static in the presence of L-NAME (100 μM). P_{O2} vs. time was measured on EC suspensions (10^7/ml) using EPR oximetry, and representative data are shown. The slope of the linear portion represents the O_2 consumption rate. (B) HUVECs were preincubated with mitoSOX (2 μM, 10 min) and fluorescence images (510 nm excitation/580 nm emission) were obtained in real-time during shear (10 dynes/cm^2, 60 min, 21% O_2) or static exposure using an inverted Nikon microscope (40x). Some monolayers were preincubated and either sheared or left static in the presence of L-NAME (500 μM). Digital images from $\geq$3 fields of view were collected per experiment. The mean fluorescence/image was calculated with Nikon Elements software, averaged over the images from the same experiment, and normalized with respect to static control. Data from a characteristic experiment are shown as mean $\pm$ SE. On the right, representative digital images collected at 60 min of shear, shear + L-NAME and static are shown (static + L-NAME was the same as static).

(Kissner *et al.*, 1997)) than with MnSOD ($k_2 = 2.3 \times 10^9\,M^{-1}\,s^{-1}$ (Klug *et al.*, 1972)), transfection with Ad.MnSOD may result in high enough MnSOD levels to allow for MnSOD to outcompete NO and prevent $ONOO^-$ formation.

MitoSOX red (a commercially available mitochondria-targeted $O_2^{\cdot-}$-specific probe) fluorescence showed that mitochondrial $O_2^{\cdot-}$ levels are increased in parallel with the P_{O2} during shear exposure, and the shear-induced NO is, at least in part, responsible for the generation of $O_2^{\cdot-}$ by the ETC ((Jones *et al.*, 2008); Fig. 3B shows the effect of L-NAME on the mitochondrial $O_2^{\cdot-}$ levels of sheared ECs). Both findings agree with the literature: Hyperoxia is known to increase the $O_2^{\cdot-}$ generation by the ETC (Brueckl *et al.*, 2006; Sanders *et al.*, 1993). Mitochondrial utilization of excess NO is known to involve QH_2 oxidation that increases the $O_2^{\cdot-}$ production, and $ONOO^-$ formation that, via inhibition of the ETC at multiple sites, further amplifies the $O_2^{\cdot-}$ generation (Carreras and Poderoso, 2007; Poderoso *et al.*, 1996; Poderoso *et al.*, 1999). Measurements of the levels of NO metabolites in the perfusate (an index of NO production), using a NO chemiluminescence analyzer, showed that NO production is slightly increased when ECs are sheared at 21% O_2 compared to when they are sheared at 5% or 10% O_2 (Jones *et al.*, 2008). Higher NO levels at the higher P_{O2} may contribute to the increased $O_2^{\cdot-}$ generation by the ETC, primarily because they would enhance the shear-induced $ONOO^-$ formation inside the mitochondria.

4. Shear-Induced Mitochondrial ROS Initiate Intracellular Signaling

Although the functional significance of mitochondrial ROS in ECs has received little attention, it is well documented that EC mitochondrial $O_2^{\cdot-}$ production from ETC complexes I and III is responsible for the shear-induced dilation in human coronary arterioles (Liu *et al.*, 2003; Zhang and Gutterman, 2007). It is also known that, during cultured EC exposure to cyclic strain, mitochondrial ROS mediate the activation of nuclear factor-kB and upregulation of vascular cell adhesion molecule-1 (Ali *et al.*, 2004). In eNOS-transfected EC lines, the regulation of respiration by NO was shown to provide protection against H_2O_2-mediated injury and death (Paxinou *et al.*, 2001) possibly due to NO-mediated maintenance of the $\Delta\Psi_m$ and prevention of apoptosis (Beltran *et al.*, 2000).

NF-E2-related factor 2 (Nrf2) is a transcription factor that, upon activation by oxidative stress, translocates to the nucleus, binds to the antioxidant response element (ARE) and activates transcription of the cytoprotective phase II genes, including heme oxygenase-1 (HO-1). Under physiological conditions, Kelch-like ECH-associated protein 1 (Keap1), a suppressor that binds to Nrf2, retains it in the cytoplasm and promotes its proteasomal degradation. Under oxidative stress, lipid oxidation products, such as the electrophilic lipid 15-deoxy-$\Delta^{12,14}$-prostaglandin J_2 (15d-PGJ_2), are thought to bind to Keap1 and cause alkylation of its critical cysteine thiols rendering it unable to repress Nrf2. Nrf2 activation may also occur when the inducers or their metabolites stimulate Nrf2 phosphorylation through redox-sensitive protein kinases, which triggers its dissociation from Keap1, its nuclear translocation and initiation of ARE-dependent transcription (Nguyen *et al.*, 2004; Ryter *et al.*, 2006). HO-1 expression data from sheared HUVECs suggested that xanthine oxidase-, NAD(P)H oxidase- and mitochondria-derived $O_2^{\cdot-}$, but not NO, mediates HO-1 expression (Warabi *et al.*, 2007).

Our group showed that, in sheared BAECs, both the endogenous NO and the mitochondria-derived H_2O_2 play an important role in the signaling pathways leading to HO-1 upregulation (Han *et al.*, 2009). ECs were sheared (10 dynes/cm^2, 6 h, 21% O_2) in the presence of L-NAME, the ROS scavengers N-acetyl-L-cysteine (NAC) and ebselen, the mitochondrial ETC inhibitors rotenone, myxothiazol and antimycin A, and a mitochondria-targeted antioxidant peptide Szeto-Schiller (SS)-31 (D-Arg-Dmt-Lys-Phe-NH_2; Dmt = 2′,6′-dimethyltyrosine) that scavenges mitochondrial $O_2^{\cdot-}$, H_2O_2, $ONOO^-$ and $OH^{\cdot}$ (Szeto, 2008). Based on the effects of these compounds on shear-induced mitoSOX fluorescence and HO-1 protein expression, it was concluded that the EC mitochondria-derived H_2O_2 diffuses to the cytosol where it initiates oxidative signaling leading to HO-1 upregulation (Han *et al.*, 2009). Besides its effect on the ETC, NO may also directly contribute to Nrf2 activation by modifying the Keap1 critical thiols via *S*-nitrosylation (Buckley *et al.*, 2008).

5. Cultured EC Exposure to H/RO Causes Mitochondrial and Cell Dysfunction

I/RP-induced EC injury is believed to be self-inflicted resulting from a burst of $ONOO^-$ formation upon the onset of RP and, due to decreased bioavailable NO, it predisposes ECs to increased neutrophil adhesion (Ferdinandy and Schulz, 2003; Wang and Zweier, 1996). In agreement to that, bolus injections of $ONOO^-$ into isolated hearts were shown to acutely inhibit EC-dependent coronary vasodilation (Villa *et al.*, 1994). Furthermore, in a rat model of splanchnic artery occlusion/RP, use of an $ONOO^-$ decomposition catalyst was shown to limit the post-ischemic EC inflammatory response (Cuzzocrea *et al.*, 2000).

The specific contribution of mitochondrial ROS/RNS in the EC dysfunction can only be derived from studies with H (1–3% O_2) or anoxia (A; 0% O_2)/RO (21% O_2)-treated cells (an *in vitro* equivalent of the *in vivo* I/RP). In H or A/RO-exposed ECs, the cytosolic xanthine oxidase (XO) and the plasma membrane-bound NAD(P)H oxidase were identified as the major sources of cellular $O_2^{\cdot-}$ production (Ng *et al.*, 2002; Zulueta *et al.*, 1997; Zweier *et al.*, 1994). However, more recent evidence suggested that the mitochondria are also responsible for ROS production following H or A (1–2 h)/RO (1 h) of cultured ECs, the ROS release site is the ETC complex III, and the neutrophil-EC adhesion at prolonged RO (10 h) is mediated by the EC mitochondrial ROS production (Ichikawa *et al.*, 1997; Ichikawa *et al.*, 2004; Therade-Matharan *et al.*, 2004). RO following H (4 h) induced loss of mitochondrial $\Delta\Psi_m$ and cytochrome c release (the latter at 18 h of RO) suggesting the mitochondria as the initiation site of H/RO-induced EC apoptosis (Dhar-Mascareno *et al.*, 2005). Even during H, cultured ECs paradoxically generate mitochondrial ROS (Pearlstein *et al.*, 2002; Sanders *et al.*, 1993). It seems that, under H, low concentrations of NO are still produced and NO inhibits complex IV resulting in increased $O_2^{\cdot-}$ generation by the ETC (Palacios-Callender *et al.*, 2004; Quintero *et al.*, 2006). The NO-dependent mitochondrial ROS were shown to activate the AMP-activated protein kinase, a key regulator of cellular bioenergetics (Quintero *et al.*, 2006).

6. I/RP-Induced Mitochondrial Oxidative Stress Leads to Cardiomyocyte/Heart Injury

Ischemic heart disease secondary to acute myocardial infarction is among the most prevalent health problems in the world and a major cause of morbidity and mortality. While timely RP of ischemic myocardium is essential for myocardial salvage, RP results in myocardial damage associated with EC dysfunction in the microcirculation (Carden and

Granger, 2000; Granger and Korthuis, 1995). In arterioles, the dysfunction is manifested as an impaired NO-mediated relaxation of smooth muscle cells, due to reduced NO bioactivity. In capillaries, it is manifested as increased filtration of fluid to the interstitium, a result of reduced bioavailable NO, and as a reduction in the number of perfused capillaries. The latter results from plugging of capillaries ("no reflow") due to trapping of activated neutrophils and microvasculature compression due to accumulation of interstitial fluid in the tissue (Carden and Granger, 2000; Granger and Korthuis, 1995). Neutrophil adhesion and transmigration occurs in postcapillary venules, and inhibition of neutrophil adhesion is known to reduce myocardial injury (Entman and Smith, 1994; Hawkins *et al.*, 1996; Jordan *et al.*, 1999; Ma *et al.*, 1992; Weyrich *et al.*, 1993).

The most likely mechanism for EC dysfunction is that of reduced NO bioavailability as a result of its interaction with $O_2^{\cdot-}$ (Moncada and Higgs, 2006; Zweier and Talukder, 2006). Using direct EPR methods, Wang and Zweier were the first to measure NO and $O_2^{\cdot-}$ production in the postischemic rat heart: They showed that production of both NO and $O_2^{\cdot-}$ is increased and that these react to form $ONOO^-$ resulting in protein nitration and cell injury (Wang and Zweier, 1996). In *in vivo* rat and dog I/RP models and in human hearts following cardiopulmonary bypass, the concentration of nitrotyrosine, a footprint of $ONOO^-$ formation, is increased and blocking its formation is cardioprotective (Hayashi *et al.*, 2000; Liu *et al.*, 1997; Yasmin *et al.*, 1997; Zhang *et al.*, 2001). It is thought that small amounts of NO released by eNOS are beneficial; high NO doses released following the expression of an inducible NOS (iNOS) in postischemic myocardium lead to enhanced $ONOO^-$ formation and are harmful (Feng *et al.*, 2001; Jugdutt, 2002; Kim *et al.*, 1999). However, there is controversy even regarding the effect of eNOS-derived NO on myocardial I/RP injury with some studies finding protection in eNOS knockout mice and some cardiac injury (Janssens *et al.*, 2004; Sharp *et al.*, 2002). Zweier's group recently showed that eNOS-derived NO during the early phase of RP following coronary ligation in mice inhibits tissue respiratory complex I activity, suppresses O_2 consumption and is responsible for $ONOO^-$-mediated protein tyrosine nitration (Zhao *et al.*, 2005).

Since inactivation of respiratory complex I is found to be associated with I/RP, complex I is a source of mitochondrial ROS upon RP (Ambrosio *et al.*, 1993; Hardy *et al.*, 1990; Paradies *et al.*, 2004). The conditions that form during early RP (characterized by high NADH, high

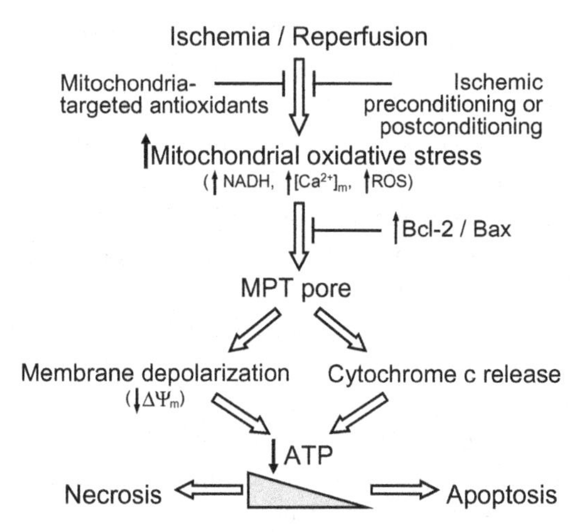

Fig. 4. Overview of the I/RP-induced signaling pathway and cell fate. Early at RP, mitochondrial oxidative stress activates the MPT pore, which leads to either cell necrosis or apoptosis depending on the availability of ATP.

intramitochondrial Ca^{2+} levels, NO/RNS-mediated inhibition of the ETC and ROS production) induce the mitochondrial permeability transition (MPT) pore opening (Halestrap *et al.*, 2004; Kim *et al.*, 2003) (Fig. 4). The MPT pore is a high conductance channel under the control of the anti- and pro-apoptotic members of the Bcl-2/Bax family. Its opening causes an increase in the permeability of the inner membrane (depolarization), inhibition of ATP synthesis, swelling of the matrix and cytochrome c release. If the onset of the MPT is widespread and glycolytic ATP sources are unavailable, the cell becomes profoundly ATP depleted, which leads to necrotic cell death. If the MPT progresses slowly or it does not involve all mitochondria in a cell and ATP partially recovers due to glycolysis, then apoptosis develops (Halestrap *et al.*, 2004; Kim *et al.*, 2003). Mitochondrial oxidative damage due to low $ONOO^-$ fluxes can be repaired, but, at large fluxes, oxidation/nitration reactions of critical targets predominate (inactivation of ETC complexes and ATP synthase) initiating a cascade of events leading to MTP pore opening, which promotes mitochondrial signaling of cell death (Radi *et al.*, 2002).

Minimization of mitochondrial $ONOO^-$ formation is critical because $ONOO^-$ irreversibly inhibits respiration, especially at the level of complex I leading to enhanced ROS formation and mitochondrial oxidative stress.

This agrees with the fact that MnSOD overexpression prevented protein nitration and neural apoptosis in cerebral ischemia in transgenic mice (Keller *et al.*, 1998) and protected cardiomyocytes from cell death following coronary artery I/RP in rats (Yang *et al.*, 2003). Incubating cells or administering general antioxidants, such as vitamin E, to animals and humans may fail to achieve significant concentrations inside the mitochondria. Research efforts to reduce the mitochondrial oxidative stress are currently being directed towards (Fig. 4): (a) Testing mitochondria-targeted antioxidants (Murphy, 2001; Sheu *et al.*, 2006; Szeto, 2006) that have shown promise in *ex vivo* heart models of I/RP (Adlam *et al.*, 2005; Wu *et al.*, 2002; Zhao *et al.*, 2004). (b) Understanding the mechanisms of cardioprotection of ischemic postconditioning (brief periods of RP/I following I and prior to prolonged RP), a therapy that is clinically feasible and was found by some groups to preserve cardiac function in animal I/RP models (Zhao *et al.*, 2003). Ischemic preconditioning (brief periods of I/RP prior to prolonged I/RP) has been studied extensively, and it is thought that it attenuates the NO formation during I/RP (Csonka *et al.*, 1999), and the NO and mitochondrial ROS formed during preconditioning protect the myocardium during I/RP (Das and Sarkar, 2003; Lebuffe *et al.*, 2003; Pain *et al.*, 2000).

7. Understanding the Mechanisms of EC Dysfunction in Cardiac I/RP

The conditions that lead to $O_2^{\cdot -}$ production by the mitochondrial ETC require reduced e^- transport centers in complexes I, II and III and the presence of O_2 to allow 1 e^- reduction to $O_2^{\cdot -}$. During ischemia, the supply of O_2 is diminished, e^- flux through the ETC stumbles, and NADH accumulates. Excess NADH inhibits the entry of pyruvate into the tricarboxylic acid (TCA) cycle and oxidative phosphorylation ceases, such that, when RP delivers O_2 in excess, the $O_2^{\cdot -}$ production by the ETC accelerates (Murphy, 2009; Riess *et al.*, 2002).

EC dysfunction appears to occur very early after cardiac RP. It is thought to be preceded by endogenous $O_2^{\cdot -}$ generation, and it is followed by a decrease in endothelium-dependent dilation suggesting that endothelial ROS may trigger the EC injury (Carden and Granger, 2000; Tsao *et al.*, 1990). In later times, neutrophils adhere to the postischemic endothelium, and the EC dysfunction is amplified by neutrophil-released products, such as ROS, cytokines, proteases and lipid mediators (Carden and Granger, 2000). Immunohistological studies using antibodies against activated caspases 8 and 9 showed that the mitochondrial pathway of apoptosis was activated in postischemic ECs of isolated rat hearts suggesting that the EC injury may be a consequence of mitochondrial oxidative stress (Scarabelli *et al.*, 2002). However, using either I/RP-exposed buffer-perfused hearts or *in vivo* hearts of anesthetized or awake animals, it is very difficult to understand the role of mitochondrial ROS in the EC dysfunction, because ROS originate from various sources besides mitochondria and also from different cell types in myocardial tissue (Davidson and Duchen, 2007). Another reason why postischemic EC mitochondria have been overlooked is that isolation protocols yield primarily mitochondria from cardiomyocytes. Similarly, it is difficult to determine the role of eNOS-derived NO in the EC dysfunction, because different NOS isoforms from various cell types are involved in determining the I/RP outcome, and eNOS gene knockouts in mice are counteracted by compensatory changes in other NOS isoforms (Schulz *et al.*, 2004).

By exposing cultured ECs to shear stress at atmospheric or lower P_{O2} and quantifying mitochondrial respiration and $O_2^{\cdot -}$ production (Han *et al.*, 2007; Jones *et al.*, 2008), we found that flow reproduces some aspects of the RP-induced EC injury, namely the $NO/ONOO^-$-mediated inhibition of respiration and resultant mitochondrial $O_2^{\cdot -}$ generation. H/RO studies of cultured ECs do not include the flow component that is essential in the RP phase of I/RP, and, as a result, do not reproduce the shear-induced NO generation and mitochondrial ROS/RNS production upon RP. It seems appropriate to develop and study *in vitro* equivalents of I/RP, where ECs will be exposed to ischemia, defined by no flow, no/low O_2, no glucose/nutrients, with or without acidosis, followed by RP, defined by reintroduction of flow and O_2, in the presence of glucose/nutrients and physiologic pH. Even better, the ECs should be flow-preconditioned at physiologic P_{O2}, and the RP phase of I/RP should also be at physiologic P_{O2}. When we exposed ECs to *in vitro* ischemia (no flow, A, no glucose/serum for 2 h)/RP (10 dynes/cm^2, 21% O_2, regular media for 1 h), I/RP resulted in much higher nitrotyrosine staining ($ONOO^-$ levels) in the mitochondria compared to shear alone (Fig. 5) suggesting that the inclusion of the flow upon RP may better simulate the I/RP-induced EC injury.

Consistent with the idea that carefully designed *in vitro* flow studies may provide useful cellular/subcellular information, our finding that flow

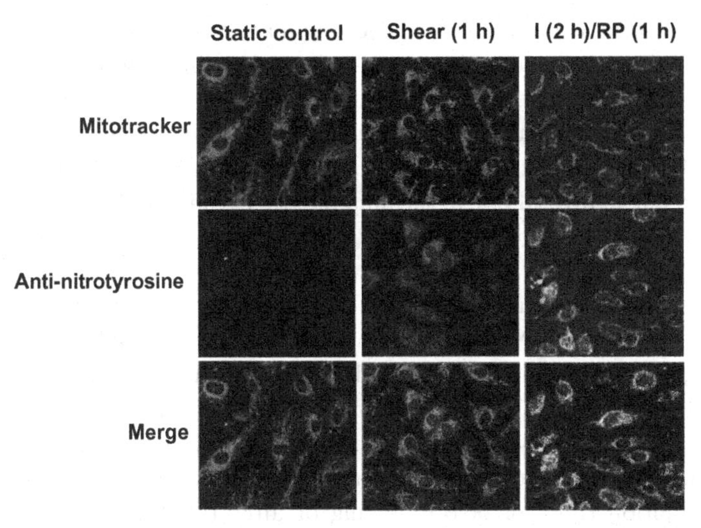

Fig. 5. Either shear stress or *in vitro* I/RP causes $ONOO^-$ formation (nitrotyrosine staining) in EC mitochondria, but I/RP causes much higher levels of $ONOO^-$ formation compared to shear stress. At the end of each treatment, either static incubation in basal medium for 1 h, shear at 10 dynes/cm^2 for 1 h under 21% O_2, or I (static incubation under A and glucose deprivation for 2 h) followed by RP (shear at 10 dynes/cm^2 for 1 h under 21% O_2), HUVEC monolayers were loaded with Mitotracker Deep Red (that stains mitochondria), fixed and stained for nitrotyrosine (the secondary antibody was Alexa 488-conjugated). Fluorescence images were acquired using confocal microscopy (40×) and were merged in order to determine whether the increase in nitrotyrosine signal colocalized in mitochondria.

at hyperoxic P_{O2} causes nitrosative stress to the EC mitochondria and inhibition of respiration (Jones *et al.*, 2008) agrees with findings from: (a) A mouse model of regional I, where the myocardial O_2 consumption in the risk region during RP was decreased because of NO-mediated inhibition of mitochondrial function (Zhao *et al.*, 2005). (b) Reperfused isolated heart models, where lowering the P_{O2} during early RP had a beneficial effect on mitochondrial bioenergetic parameters such as O_2 consumption, ETC complex activities, mitochondrial ROS production and lipid peroxidation, and improved cardiac performance (Massoudy *et al.*, 1999; Petrosillo *et al.*, 2005). (c) Animal models of brain injury caused by cardiac arrest, where the use of lower P_{O2} during resuscitation improved neurologic outcomes (Fiskum *et al.*, 2008).

Similarly to our studies with HUVECs or BAECs exposed to low arterial shear stress, cultured human microvascular ECs exposed to a shear stress level that is encountered in postcapillary venules (4 dynes/cm^2), at 21% O_2, were observed to have a NO-dependent increase in intracellular ROS generation (Jones *et al.*, 2007); the origin/subcellular localization of ROS was not examined. This would suggest that flow may be of importance even in the case of postcapillary venular ECs at the onset of RP. ROS are known to play a pivotal role in the inflammatory response that characterizes the I/RP-induced endothelial dysfunction in postcapillary venules (Carden and Granger, 2000; Granger and Korthuis, 1995).

Future work in our laboratory is aimed at increasing our knowledge of how endogenous NO regulates the EC death cascades (apoptosis, necrosis, and autophagy) via its effect on the mitochondria and other intracellular targets, by using *in vitro* I/RP experimental models. Only after we better understand these processes, can we decide on specifics of NO and/or antioxidant targeted therapy, such as the subcellular organelle, or intervention times of before, during or after I/RP, in order to better protect the vascular endothelium and preserve myocardial function.

Acknowledgments

We would like to thank Dr. J. L. Zweier from the Davis Heart & Lung Research Institute, Ohio State University, for a critical review of the manuscript, the previous and current members of our lab, Drs. Z. Han and G. Steinbaugh, for their scientific contributions, and the National Institutes of Health for funding (HL-91417 to B. R. Alevriadou).

References

1. Adlam, V. J., Harrison, J. C., Porteous, C. M., James, A. M., Smith, R. A., Murphy M. P., and Sammut I. A. (2005) Targeting an antioxidant to mitochondria decreases cardiac ischemia-reperfusion injury. *Faseb J* **19**, 1088–1095.
2. Ali, M. H., Pearlstein, D. P., Mathieu, C. E., and Schumacker, P. T. (2004) Mitochondrial requirement for endothelial responses to cyclic strain: implications for mechanotransduction. *Am J Physiol Lung Cell Mol Physiol* **287**, L486–496.
3. Ambrosio, G., Zweier, J. L., Duilio, C., Kuppusamy, P., Santoro, G., Elia, P. P., Tritto, I., Cirillo, P., Condorelli, M., Chiariello, M., *et al.* (1993) Evidence that mitochondrial respiration is a source of potentially toxic oxygen free radicals in intact rabbit hearts subjected to ischemia and reflow. *J Biol Chem* **268**, 18532–18541.

4. Azarov, I., Huang, K. T., Basu, S., Gladwin, M. T., Hogg, N., and Kim-Shapiro, D. B. (2005). Nitric oxide scavenging by red blood cells as a function of hematocrit and oxygenation. *J Biol Chem* **280**, 39024–39032.
5. Beltran, B., Mathur, A., Duchen, M. R., Erusalimsky, J. D., and Moncada, S. (2000) The effect of nitric oxide on cell respiration: A key to understanding its role in cell survival or death. *Proc Natl Acad Sci U S A* **97**, 14602–14607.
6. Boveris, A., and Cadenas, E. (2000) Mitochondrial production of hydrogen peroxide regulation by nitric oxide and the role of ubisemiquinone. *IUBMB Life* **50**, 245–250.
7. Brookes, P. S. (2004) Mitochondrial nitric oxide synthase. *Mitochondrion* **3**, 187–204.
8. Brown, G. C., and Borutaite, V. (2002) Nitric oxide inhibition of mitochondrial respiration and its role in cell death. *Free Radic Biol Med* **33**, 1440–1450.
9. Brown, G. C., and Borutaite, V. (2004) Inhibition of mitochondrial respiratory complex I by nitric oxide, peroxynitrite and S-nitrosothiols. *Biochim Biophys Acta* **1658**, 44–49.
10. Brueckl, C., Kaestle, S., Kerem, A., Habazettl, H., Krombach, F., Kuppe, H., and Kuebler, W. M. (2006). Hyperoxia-induced reactive oxygen species formation in pulmonary capillary endothelial cells *in situ*. *Am J Respir Cell Mol Biol* **34**, 453–463.
11. Buckley, B. J., Li, S., and Whorton, A. R. (2008) Keap1 modification and nuclear accumulation in response to S-nitrosocysteine. *Free Radic Biol Med* **44**, 692–698.
12. Cadenas, E. (2004) Mitochondrial free radical production and cell signaling. *Mol Aspects Med* **25**, 17–26.
13. Carden, D. L., and Granger, D. N. (2000) Pathophysiology of ischaemia-reperfusion injury. [Review]. *J Pathol* **190**, 255–266.
14. Carreras, M. C., and Poderoso, J. J. (2007) Mitochondrial nitric oxide in the signaling of cell integrated responses. *Am J Physiol Cell Physiol* **292**, C1569–1580.
15. Cassina, A., and Radi, R. (1996) Differential inhibitory action of nitric oxide and peroxynitrite on mitochondrial electron transport. *Arch Biochem Biophys* **328**, 309–316.
16. Cleeter, M. W., Cooper, J. M., Darley-Usmar, V. M., Moncada, S., and Schapira, A. H. (1994) Reversible inhibition of cytochrome c oxidase, the terminal enzyme of the mitochondrial respiratory chain, by nitric oxide. Implications for neurodegenerative diseases. *FEBS Lett* **345**, 50–54.
17. Clementi, E., Brown, G. C., Foxwell, N., and Moncada, S. (1999) On the mechanism by which vascular endothelial cells regulate their oxygen consumption. *Proc Natl Acad Sci U S A* **96**, 1559–1562.
18. Csonka, C., Szilvassy, Z., Fulop, F., Pali, T., Blasig, I. E., Tosaki, A., Schulz, R., and Ferdinandy, P. (1999) Classic preconditioning decreases the harmful accumulation of nitric oxide during ischemia and reperfusion in rat hearts. *Circulation* **100**, 2260–2266.

19. Cuzzocrea, S., Misko, T. P., Costantino, G., Mazzon, E., Micali, A., Caputi, A. P., Macarthur, H., and Salvemini, D. (2000) Beneficial effects of peroxynitrite decomposition catalyst in a rat model of splanchnic artery occlusion and reperfusion. *Faseb J* **14**, 1061–1072.
20. Das, B., and Sarkar, C. (2003) Cardiomyocyte mitochondrial KATP channels participate in the antiarrhythmic and antiinfarct effects of KATP activators during ischemia and reperfusion in an intact anesthetized rabbit model. *Pol J Pharmacol* **55**, 771–786.
21. Davidson, S. M., and Duchen, M. R. (2007) Endothelial mitochondria: contributing to vascular function and disease. *Circ Res.* **100**, 1128–1141.
22. Dhar-Mascareno, M., Carcamo, J. M., and Golde, D. W. (2005) Hypoxia-reoxygenation-induced mitochondrial damage and apoptosis in human endothelial cells are inhibited by vitamin C. *Free Radic Biol Med* **38**, 1311–1322.
23. Entman, M. L., and Smith, C. W. (1994) Postreperfusion inflammation: a model for reaction to injury in cardiovascular disease. *Cardiovasc Res* **28**, 1301–1311.
24. Feng, Q., Lu, X., Jones, D. L., Shen, J., and Arnold, J. M. (2001) Increased inducible nitric oxide synthase expression contributes to myocardial dysfunction and higher mortality after myocardial infarction in mice. *Circulation* **104**, 700–704.
25. Ferdinandy, P., and Schulz, R. (2003) Nitric oxide, superoxide, and peroxynitrite in myocardial ischaemia-reperfusion injury and preconditioning. *Br J Pharmacol* **138**, 532–543.
26. Fiskum, G., Danilov, C. A., Mehrabian, Z., Bambrick, L. L., Kristian, T., McKenna, M. C., Hopkins, I., Richards, E. M., and Rosenthal, R. E. (2008) Postischemic oxidative stress promotes mitochondrial metabolic failure in neurons and astrocytes. *Ann N Y Acad Sci* **1147**, 129–138.
27. Granger, D. N., and Korthuis, R. J. (1995) Physiologic mechanisms of post-ischemic tissue injury. [Review]. *Annu Rev Physiol* **57**, 311–332.
28. Gutteridge, J. M., and Halliwell, B. (2000) Free radicals and antioxidants in the year 2000. A historical look to the future. *Ann N Y Acad Sci* **899**, 136–147.
29. Halestrap, A. P., Clarke, S. J., and Javadov, S. A. (2004) Mitochondrial permeability transition pore opening during myocardial reperfusion–a target for cardioprotection. *Cardiovasc Res* **61**, 372–385.
30. Han, Z., Chen, Y. R., Jones, C. I. 3rd, Meenakshisundaram, G., Zweier, J. L., and Alevriadou, B. R. (2007) Shear-induced reactive nitrogen species inhibit mitochondrial respiratory complex activities in cultured vascular endothelial cells. *Am J Physiol Cell Physiol* **292**, C1103–1112.
31. Han, Z., Varadharaj, S., Giedt, R. J., Zweier, J. L., Szeto, H. H., and Alevriadou, B. R. (2009) Mitochondria-derived reactive oxygen species mediate heme oxygenase-1 expression in sheared endothelial cells. *J Pharmacol Exp Ther* **329**, 94–101.

32. Hardy, D. L., Clark, J. B., Darley-Usmar, V. M., and Smith, D. R. (1990) Reoxygenation of the hypoxic myocardium causes a mitochondrial complex I defect. *Biochem Soc Trans* **18**, 549.
33. Hawkins, H. K., Entman, M. L., Zhu, J. Y., Youker, K. A., Berens, K., Dore, M., and Smith, C. W. (1996) Acute inflammatory reaction after myocardial ischemic injury and reperfusion. Development and use of a neutrophil-specific antibody. *Am J Pathol* **148**, 1957–1969.
34. Hayashi, Y., Sawa, Y., Nishimura, M., Tojo, S. J., Fukuyama, N., Nakazawa, H., and Matsuda, H. (2000) P-selectin participates in cardiopulmonary bypass-induced inflammatory response in association with nitric oxide and peroxynitrite production. *J Thorac Cardiovasc Surg* **120**, 558–565.
35. Huddleson, J. P., Ahmad, N., Srinivasan, S., and Lingrel, J. B. (2005) Induction of KLF2 by fluid shear stress requires a novel promoter element activated by a phosphatidylinositol 3-kinase-dependent chromatin-remodeling pathway. *J Biol Chem* **280**, 23371–23379.
36. Ichikawa, H., Flores, S., Kvietys, P. R., Wolf, R. E., Yoshikawa, T., Granger, D. N., and Aw, T. Y. (1997) Molecular mechanisms of anoxia/reoxygenation-induced neutrophil adherence to cultured endothelial cells. *Circ Res* **81**, 922–931.
37. Ichikawa, H., Kokura, S., and Aw, T. Y. (2004) Role of endothelial mitochondria in oxidant production and modulation of neutrophil adherence. *J Vasc Res* **41**, 432–444.
38. Ilangovan, G., Zweier, J. L., and Kuppusamy, P. (2004) Microximetry: simultaneous determination of oxygen consumption and free radical production using electron paramagnetic resonance spectroscopy. *Methods Enzymol* **381**, 747–762.
39. Janssens, S., Pokreisz, P., Schoonjans, L., Pellens, M., Vermeersch, P., Tjwa, M., Jans, P., Scherrer-Crosbie, M., Picard, M. H., Szelid, Z., Gillijns, H., Van de Werf, F., Collen, D., and Bloch, K. D. (2004) Cardiomyocyte-specific overexpression of nitric oxide synthase 3 improves left ventricular performance and reduces compensatory hypertrophy after myocardial infarction. *Circ Res* **94**, 1256–1262.
40. Jin, Z.-G., Ueba, H., Tanimoto, T., Lungu, A. O., Frame, M. D., and Berk, B. C. (2003) Ligand-independent activation of vascular endothelial growth factor receptor 2 by fluid shear stress regulates activation of endothelial nitric oxide synthase. *Circ Res* **93**, 354–363.
41. Jones, C. I. 3rd, Han, Z., Presley, T., Varadharaj, S., Zweier, J. L., Ilangovan, G., and Alevriadou, B. R. (2008) Endothelial cell respiration is affected by the oxygen tension during shear exposure: role of mitochondrial peroxynitrite. *Am J Physiol Cell Physiol* **295**, C180–191.
42. Jones, C. I. 3rd, Zhu, H., Martin, S. F., Han, Z., Li, Y., and Alevriadou, B. R. (2007) Regulation of antioxidants and phase 2 enzymes by shear-induced reactive oxygen species in endothelial cells. *Ann Biomed Eng* **35**, 683–693.

43. Jordan, J. E., Zhao, Z. Q., and Vinten-Johansen, J. (1999) The role of neutrophils in myocardial ischemia-reperfusion injury [Review]. *Cardiovasc Res* **43**, 860–878.
44. Jugdutt, B. I. (2002) Nitric oxide and cardioprotection during ischemia-reperfusion. *Heart Fail Rev* **7**, 391–405.
45. Keller, J. N., Kindy, M. S., Holtsberg, F. W., St Clair, D. K., Yen, H. C., Germeyer, A., Steiner, S. M., Bruce-Keller, A. J., Hutchins, J. B., and Mattson, M. P. (1998) Mitochondrial manganese superoxide dismutase prevents neural apoptosis and reduces ischemic brain injury: suppression of peroxynitrite production, lipid peroxidation, and mitochondrial dysfunction. *J Neurosci* **18**, 687–697.
46. Kim, J. S., He, L., and Lemasters, J. J. (2003) Mitochondrial permeability transition: a common pathway to necrosis and apoptosis. *Biochem Biophys Res Commun* **304**, 463–470.
47. Kim, Y. M., Bombeck, C. A., and Billiar, T. R. (1999) Nitric oxide as a bifunctional regulator of apoptosis. *Circ Res.* **84**, 253–256.
48. Kissner, R., Nauser, T., Bugnon, P., Lye, P. G., and Koppenol, W. H. (1997) Formation and properties of peroxynitrite as studied by laser flash photolysis, high-pressure stopped-flow technique, and pulse radiolysis. *Chem Res Toxicol* **10**, 1285–1292.
49. Klug, D., Rabani, J., and Fridovich, I. (1972) A direct demonstration of the catalytic action of superoxide dismutase through the use of pulse radiolysis. *J Biol Chem* **247**, 4839–4842.
50. Kuchan, M. J., and Frangos, J. A. (1994) Role of calcium and calmodulin in flow-induced nitric oxide production in endothelial cells. *Am J Physiol* **266**, C628–636.
51. Lebuffe, G., Schumacker, P. T., Shao, Z. H., Anderson, T., Iwase, H., and Vanden Hoek, T. L. (2003) ROS and NO trigger early preconditioning: relationship to mitochondrial KATP channel. *Am J Physiol Heart Circ Physiol* **284**, H299–308.
52. Lenaz, G. (1998) Role of mitochondria in oxidative stress and ageing. *Biochim Biophys Acta* **1366**, 53–67.
53. Liu, P., Hock, C. E., Nagele, R., and Wong, P. Y. (1997) Formation of nitric oxide, superoxide, and peroxynitrite in myocardial ischemia-reperfusion injury in rats. *Am J Physiol* **272**, H2327–2336.
54. Liu, Y., Zhao, H., Li, H., Kalyanaraman, B., Nicolosi, A. C., and Gutterman, D. D. (2003) Mitochondrial sources of H_2O_2 generation play a key role in flow-mediated dilation in human coronary resistance arteries. *Circ Res* **93**, 573–580.
55. Loke, K. E., McConnell, P. I., Tuzman, J. M., Shesely, E. G., Smith, C. J., Stackpole, C. J., Thompson, C. I., Kaley, G., Wolin, M. S., and Hintze, T. H. (1999) Endogenous endothelial nitric oxide synthase-derived nitric oxide is a physiological regulator of myocardial oxygen consumption. *Circ Res* **84**, 840–845.

56. Ma, X. L., Lefer, D. J., Lefer, A. M., and Rothlein, R. (1992) Coronary endothelial and cardiac protective effects of a monoclonal antibody to intercellular adhesion molecule-1 in myocardial ischemia and reperfusion. *Circulation* **86**, 937–946.
57. Martin, S. F., Chatterjee, S. Parinandi, N., and Alevriadou, B. R. (2005) Rac1 inhibition protects against hypoxia/reoxygenation-induced lipid peroxidation in human vascular endothelial cells. *Vascul Pharmacol* **43**, 148–156.
58. Massoudy, P., Mempel, T., Raschke, P., and Becker, B. F. (1999) Reduction of oxygen delivery during post-ischemic reperfusion protects the isolated guinea pig heart. *Basic Res Cardiol* **94**, 231–237.
59. Moncada, S., and Higgs, E. A. (2006) The discovery of nitric oxide and its role in vascular biology. *Br J Pharmacol* **147**(Suppl 1), S193–201.
60. Muller, F. L., Liu, Y., and Van Remmen, H. (2004) Complex III releases superoxide to both sides of the inner mitochondrial membrane. *J Biol Chem* **279**, 49064–49073.
61. Murphy, M. P. (2001) Development of lipophilic cations as therapies for disorders due to mitochondrial dysfunction. *Expert Opin Biol Ther* **1**, 753–764.
62. Murphy, M. P. (2009) How mitochondria produce reactive oxygen species. *Biochem J* **417**, 1–13.
63. Ng, C. K., Deshpande, S. S., Irani, K., and Alevriadou, B. R. (2002) Adhesion of flowing monocytes to hypoxia-reoxygenation-exposed endothelial cells: role of Rac1, ROS, and VCAM-1. *Am J Physiol Cell Physiol* **283**, C93–102.
64. Nguyen, T., Yang, C. S., and Pickett, C. B. (2004) The pathways and molecular mechanisms regulating Nrf2 activation in response to chemical stress. *Free Radic Biol Med* **37**, 433–441.
65. Pain, T., Yang, X. M., Critz, S. D., Yue, Y., Nakano, A., Liu, G. S., Heusch, G., Cohen, M. V., and Downey, J. M. (2000) Opening of mitochondrial K(ATP) channels triggers the preconditioned state by generating free radicals. *Circ Res* **87**, 460–466.
66. Palacios-Callender, M., Quintero, M., Hollis, V. S., Springett, R. J., and Moncada, S. (2004) Endogenous NO regulates superoxide production at low oxygen concentrations by modifying the redox state of cytochrome c oxidase. *Proc Natl Acad Sci U S A* **101**, 7630–7635.
67. Paradies, G., Petrosillo, G., Pistolese, M., Di Venosa, N., Federici, A., and Ruggiero, F. M. (2004) Decrease in mitochondrial complex I activity in ischemic/reperfused rat heart: involvement of reactive oxygen species and cardiolipin. *Circ Res* **94**, 53–59.
68. Paxinou, E., Weisse, M., Chen, Q., Souza, J. M., Hertkorn, C., Selak, M., Daikhin, E., Yudkoff, M., Sowa, G., Sessa, W. C., and Ischiropoulos, H. (2001) Dynamic regulation of metabolism and respiration by endogenously produced nitric oxide protects against oxidative stress. *Proc Natl Acad Sci U S A* **98**, 11575–11580.

69. Pearlstein, D. P., Ali, M. H., Mungai, P. T., Hynes, K. L., Gewertz, B. L., and Schumacker, P. T. (2002) Role of mitochondrial oxidant generation in endothelial cell responses to hypoxia. *Arterioscler Thromb Vasc Biol* **22**, 566–573.
70. Petrosillo, G., Di Venosa, N., Ruggiero, F. M., Pistolese, M., D'Agostino, D., Tiravanti, E., Fiore, T., and Paradies, G. (2005) Mitochondrial dysfunction associated with cardiac ischemia/reperfusion can be attenuated by oxygen tension control. Role of oxygen-free radicals and cardiolipin. *Biochim Biophys Acta* **1710**, 78–86.
71. Poderoso, J. J., Carreras, M. C., Lisdero, C., Riobo, N., Schopfer, F., and Boveris, A. (1996) Nitric oxide inhibits electron transfer and increases superoxide radical production in rat heart mitochondria and submitochondrial particles. *Arch Biochem Biophys* **328**, 85–92.
72. Poderoso, J. J., Lisdero, C., Schopfer, F., Riobo, N., Carreras, M. C., Cadenas, E., and Boveris, A. (1999) The regulation of mitochondrial oxygen uptake by redox reactions involving nitric oxide and ubiquinol. *J Biol Chem* **274**, 37709–37716.
73. Quintero, M., Colombo, S. L., Godfrey, A., and Moncada, S. (2006) Mitochondria as signaling organelles in the vascular endothelium. *Proc Natl Acad Sci U S A* **103**, 5379–5384.
74. Radi, R., Cassina, A., Hodara, R., Quijano, C., and Castro, L. (2002) Peroxynitrite reactions and formation in mitochondria. *Free Radic Biol Med* **33**, 1451–1464.
75. Riess, M. L., Camara, A. K., Chen, Q., Novalija, E., Rhodes, S. S., and Stowe, D. F. (2002). Altered NADH and improved function by anesthetic and ischemic preconditioning in guinea pig intact hearts. *Am J Physiol Heart Circ Physiol* **283**, H53–60.
76. Riobo, N. A., Clementi, E., Melani, M., Boveris, A., Cadenas, E., Moncada, S., and Poderoso, J. J. (2001) Nitric oxide inhibits mitochondrial NADH:ubiquinone reductase activity through peroxynitrite formation. *Biochem J* **359**, 139–145.
77. Ryter, S. W., Alam, J., and Choi, A. M. (2006) Heme oxygenase-1/carbon monoxide: from basic science to therapeutic applications. *Physiol Rev* **86**, 583–650.
78. Sanders, S. P., Zweier, J. L., Kuppusamy, P., Harrison, S. J., Bassett, D. J., Gabrielson, E. W., and Sylvester, J. T. (1993) Hyperoxic sheep pulmonary microvascular endothelial cells generate free radicals via mitochondrial electron transport. *J Clin Invest* **91**, 46–52.
79. Scarabelli, T. M., Stephanou, A., Pasini, E., Comini, L., Raddino, R., Knight, R. A., and Latchman, D. S. (2002) Different signaling pathways induce apoptosis in endothelial cells and cardiac myocytes during ischemia/reperfusion injury. *Circ Res* **90**, 745–748.
80. Schulz, R., Kelm, M., and Heusch, G. (2004) Nitric oxide in myocardial ischemia/reperfusion injury. *Cardiovasc Res* **61**, 402–413.

81. Sharp, B. R., Jones, S. P., Rimmer, D. M., and Lefer, D. J. (2002) Differential response to myocardial reperfusion injury in eNOS-deficient mice. *Am J Physiol Heart Circ Physiol* **282**, H2422–2426.
82. Shen, W., Hintze, T. H., and Wolin, M. S. (1995) Nitric oxide. An important signaling mechanism between vascular endothelium and parenchymal cells in the regulation of oxygen consumption. *Circulation* **92**, 3505–3512.
83. Sheu, S. S., Nauduri, D., and Anders, M. W. (2006) Targeting antioxidants to mitochondria: a new therapeutic direction. *Biochim Biophys Acta* **1762**, 256–265.
84. Szeto, H. H. (2006) Mitochondria-targeted peptide antioxidants: novel neuroprotective agents. *Aaps J* **8**, E521–531.
85. Szeto, H. H. (2008) Mitochondria-targeted cytoprotective peptides for ischemia-reperfusion injury. *Antioxid Redox Signal* **10**, 601–619.
86. Therade-Matharan, S., Laemmel, E., Duranteau, J., and Vicaut, E. (2004) Reoxygenation after hypoxia and glucose depletion causes reactive oxygen species production by mitochondria in HUVEC. *Am J Physiol Regul Integr Comp Physiol* **287**, R1037–1043.
87. Tsai, A. G., Johnson, P. C., and Intaglietta, M. (2003) Oxygen gradients in the microcirculation. *Physiol Rev* **83**, 933–963.
88. Tsao, P. S., Aoki, N., Lefer, D. J., Johnson, G. 3rd, and Lefer, A. M. (1990) Time course of endothelial dysfunction and myocardial injury during myocardial ischemia and reperfusion in the cat. *Circulation* **82**, 1402–1412.
89. Turrens, J. F., and Boveris, A. (1980) Generation of superoxide anion by the NADH dehydrogenase of bovine heart mitochondria. *Biochem J* **191**, 421–427.
90. Turrens, J. F., Freeman, B. A., Levitt, J. G., and Crapo, J. D. (1982) The effect of hyperoxia on superoxide production by lung submitochondrial particles. *Arch Biochem Biophys* **217**, 401–410.
91. Villa, L. M., Salas, E., Darley-Usmar, V. M., Radomski, M. W., and Moncada, S. (1994) Peroxynitrite induces both vasodilatation and impaired vascular relaxation in the isolated perfused rat heart. *Proc Natl Acad Sci U S A* **91**, 12383–12387.
92. Wallace, D. C. (2005) A mitochondrial paradigm of metabolic and degenerative diseases, aging, and cancer: a dawn for evolutionary medicine. *Annu Rev Genet* **39**, 359–407.
93. Wang, P., and Zweier, J. L. (1996) Measurement of nitric oxide and peroxynitrite generation in the postischemic heart. *J Biol Chem* **271**, 29223–29230.
94. Warabi, E., Takabe, W., Minami, T., Inoue, K., Itoh, K., Yamamoto, M., Ishii, T., Kodama, T., and Noguchi, N. (2007) Shear stress stabilizes NF-E2-related factor 2 and induces antioxidant genes in endothelial cells: Role of reactive oxygen/nitrogen species. *Free Radic Biol Med* **42**, 260–269.

95. Weyrich, A. S., Ma, X. L., Lefer, D. J., Albertine, K. H., and Lefer, A. M. (1993) In vivo neutralization of P-selectin protects feline heart and endothelium in myocardial ischemia and reperfusion injury. *J Clin Invest* **91**, 2620–2629.
96. Wu, D., Soong, Y., Zhao, G. M., and Szeto, H. H. (2002) A highly potent peptide analgesic that protects against ischemia-reperfusion-induced myocardial stunning. *Am J Physiol Heart Circ Physiol* **283**, H783–791.
97. Xie, Y. W., and Wolin, M. S. (1996) Role of nitric oxide and its interaction with superoxide in the suppression of cardiac muscle mitochondrial respiration. Involvement in response to hypoxia/reoxygenation. *Circulation* **94**, 2580–2586.
98. Yang, J., Marden, J. J., Fan, C., Sanlioglu, S., Weiss, R. M., Ritchie, T. C., Davisson, R. L., and Engelhardt, J. F. (2003) Genetic redox preconditioning differentially modulates AP-1 and NF kappa B responses following cardiac ischemia/reperfusion injury and protects against necrosis and apoptosis. *Mol Ther* **7**, 341–353.
99. Yasmin, W., Strynadka, K. D., and Schulz, R. (1997) Generation of peroxynitrite contributes to ischemia-reperfusion injury in isolated rat hearts. *Cardiovasc Res.* **33**, 422–432.
100. Yeh, L. H., Kinsey, A. M., Chatterjee, S., and Alevriadou, B. R. (2001) Lactosylceramide mediates shear-induced endothelial superoxide production and intercellular adhesion molecule-1 expression. *J Vasc Res* **38**, 551–559.
101. Yeh, L. H., Park, Y. J., Hansalia, R. J., Ahmed, I. S., Deshpande, S. S., Goldschmidt-Clermont, P. J., Irani, K., and Alevriadou, B. R. (1999) Shear-induced tyrosine phosphorylation in endothelial cells requires Rac1-dependent production of ROS. *Am J Physiol* **276**, C838–847.
102. Zhang, D. X., and Gutterman, D. D. (2007) Mitochondrial reactive oxygen species-mediated signaling in endothelial cells. *Am J Physiol Heart Circ Physiol* **292**, H2023–2031.
103. Zhang, Y., Bissing, J. W., Xu, L., Ryan, A. J., Martin, S. M., Miller, F. J. Jr., Kregel, K. C., Buettner, G. R., and Kerber, R. E. (2001) Nitric oxide synthase inhibitors decrease coronary sinus-free radical concentration and ameliorate myocardial stunning in an ischemia-reperfusion model. *J Am Coll Cardiol* **38**, 546–554.
104. Zhao, K., Zhao, G. M., Wu, D., Soong, Y., Birk, A. V., Schiller, P. W., and Szeto, H. H. (2004) Cell-permeable peptide antioxidants targeted to inner mitochondrial membrane inhibit mitochondrial swelling, oxidative cell death, and reperfusion injury. *J Biol Chem* **279**, 34682–34690.
105. Zhao, X., He, G., Chen, Y. R., Pandian, R. P., Kuppusamy, P., and Zweier, J. L. (2005) Endothelium-derived nitric oxide regulates postischemic myocardial oxygenation and oxygen consumption by modulation of mitochondrial electron transport. *Circulation* **111**, 2966–2972.
106. Zhao, Z. Q., Corvera, J. S., Halkos, M. E., Kerendi, F., Wang, N. P., Guyton, R. A., and Vinten-Johansen, J. (2003) Inhibition of myocardial injury by ischemic postconditioning during reperfusion: comparison

with ischemic preconditioning. *Am J Physiol Heart Circ Physiol* **285**, H579–588.

107. Zulueta, J. J., Sawhney, R., Yu, F. S., Cote, C. C., and Hassoun, P. M. (1997) Intracellular generation of reactive oxygen species in endothelial cells exposed to anoxia-reoxygenation. *Am J Physiol* **272**, L897–902.
108. Zweier, J. L., Kuppusamy, P., Thompson-Gorman, S., Klunk, D., and Lutty, G. A. (1994) Measurement and characterization of free radical generation in reoxygenated human endothelial cells. *Am J Physiol* **266**, C700–708.
109. Zweier, J. L., and Talukder, M. A. (2006) The role of oxidants and free radicals in reperfusion injury. *Cardiovasc Res* **70**, 181–190.

Chapter 7

GENOMIC APPROACHES TO ENDOTHELIAL CELL PHENOTYPING

ANTHONY G. PASSERINI
Department of Biomedical Engineering, University of California, Davis,
451 E. Health Sciences Dr. (GBSF 3319), Davis, CA 95616
agpasserini@ucdavis.edu

In this chapter we highlight the contributions of genomics approaches to our understanding of endothelial phenotypic heterogeneity, particularly with respect to the influence of arterial hemodynamics and endothelial mechanobiology on normal vascular physiology and susceptibility to disease. Microarray approaches, experimental design and data analysis are reviewed so far as necessary to introduce the reader to the most important considerations, and a case study is presented to illustrate a typical workflow and analysis.

1. Introduction

Rapid advances in biotechnology, spurred in part by efforts to sequence the human genome at the turn of the century, have led to the development of powerful high-throughput approaches to evaluate gene expression, protein expression and activity that serve as valuable tools for diagnostic and research use. Over the past several years, researchers have applied these genomics-based tools to the study of endothelial cell heterogeneity with the goals of understanding the molecular basis of endothelial physiology and pathophysiology, including the role that mechanobiology plays in endothelial function and disease.

The use of genomics approaches is a bit of a double-edged sword. On the one hand, these approaches provide the opportunity to rapidly gain a global perspective on the state of the cell–providing insight into how genes vary together, how pathways are recruited, etc. On the other hand, they result in large amounts of data from which to extract biological meaning, requiring considerable effort and the use of complex analyses. Compared to single gene approaches like qPCR, microarray data are messy and can present a formidable statistical challenge. The rapid concomitant evolution of bioinformatics tools has been necessary to support the analysis of the large data sets and address the unique statistical challenges presented by these approaches. Careful consideration must also be given *a priori* to the design of such experiments in order to maximize the probability of extracting statistically useful information that reflects biology.

Studies involving microarrays and other high-throughput approaches are often criticized for being too discovery-based, thus failing to provide any detailed mechanistic insight into the biology of the cell. In fact it is true that many early microarray experiments were poorly designed and executed, resulting in nothing more than extended lists of genes chosen on the basis of limited observation and without any sort of statistical confidence. The field of bioinformatics has provided researchers with the tools for processing these data and extracting differentially expressed genes with statistical confidence. It is now also well recognized that microarray studies as a discovery tool can no longer stand alone, but must be followed-up by validation of the most promising gene candidates (e.g. using the gold standard for single gene expression analysis of qPCR) and by more mechanistically-driven studies to evaluate protein expression and activity, signaling pathways and their inhibition. More recently, increasingly user friendly data analysis and pathway mining approaches are making it easier for the researcher to focus in on key genes or pathways for follow-up mechanistic analysis. These approaches thus make for powerful hypothesis-generating tools. Furthermore, the global analysis approach provides a useful perspective for making observations related to cell function that would otherwise be missed. One goal of this chapter is to highlight some of the insights gained into endothelial function through the use of such approaches.

The purpose of this chapter is to review how the use of microarrays and other genomics approaches have led to recent insight into endothelial heterogeneity, physiology and susceptibility to disease. We start with a brief introduction of microarrays and other high-throughput methods, along with considerations for experimental design and data analysis. We will make use of a case study to illustrate a typical workflow and analysis. Specifically, we will demonstrate how the results of analysis of microarray data for TNFα-stimulated endothelial cells reflect the well-characterized biology of this inflammatory cytokine. Finally, we document some of the recent observations that genomics approaches have provided with respect to the importance of endothelial heterogeneity, hemodynamics and mechanobiology in normal vascular function and in disease. Observations such as these are facilitated by and can only be fully appreciated in the context of the global approach.

2. Introduction to Microarray Technologies

Microarrays are now a commonly used high-throughput approach to profiling gene expression in a population of cells in a highly parallel manner.[1] The basic principle is to have a large number of probes, each specific for a particular gene of interest, arrayed on a planar substrate such that each probe has a specific known address. RNA isolated from a cell or tissue sample is converted to a cDNA or cRNA probe, and labeled with a radioisotope or fluorophore. The labeled sample (target) is hybridized to the array where individual transcripts bind to their specific probes in proportion to the amount present. This is often done as a competitive hybridization where two cell samples (e.g. treated vs. control, diseased vs. normal) are labeled with different fluorophores and cohybridized. The array is washed to remove non-specifically bound targets and scanned. The resulting image contains information on which transcripts are present and in what amount. This information tends to be most useful when considered in a relative sense–e.g. which genes are upregulated or downregulated in a diseased cell population vs. a normal one. The array can represent a targeted pathway or disease, a random sampling of known genes (or even ones with unknown function), or even in theory an entire genome. Applications include transcriptional profiling to get a global snapshot or fingerprint of the state of gene expression in a cell at a given time, to SNP detection, to individualized medicine.

A linear amplification step is often incorporated into the transcript labeling step in an approach first described by Eberwine and colleagues.[2] This can be an enabling technology when the researcher is using a small number of cells (and therefore, a small amount of RNA) as micrograms of material are generally required to go to microarray. However, it is also a common step in target preparation for many platforms, including Affymetrix. The method seems to enhance the discovery potential of microarray studies, in part by improving the signal-to-noise ratio of the array data, allowing additional differential expression calls. However, there is a tradeoff in that there appear to be some transcript dependent biases and a higher false positive rate associated with these additional calls.[3]

There have been many microarray platforms developed both commercially and in house over the past decade and the probes that are used to make the array can vary from short oligonucleotide sequences to full length cDNAs.[1] Most commonly, each transcript is represented by a single, longer oligo probe (50–70 bp) or sometimes a cDNA. Traditionally microarrays have been manufactured by spotting functionalized glass slides or membranes with specialized print tips from multiwell plates containing probe libraries.

The alternative approach to microarray manufacturing uses the techniques of photolithography taken from the semiconductor industry to assemble the probes directly on the substrate. One of the industry standards for microarrays has been Affymetrix (see web resources) which pioneered the use of photolithography to synthesize the oligonucleotide probes *in situ*. On these arrays, each gene is represented by a series of short (25 bp) oligonucleotide sequence pairs (a perfect *match* and a *mismatch* which differ by one nucleotide) over the entire transcript. An algorithm is used to calculate an expression value for the transcript from the set of probe pairs. Affymetrix offers a wide range of solutions, with arrays covering many species and applications such as whole genome analysis, alternative exon splicing, and SNP detection.

A newer platform by Illumina (see web resources) uses a novel high density bead-array technology to screen ~48,000 human feature from the RefSeq and Unigene databases with ~30-fold redundancy. Each bead is coated with oligos that consist of a 50 bp gene specific capture sequence that is concatenated to a 29 bp address sequence, which is recognized by a complementary decoder sequence. The 3 micron silica beads self assemble at random into microwells and a series of hybridizations with fluorescently labeled decoder sequences is used to map and decode the array prior to measuring the gene specific signal. It might be helpful to think of it as if each bead contained a *barcode* that identified the specific gene it was designed to measure. This approach seems to have been useful in eliminating a lot of the positional biases that have long been associated with microarrays (e.g. print tip effects, edge effects, etc).

Bead-based technologies are also being used for high-throughput analyses beyond the level of the transcriptome. Luminex (see web resources) offers a bead-based platform for use in multiplexing assays for up to 100 analytes in a single sample. Microspheres are internally labeled with a dye combination that distinguishes the individual bead set with a unique spectral signature. Each of these can be specifically modified for the capture and detection of a particular analyte in solution. The surface chemistry of the beads allows the coupling of a range of possible capture reagents including antibodies, oligonucleotides, peptides, and receptors. Thus a number of high-throughput solution phase assays are possible including DNA assays, immunoassays, receptor-ligand assays, and enzyme assays. The principles of flow cytometry are used for detection. Two lasers are necessary: one for detecting the spectral signature of the bead and one to detect the fluorescence associated with binding of the analyte.

It is worth mentioning that the current state of the art is such that next-generation rapid DNA sequencing techniques seem poised to ultimately replace microarrays as a cost effective means of transcriptional profiling.[4] However, these come with their own challenges with respect to managing large amounts of data, experimental design and analysis, and do not impact the discussion to follow.

3. Experimental Design and Data Analysis

To researchers in the biomedical sciences, the microarray is a discovery tool to elucidate the molecular biology of the cell in order to understand normal function or disease. The most relevant question is one of extracting biologically interesting and meaningful observations from a large data set. However, data analysis often becomes a daunting and time consuming task that leaves one with the impression that it is necessary to have a bioinformaticist on staff. Fortunately, the field of bioinformatics has evolved with high-throughput technologies to provide researchers with the tools to probe the underlying biology. Software has become increasingly user friendly to the point where that staff bioinformaticist might not be strictly necessary (though consultation and collaboration with one can be extremely useful and is highly recommended). We don't attempt here to exhaustively cover the nuances of experimental design or of the subsequent data analysis which have been the subjects of other excellent reviews[5–6] and inspire much of the following discussion. We refer the reader to these for more detailed treatment of the following topics and some commonly accepted best practices, with the understanding that techniques continue to evolve and that there is often no consensus on the *best* way to do a particular step. As we will see below, analysis decisions are often dependent upon the platform and the data set, and require tradeoffs, depending on the amount of risk the user is willing to take.

3.1. *Experimental Design*

Careful consideration must be given *a priori* to the design of microarray experiments in order to maximize the probability of extracting statistically useful information that reflects biology.[5–6] Among the considerations are which platform and experimental model to use and how to define replication for the study, recognizing that there is a distinction between *technical* and *biological* replication. Perhaps the most important consideration is the design of the experiment to avoid (or at least be able to account for) factors other than the experimental variables. Microarrays were once notorious for positional artifacts, batch and operator effects that confounded the analysis. The author has witnessed first-hand data sets consisting of large numbers of arrays where the experimental variable was hopelessly confounded with batch and operator effects that were larger than the anticipated treatment effect. Though the situation seems to have improved with recent years, especially with the introduction of platforms such as Illumina, it can be very useful to consult with a biostatistician or bioinformaticist at this stage.

Quality control of samples is of particular importance in the experimental workflow as RNA is susceptible to degradation from rather ubiquitous RNAase enzymes and the *garbage in — garbage out* maxim applies to microarrays when starting with a degraded sample for labeling. In our experience, we have had few issues with RNA degradation from exogenous sources when applying RNAase free technique and using commercially available kits and consumables. We have found degradation from endogenous sources to be more common, e.g. when processing samples from tissues that take considerable time to harvest. We routinely monitor RNA quality using the Agilent Bioanalyzer and Lab Chip assay, which is a microfluidics based alternative to gel electrophoresis that is particularly useful when working with small numbers of cells (small quantities of RNA) and there is a need to conserve precious sample. Similarly, we quantify our samples using a Nanodrop spectrophotometer, which allows full spectrum absorbance measurements to be made in as little as 1 μl of undiluted sample.

Moreover, it is also important to note that standards have been developed for the documentation and archiving of microarray experiments which have been adopted as requirements for publishing in many journals. The Microarray Gene Expression Data (MGED) Society has been responsible for defining these standards called Minimal Information About a Microarray Experiment (MIAME).[7–8] It is useful to know what information will be required and to keep careful documentation in anticipation of this (see web resources).

3.2. *Data Analysis*

In general, the problem of data analysis can be broken down into several stages: preprocessing, differential expression analysis, and data mining.[6] Preprocessing includes feature extraction, background correction, quality control, filtering, and normalization. Differential expression analysis is the method by which a list of genes is determined that is different between the experimental groups within a certain statistical confidence. Data mining includes classification approaches, gene set and pathway analysis that go beyond a gene-centric approach to look at how genes vary together in non-random ways that might implicate the involvement of particular gene classes or pathways.

3.2.1. *Preprocessing*

As the reader is already aware from our previous discussion, microarray data analysis is non-trivial and presents some unique challenges.[5–6] At the level of preprocessing one must decide how to remove array artifacts, whether or not to background subtract (as background can be nonuniform, subtraction can increase variability and present a problem with negative expression values), whether and how to remove outliers, whether and how to remove non- or poorly expressed genes from the analysis, and how to normalize. Normalization attempts to identify and remove systematic sources of variation and is generally different for one vs. two channel arrays.[6]

3.2.2. *Differential Expression*

When determining differential expression, the data present some formidable statistical challenges including unequal variances across genes, the possibility of non-normally distributed intensities, and the problem of a conducting a large number of comparisons with small sample size.[5–6] This is quite the opposite of the ideal data set with few comparisons and large sample size. To illustrate the problem, consider an experiment using an array of 10,000 genes, each of which will be subjected to a statistical test to determine if it can be considered differentially expressed between two conditions with confidence. This is analogous to doing 10,000 t-tests. Using a commonly accepted *family-wise error rate* (FWER) of 0.05 (i.e. *alpha error*, 5% chance of a false positive call) on a per gene basis, one can see that very soon the false positive rate becomes prohibitively high. Indeed, for our example, if we were wrong only 5% of the time, we might expect as many as 500 genes to be called differentially expressed by chance alone. Clearly this is unacceptable and some sort of correction for multiple testing is required.

There are several approaches to multiple test correction that vary in the stringency by which they adjust for false positives in a data set (genes being called differentially expressed when they are not), the trade off being false negatives (missed genes that are truly differentially expressed). Practically speaking, these approaches result in a cutoff for significance at p-values considerably lower than the typical 0.05. It is possible to err too much on the side of caution, resulting in a data set with essentially no false positives at the expense of a large number of missed genes that are truly differentially expressed. This sort of approach might be preferred for example in a diagnostic application, where a small number of markers detected with a high degree of confidence would distinguish a disease subtype. Generally, a very small gene list is of little use to the researcher for discovery based-studies, and the user would be happy to have a more extended list for a global analysis and data mining, recognizing that the tradeoff for this is an increased likelihood of false positives. A widely used method of multiple test correction that strikes a balance between the false positive and false negative calls within a gene list is the false discovery rate (FDR). In the FDR approach, the expected proportion of false positives among the set of all predictions is controlled, whereas in the classic family-wise type I error approach, the probability that there is at least one false prediction is controlled.[9] For example, setting a FDR of 5% results in the identification of a gene set of which 95% are expected to be truly differentially expressed. Some researchers choose to set the FDR even higher at 10% or even 25% depending on their needs. We have used differential expression algorithms such as that found in Patterns from Gene Expression (PaGE),[10] which utilizes a permutation estimation approach that makes fewer assumptions about the data than other methods (see web resources).

It is important to note that in order to control the error rate across the multiple parallel tests, even with the FDR approach, we sacrifice some power in considering individual genes.[6] On an individual gene basis, FDR adjusted p-values might be quite small (e.g. we have commonly seen these at ~0.001). The way the statistics work, failure of an individual gene to be called differentially expressed does not mean that it necessarily is not. It simply means that there is insufficient evidence to determine this, and clearly this is complicated by the need for multiple test correction. The researcher must be given some latitude here. For example, let's say that we have a particular interest in *Gene A* which did not make our list of differentially expressed genes selected with a FDR of 5%. It is highly unlikely that we will ignore this gene if we mine further and find that the FDR adjusted p-value is 0.01. Rather, we would follow-up this observation with a technique like qPCR to validate this finding. Indeed we endorse a two-fold approach to the analysis of microarray data, both using data mining strategies to search for biological meaning *post priori*, and also considering *a priori* genes and pathways likely to be important and worthy of consideration.

Despite the challenges associated with statistical tests and multiple test corrections applied to differential expression analysis of microarray data, the merit of such an approach, where each gene is evaluated based on its own variance, is clear. This is far superior to the once commonly applied heuristic approach which set an arbitrary cutoff in expression ratios (usually 2-fold) to determine differential expression based on a sample size of 1–2. Using the statistical approach, some genes which appear to be different by 2-fold or greater are too highly variable in their expression and can be excluded from the analysis. On the other hand, it is possible to routinely identify relatively small changes in gene expression which are *statistically significant* with high probability. The question commonly arises as to whether or not these small changes are *biologically significant.* It is likely that the answer to this question is different for each individual gene, given the levels of complexity involved in biological regulation. For example, differences at the transcript level are not necessarily reflected at the protein level. A very small difference in transcript levels may have a large impact in one case, while relatively large differences may not translate to a meaningful effect in another. Still, differences at the transcript level reflect the state of the cell which might provide insight into mechanisms even in the absence of other changes (e.g. *priming* the cell for a response under the right conditions as we will see with some of our examples below). It should be emphasized here that microarray observations are most useful when followed-up by validation of the most promising gene candidates (e.g. using the gold standard for single gene expression analysis of qPCR) and by more mechanistically-driven studies to evaluate protein expression and activity, signaling pathways and their inhibition.

3.2.3. *Data Mining Strategies*

Perhaps one of the most significant challenges associated with the analysis of microarray data is how to attach meaning to a large list of differentially expressed genes, no matter how rigorously obtained. Genes are part of networks and pathways and their expression will not be completely independent from that of other genes. This can not typically be appreciated simply by glancing at the most regulated features from an ordered gene list. It is also complicated by the gene annotations, which are not always intuitive and have been something of a moving target as genome data has been updated and refined. For example, one might be hard-pressed to determine the importance of a gene named *son of sevenless* that appeared in a study of human endothelium. The MGED Society is working to help standardize annotation and naming conventions (see web resources).

Fortunately, data mining tools have emerged which facilitate the analysis of high-throughput expression data, allowing the user to more rapidly and objectively assess the functionality underlying sets of differentially expressed genes. These tools go beyond the preliminary gene-by-gene analysis to identify themes in biological data and illustrate the data in the context of biological pathways. Highly interactive formats provide quick links to annotation, gene-specific information, the nature of biological interaction and the scientific literature. An additional level of confidence in the biological importance of selected differentially expressed genes can be realized through the identification of themes and pathways where patterns involving many genes are identified. These methods are valuable for identifying targets for validation, and pathways for functional analysis, using tools such as qPCR, RNAi, and immunoassays.

Expression Analysis Systematic Explorer (EASE) is a freely available online tool that aides the researcher in exploring the biological significance of groups of genes identified in an experiment[11] (see web resources). EASE identifies potentially interesting themes in biological data by highlighting over-represented categories in a gene list relative to an array or genome. Gene IDs are mapped to primary (non-redundant) gene identifiers (i.e. LocusLink numbers) and then to gene categories in one of various biological classification schemes. EASE then calculates a probability of finding a certain number of genes with a given biological annotation in a gene list given a frequency of genes in that biological category represented on the array. A ranked list of gene categories is presented based on this probability calculation which can be subjected to various multiple test corrections. The interface includes link-out tools which create custom URLs with gene specific information, annotations, etc.

Ingenuity Pathways Analysis (IPA) compares a user defined list of "focus" genes to a vast biological database consisting of a network of gene products and interactions between them (see web resources). It looks for subsets of these focus genes that "cluster" together in a non-random way when superimposed upon the knowledgebase. The result is a ranked set of "virtual" networks consisting of interacting sets of focus genes. The networks are scored by the likelihood of the focus genes in a network being found together by random chance. The interface is very interactive allowing the user to link to gene specific information, details on interactions, relevant literature, etc. A set of tools are provided to assess the functionality underlying groups of genes in a network. These include an EASE-like functional analysis and visualizations of known metabolic and cell signaling (canonical) pathways, drug targets, and subcellular localization of gene products.

In contrast to the methods of EASE and IPA, which are *post priori* analyses conducted on a pre-identified set of differentially expressed genes, many researchers are now using an *a priori* method for analyzing sets of genes called Gene Set Enrichment Analysis (GSEA)[12] (see web resources). An enrichment score is calculated that reflects the extent to which a predefined set of genes is overrepresented at the extremes of the entire ranked list of genes, and thus likely to be different between the biological states defined by the experiment. The statistical significance of the enrichment score is determined by a permutation-based test and FDR multiple test correction. One potential advantage of GSEA is the additional power gained from looking at how sets of genes that are part of a common biological classification vary as a whole, since individual genes might be lost in a single gene analysis.

Hierarchical clustering is one of a number of commonly used class discovery methods which we introduce only briefly here for the purposes of understanding our examples below. It can be done for arrays, for genes, or for both together. This is basically a way of grouping together samples based on their similarity to each other such that samples which share a common node are considered more similar to each other than to those outside the node. A metric such as the centered Pearson correlation coefficient is used as the basis for this similarity measurement. This is done in an iterative fashion until everything is attached in a tree-like structure. The method can be particularly useful for quality control purposes (such as visualizing experimental biases) and for illustrating trends in the data. There are freely available online tools for hierarchical clustering such as XCluster[13] (see web resources).

4. Case Study

4.1. *Introduction*

Tumor necrosis factor alpha (TNFα) is an inflammatory cytokine, the biology of which has been well studied and characterized in the context of the endothelium and atherosusceptibility.[3,14–18] TNFα binding to its receptor activates a variety of map kinase (MAPK) pathways and leads to activation of the redox-sensitive transcription factor NFκB, which subsequently binds the promoter region of a host of genes involved in inflammation, inducing their transcription. These include cell adhesion molecules involved in leukocyte recruitment to the site of inflammation (VCAM, ICAM, SELE), chemokines (MCP1), and cytokines (TNF, IL8, IL1α, IL1β). However, the NFκB pathway is a highly regulated one, and is feedback inhibited via upregulation of its inhibitors (IκBs).[14] The detrimental effects of inflammation are also held in check by the induction of genes that encode for such proteins as inhibitors of apoptosis (IAPs) and antioxidants such as SOD. In part due to the importance of TNFα as a cytokine driving inflammation in endothelium and its relationship to atherogenesis, and in part due to its well characterized nature *a priori*, we use it as an example here to trace through a typical microarray study and dataset analysis. In demonstrating the reliability of such a study to highlight the known biology, we hope to instill confidence in the ability of such studies to direct the researcher to important aspects of the biology when there is the much larger element of the unknown.

4.2. *Study Design and Methods*

The results presented here are derived from an American Heart Association sponsored study to investigate the effects of endothelial aging on inflammation and athero-susceptibility. Seventeen lots of human aortic endothelial cells (HAEC) from a range of donors aged 18–65 were characterized for their inflammatory response to TNFα (10 ng/ml, 4 hr) compared to untreated controls. The results presented here focus on the common response to TNFα across all HAEC lots, rather than age-associated differences which are presented elsewhere.

Total RNA was isolated using the Absolutely RNA Miniprep Kit (Stratagene) which includes a DNAse digestion step to remove contaminating genomic DNA. Samples were monitored for quality and quantity using an Agilent 2100 Bioanalyzer/ LabChip assay and a Nanodrop ND-1000 Spectrophotometer. RNA samples were then used to generate biotinylated, amplified RNA probes for hybridization with the Illumina Human HT-12 Expression BeadChip arrays in the UC Davis Expression Analysis Core. As described previously, this novel high density bead-array technology uses 50-mer probes to screen ~48,000 human features from the RefSeq and Unigene databases with ~30-fold redundancy.

Data analysis was performed in consultation with the UCD Bioinformatics Core. Briefly, analysis was done using the "beadarray"[19] and "limma"[20] packages for Bioconductor (an open source software project for the analysis of genomic data using the *R* programming language for statistical computing, see web resources). Data were background corrected using a normal exponential convolution method (similar to the approach used in RMA for Affymetrix data), quantile normalized and $\log_2$ — transformed.[19] Differential expression was determined using a Bayesian model and a FDR correction applied.[21]

4.3. *Results and Conclusions*

Figure 1 is a *ratio-intensity (RI) plot* of the data for ~48,000 features represented on the Illumina Human HT-12 BeadChip. These plots (also referred to as MA plots) are useful in providing an overall view of the data for quality control purposes.[22] One can gain a sense of how closely the data track between experimental conditions, and also look for intensity dependent biases, observe the effects of normalization, background

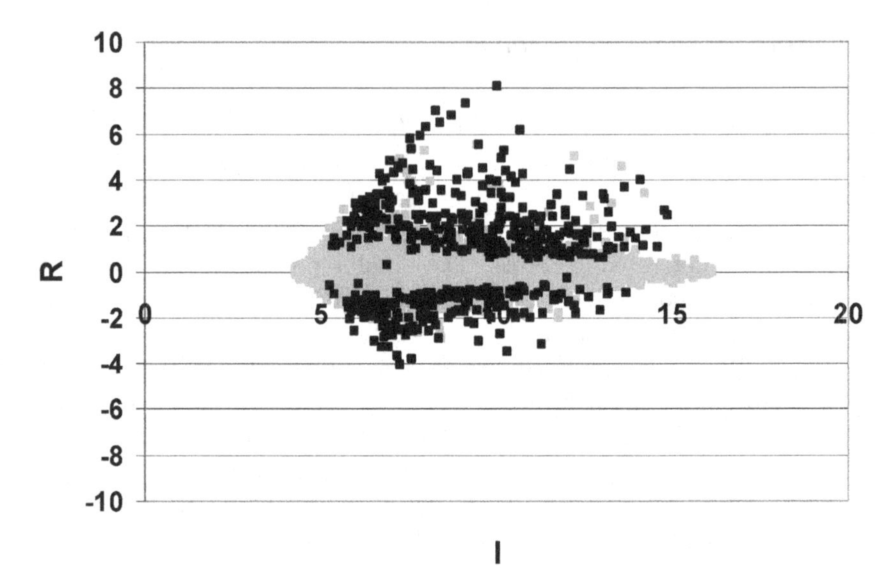

Fig. 1. Ratio-Intensity (RI) Plot of preprocessed data for the case study using the Illumina Human HT-12 BeadChip platform. Highlighted (black squares) are 538 features determined to be differentially expressed between TNFα and untreated cells at a FDR of 1%, and held in common by HAEC binned into 3 age categories (n = 5–7 each). $R = \log_2 I_1 - \log_2 I_2$, and $I = (\log_2 I_1 + \log_2 I_2)/2$, where I_1 is the average intensity for TNFα treated HAEC and I_2 is that for untreated HAEC. (AGP, unpublished data)

correction, etc. $R = \log_2 I_1 - \log_2 I_2$, and $I = (\log_2 I_1 + \log_2 I_2)/2$, where I_1 is the average intensity for TNFα treated HAEC and I_2 is that for untreated HAEC. Features that remain unchanged between conditions are expected to cluster closely about the R=0 line with some random scatter. Those that fall off of this line (outliers) are likely to be differentially expressed between conditions (here, above the line = upregulated by TNFα, below the line = downregulated by TNFα). Highlighted are 538 features determined to be differentially expressed using a rather conservative FDR of 1%, and held in common by HAEC binned into 3 age categories. Note that the statistical approach, particularly when combined with multiple test correction allows the user to assign a confidence to expression calls. Here there are a number of features that are significantly differentially expressed that fall within an arbitrary 2 fold cutoff ($R = \pm 1$), but also some that are not flagged because the variance in expression was such that this could not be determined with confidence for one or more of the age categories.

Table 1 is a sampling from the set of 538 identified genes represented in the RI plot above from the *top tables* ranking them by the probability of differential expression. Highlighted are some of the well characterized gene products upregulated by TNFα, their fold change relative to untreated cells, and the FDR adjusted p-values. (Also commonly referred to as *q-values*, these actually correspond to the highest FDR at which the gene would be considered significantly differentially expressed). Of particular note are the presence of vascular adhesion molecules, chemokines, cytokines, elements of the NFκB system, inhibitors of apoptosis and antioxidative genes referred to in the introduction.

The set of differentially expressed genes identified above were used as focus genes in mapping to the IPA knowledgebase for analysis of gene networks and pathways. Figure 2 shows one of the top ranked gene networks identified by IPA as highly significant for this set of genes (Ingenuity® Systems, www.ingenuity.com). Striking about this network is the upregulation of the NFκB complex which is prominently positioned as a central node, surrounded by a host of related gene products which are upregulated, including the IKK complex and IκBs, TNF receptors, chemokines and inhibitors of apoptosis, in accordance with the known biology of NFκB.[14] Other top ranked networks focused on TNFα signaling, MAPK signaling, etc. Such networks would represent good starting points for the design of mechanistic studies and functional analyses.

Here we extend the treatment of the case study to illustrate an example of how other high-throughput approaches can be used beyond the transcript level to elucidate biological mechanisms. Figure 3 shows a subset of the results of a pilot study evaluating TNFα-induced MAPK and transcription factor activation over a time series using a Luminex bead-based multiplex assay. Phosphorylation is associated with activation and compared to total protein as a baseline. Even based on this limited sampling ($n = 2$), it is clear that TNFα induced ERK1/2, p38 and JNK MAPK activation, peaking at around 15 min. This activation was also associated with downstream IκB phosphorylation (and thus NFκB activation) and also activation of c-jun (a component of the transcription factor AP-1). Once again, these observations are consistent with known TNFα-induced signaling mechanisms. These data were acquired from a single experiment analogous to a high-throughput, solution based ELISA. In theory, as many as 100 analytes may be measured simultaneously by this technology.

Table 1. Selected genes from the list of 538 differentially expressed by TNFα at FDR = 1% and ranked by their probability of differential expression. (AGP, unpublished data)

Rank	Gene Symbol	Entrez Gene ID	Fold Change	FDR adj. p-value
1	TNFAIP2	7127	111.68	3.76E-15
4	CCL20	6364	161.81	2.67E-15
5	TNFAIP6	7130	125.49	3.89E-15
7	CSF2	1437	54.85	2.22E-15
8	ICAM1	3383	16.41	4.59E-09
10	CXCL5	6374	10.17	2.40E-10
11	SELE	6401	25.52	1.12E-10
18	SOD2	6648	10.02	5.25E-08
24	NFKBIA	4792	6.02	3.15E-08
27	TNFRSF9	3604	9.42	3.71E-08
28	TNFAIP3	7128	38.59	2.05E-12
30	CCL5	6352	14.94	4.74E-10
33	TNFAIP1	7126	3.03	1.88E-04
34	TNFRSF4	7293	9.39	2.34E-08
44	TNF	7124	8.65	5.63E-07
50	NFKB1	4790	3.51	1.70E-05
82	NFKB2	4791	10.78	8.18E-10
88	VCAM1	7412	72.69	1.14E-15
98	TRAF1	7185	10.38	1.47E-08
99	NFKBIE	4794	5.85	1.04E-07
115	BIRC3	330	5.11	2.56E-07
153	IL8	3576	6.28	8.02E-09
161	BIRC2	329	2.75	3.41E-04
187	IL6	3569	10.11	6.00E-07
206	TANK	10010	3.02	1.19E-03
218	NFKBIB	4793	2.47	1.08E-05
312	CCL2	6347	5.49	2.56E-04
350	IKBKE	9641	3.00	6.06E-05
412	RELA	5970	1.65	8.89E-04

TNFAIP2, TNFα-induced protein 2; CCL20, chemokine (C-C motif) ligand 20; TNFAIP6, TNFα-induced protein 6; CSF2, colony stimulating factor 2 (granulocyte-macrophage); ICAM1, intercellular adhesion molecule 1 (CD54); CXCL5, chemokine (C-X-C motif) ligand 5; SELE, selectin E (endothelial adhesion molecule 1); SOD2, superoxide dismutase 2, mitochondrial; NFKBIA, NFκB inhibitor, alpha; TNFRSF9, TNF receptor superfamily, member 9; TNFAIP3, TNFα-induced protein 3; CCL5, chemokine (C-C motif) ligand 5; TNFAIP1, TNFα-induced protein 1 (endothelial); TNFRSF4, TNF receptor superfamily, member 4; TNF, TNF superfamily, member 2; NFKB1, NFκB1 (p105); NFKB2, NFκB2 (p49/p100); VCAM1, vascular cell adhesion molecule 1; TRAF1, TNF receptor-associated factor 1; NFKBIE, NFκB inhibitor, epsilon; BIRC3, baculoviral IAP (inhibitor of apoptosis) repeat-containing 3; IL8, interleukin 8 (IL8); BIRC2, baculoviral IAP (inhibitor of apoptosis) repeat-containing 2; IL6, interleukin 6 (interferon, beta 2); TANK, TRAF family member-associated NFKB activator; NFKBIB, NFκB inhibitor, beta; CCL2, chemokine (C-C motif) ligand 2 (a.k.a. MCP-1); IKBKE, IκB kinase complex, epsilon; RELA, NFκB3, p65.

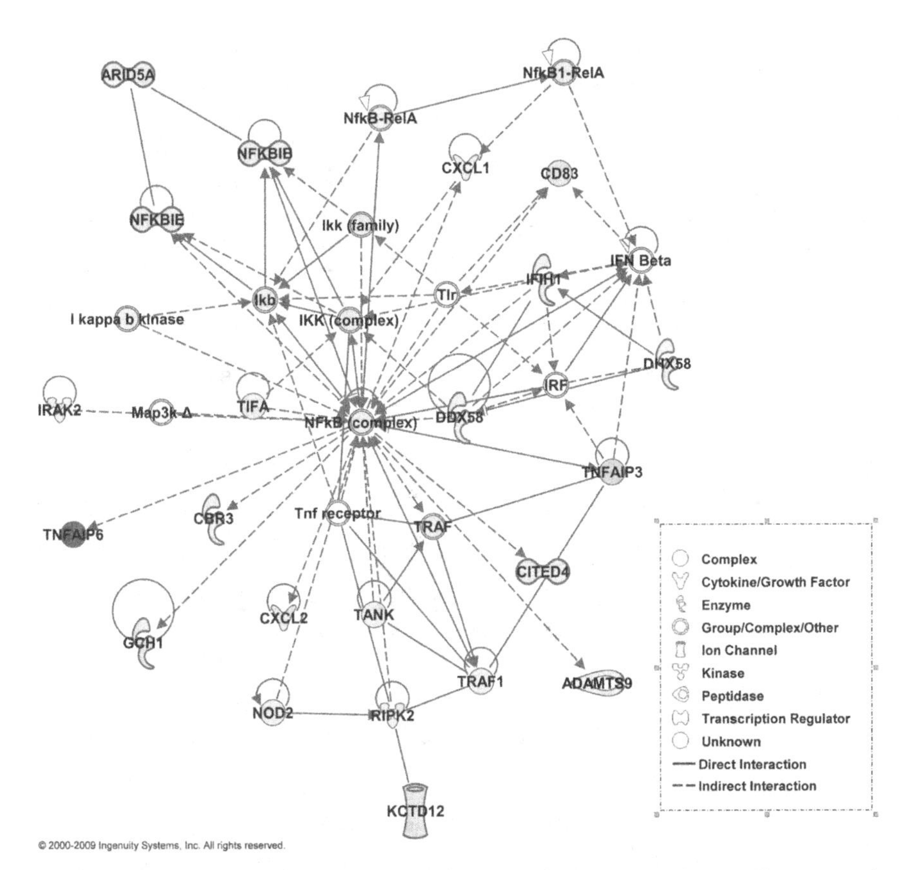

Fig. 2. A top ranked gene network associated with the set of differentially expressed genes by TNFα at FDR = 1% identified through Ingenuity Pathways Analysis as highly significant (Ingenuity® Systems, www.ingenuity.com). Shading intensity proportional to magnitude of fold change. All genes are upregulated except KCTD12. Note presence of NFκB complex as central node in close association with NFκB inhibitors (IκBs) and the IκB kinase complex (IKK), associated with degradation of IκBs and subsequent activation of NFκB. (Of particular note: NFKB1-RELA, p50-p65; NFKBIE, NFκB inhibitor, epsilon; NFKBIB, NFκB inhibitor, beta; TNFAIP3, TNFα-induced protein 3; TNFAIP6, TNFα-induced protein 6; CXCL2, chemokine (C-X-C motif) ligand 2; TRAF, TNF receptor-associated factor; TANK, TRAF family member-associated NFKB activator). (AGP, unpublished data).

4.4. *Summary*

The results presented in brief for this case study demonstrate the reliability of a well designed microarray study and carefully conducted data analysis strategy to produce results in accordance with a well documented biological

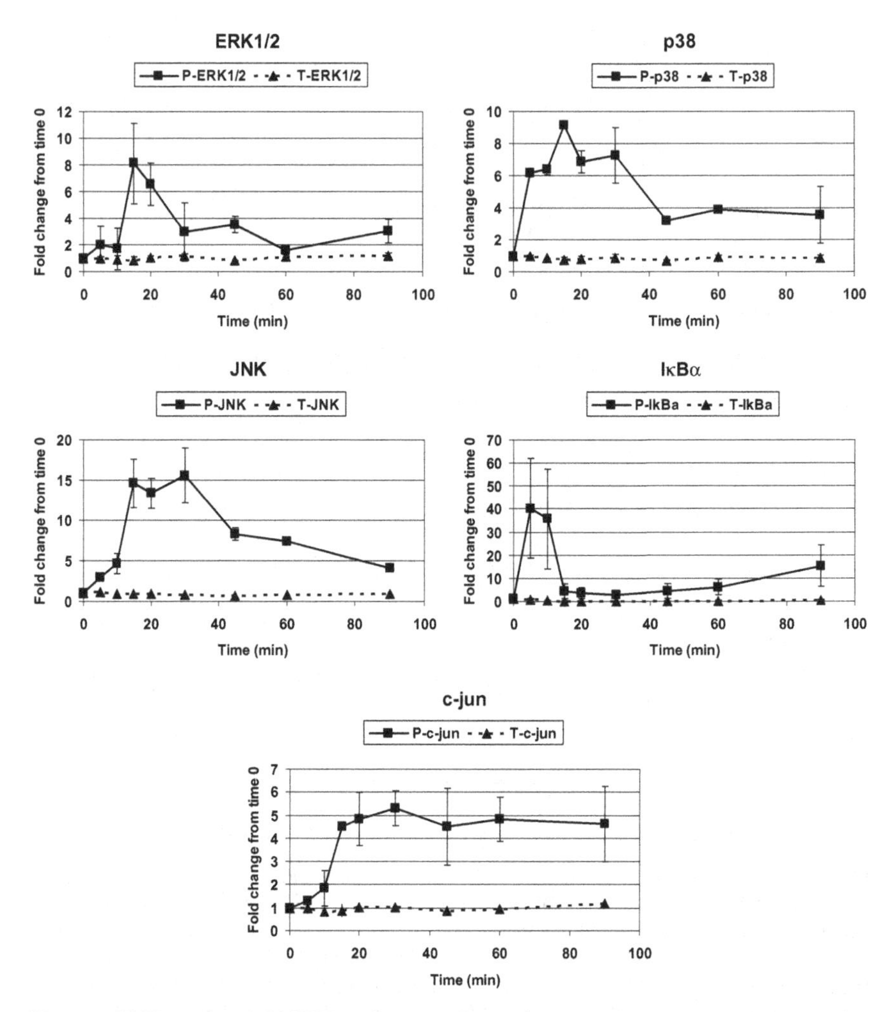

Fig. 3. TNFα-induced MAPK and transcription factor activation over a time series using a Luminex bead-based multiplex assay. Fold change in phosphorylated protein (solid line, squares) and total protein (dashed line, triangles) over a time series. (AGP, unpublished data).

response. It also serves to introduce the reader to a typical analysis workflow that might prove useful when probing a less well characterized response for the purpose of hypothesis generation and the design of follow-up mechanistic studies.

5. Genomics Studies of Endothelium

In this section we highlight the contributions of some genomics-based studies to our understanding of EC heterogeneity, hemodynamics and endothelial mechanobiology, with a particular emphasis on susceptibility to atherosclerotic disease.

5.1. *Insights into Endothelial Heterogeneity*

The importance of EC heterogeneity as influential to both normal vascular physiology and various pathologies is now perhaps widely appreciated.[23–24] One the one hand, it may seem intuitively obvious that all endothelial cells are not alike. For example, pathologies like atherosclerosis strike only the arterial system, and non-uniformly at predictable anatomic locations. But the shift from thinking of the EC as a passive lining of the vessel and purely a victim of its environment to one of an active participant with its own specialized intrinsic properties has taken some time.

Interindividual variability in endothelial phenotype plays an important role in susceptibility to disease. For example, Gargalovic *et al.*[25] in examining primary HAEC derived from multiple heart transplant donors, noted striking differences in inflammatory cytokine IL8 induction by oxidized phospholipids that were maintained upon passaging in culture. They made use of this interindividual variability in the analysis of microarray data using a technique called a gene coexpression network. By grouping genes into pathways and predicting gene–gene regulatory relationships, they illustrated that the unfolded protein response (UPR) pathway is one of the key regulators of IL-8 production. They attributed these differences in inflammatory phenotype to genetic or epigenetic regulatory differences.

The importance of EC heterogeneity observed across vascular beds was illustrated by an important study by Chi *et al.*[26] They used DNA microarrays to analyze gene expression in endothelial cells of various origin (artery, vein, and microvascular from different anatomical locations) grown in culture for several passages. Remarkably, they found that certain features persisted in culture that clearly differentiated EC origin. They observed extensive specialization by anatomic location and also noted that large vessel EC were overall more different from small vessel EC than from each other. They also found evidence that the identity of artery vs. vein might be established by divergence very early in development. The authors concluded that EC comprise many distinct differentiated cell types. These observations have important implications for research studies, tissue engineering approaches, and surgical interventions associated with autologous grafting. They also pose an interesting question as to the relative importance of intrinsic vs. extrinsic factors in the non-uniformity of vascular disease.

5.2. *Hemodynamics and Atherosusceptibility*

However, it may be important to consider a multitude of scales when it comes to understanding the contribution of endothelial phenotypic heterogeneity to disease.[27] This heterogeneity extends beyond different vascular beds to short distances within the same blood vessel and perhaps over distances of even a few cells. For example, in arteries, regional differences in cell shape and alignment reflect differences in the local hemodynamic environment. These morphological differences can be pronounced across the distance of only a few cells. There is a well recognized correlation between local blood flow characteristics and the occurrence of sclerotic diseases of arteries and heart valves, implicating arterial hemodynamics as an important determinant of endothelial phenotype underlying cardiovascular disease.

Atherosclerosis, a chronic inflammatory disease of arteries and an underlying cause of heart attack, stroke and peripheral arterial disease, remains a major cause of morbidity and mortality in the western world according to the American Heart Association.[28] It is characterized by the formation of lipid-rich plaques at focal regions on the wall of large arteries. The mechanisms of atherogenesis are complex, particularly when considered in the context of a multitude of factors associated with diet and genetics.[15,29–30] However, the strong correlation between local flow characteristics in arteries and focal susceptibility to atherosclerosis is well established.[31–32] Arterial geometries such as curvature, branches and bifurcations are associated with flows that are disturbed in nature (characterized by flow separation from the vessel wall, transient vortices, low time-averaged shear stresses (SS), but a high oscillatory shear index, and high shear stress gradients (SSG)). Conversely, straight, unbranching arteries experience relatively undisturbed flow (laminar, unidirectional, high time-averaged SS, and low SSG). Sites of disturbed flow (low SS) are considered to be susceptible to lesion formation, whereas sites of undisturbed flow (high SS) are relatively resistant.

Endothelial cells, which line the arteries and are retained throughout lesion formation,[33] actively mediate vessel tone, hemostasis, inflammation, growth and remodeling, and are responsive to molecular and mechanical stimuli, including shear stress.[34] Observations of EC responses to shear stress in culture have ranged from differences in gene transcription, to protein expression, to functional and morphological changes. The prominent role of EC heterogeneity in normal vascular physiology, coupled with the above observations, have lead to the hypothesis that they play a central role in the pathology of atherosclerosis. Specifically, it has been proposed that local biomechanical forces influence EC phenotypic heterogeneity to promote atheroresistance or atherosusceptibility.[35] One implication is that EC in a region of flow disturbance are expected to be characterized by a gene expression profile which is overall inherently pro-inflammatory, pro-oxidative and pro-adhesive when compared to a region of undisturbed flow.

The endothelium is uniquely positioned to play an important role in mediating atherogenesis by maintaining the delicate balance between inflammation and atheroprotective mechanisms. Inflammatory responses in EC involve focal activation of acute inflammatory cytokines such as tumor necrosis factor (TNFα) which activates the NFκB pathway that promotes expression of vascular adhesion molecules (e.g. VCAM-1, ICAM-1, SELE) and chemokines such as MCP-1 that guide leukocyte recruitment. In a complex multistep process, monocytes adhere to the EC, migrate through to the subintimal space, differentiate to form macrophages, and begin to uptake oxidized lipid products.[15,30,36] Physiological flow also mediates atheroprotective mechanisms in EC, perhaps through multiple synergistic mechanisms that counteract inflammatory signaling.[37] These mechanisms involve crosstalk among mitogen activate protein kinase (MAPK) pathways and transcription factors (TF) such as KLF2, NRF2, and PPARs.

5.3. *In vitro Genomics Approaches*

There is a rather large body of work characterizing endothelial gene expression in cells cultured under simulated physiological flow conditions in flow chambers of various design, primarily on a single gene basis. However, it is only more recently that genomic approaches have been used in such *in vitro* studies to explore the contributions of various aspects of flow and shear stress to conferring an "athero-resistant" or "athero-permissive" phenotype in endothelial cells.

Early microarray studies focused primarily on elucidating shear modulated endothelial gene expression on a global scale by comparing EC exposed to steady laminar shear stress (LSS) with static cultured controls. For example, McCormick *et al.*[38] exposed human umbilical vein endothelial cells (HUVEC) to steady LSS of 25 dynes/cm^2 for 6 and 24 hr., comparing them with static controls on cDNA microarrays. They used a heuristics approach to identify 52 genes that were regulated by shear and focused on potential mechanisms for shear stress induced NO production. Similarly, Wasserman *et al.*[39] compared HUVEC exposed to LSS of 10 dynes/cm^2 for 24 hr. with static controls. They used an approach called *Gene Calling* (a high-throughput expression profiling technique that combines PCR-based linear amplification of gene fragments and in silico database queries to generate a genome-wide assessment of differences in gene expression) to identify 107 genes showing 2-fold changes in expression that represented a limited number of functional clusters that included transcription factors, antioxidants, signaling molecules, cell cycle regulators, and genes involved in cellular differentiation. They concluded that the shear-modulated expression profile was enriched for gene expression so as to create an anti-oxidative, anti-inflammatory, anti-apoptotic, anti-proliferative, and differentiated environment. Furthermore, Chen *et al.*[40] exposed human aortic endothelial cells (HAEC) to 24 hr. of LSS at 12 dynes/cm^2 and compared them with static controls. They reported significant modulation of EC gene expression related to inflammatory cytokines, cell proliferation, ECM/cytoskeleton remodeling, and signal transduction. In particular, they concluded that LSS inhibited EC turnover and inflammatory responses, while promoting angiogenesis, EC remodeling, and migration.

Perhaps of more direct physiological relevance to the elucidation of the athero-permissive phenotype are *in vitro* studies that compare flow conditions analogous to those experienced by EC in regions long-adapted to the differential hemodynamic environments of DF and UF *in vivo*.

For example, the ability of endothelial cells to discriminate among different types of biomechanical stimuli in terms of global patterns of gene expression underlying functional phenotype was demonstrated by Garcia-Cardena *et al.*[41] They compared differential expression in cultured human umbilical vein endothelial cells (HUVEC) exposed to a steady laminar shear stress (LSS) of 10 dynes/cm^2, a turbulent shear stress (TSS) of comparable spatial and temporal average, and static controls using cDNA arrays. One hundred genes were identified as differentially expressed (TSS vs. LSS) at 24 hr. (68 up-regulated and 32 down-regulated). A set of genes that was down-regulated in LSS but up-regulated in TSS was identified as potentially the most pathologically relevant. They considered highly regulated genes of known or putative function in signaling, response to injury, or atherogenesis and focused on linking the protective effects of LSS to matrix biology and cell cycle.

Brooks *et al.*[42] compared gene expression in cultured human aortic endothelial cells (HAEC) under disturbed flow (pulsatile, low magnitude shear stress) conditions with steady LSS of 13 dynes/cm^2 using cDNA microarrays and subtraction cloning. They identified ~100 genes as differentially expressed at 24 h, many of which were up-regulated genes associated with mechanisms known to be pro-atherosclerotic; particularly inflammatory molecules, adhesion factors, and oxidation-related molecules. A relevance to EC inflammatory phenotype was demonstrated by increased monocyte adhesion that coincided with enhanced VCAM expression under DF. The authors also noted distinct differences in the cellular response to TNFα compared to DF, suggesting a role for different signaling pathways in their cellular activation.

Using the state-of-the-art of *in vitro* approaches, Dai *et al.*[43] used cDNA microarrays to transcriptionally profile HUVEC cultured for 24 hr under athero-prone or athero-protective shear stress waveforms in a dynamic flow system based on cone and plate viscometer. These waveforms were derived from computational fluid dynamics analysis of the carotid bifurcation, using vessel geometry and flow profiles determined by MRI and ultrasound for normal human subjects. They determined that EC could discriminate between the applied biomechanical stimuli, as demonstrated by distinct patterns of gene expression for each shear stress waveform versus untreated cells. Differential expression of many genes of putative pathophysiological importance to atherosclerosis was observed, in accordance with above hypothesis and previous *in vitro* studies. In particular, several chemokines and receptors were expressed under the atheroprone waveform consistent with a proinflammatory response. Enhanced IL-8 production, activation of the NFκB pathway and cytokine (IL-1β)-inducible cell surface expression of VCAM-1 were all observed in EC preconditioned by exposure to the athero-prone waveform compared with the athero-protective one. The group also noted dysregulation of the expression and organization of cytoskeletal and junctional proteins, where actin cytoskeletal organization and subcellular localization of C× 37 and C× 43 were regulated differentially by shear stress waveforms.

Dekker *et al.*[44] used a microarray approach and stringent fold-change cutoff to identify a set of endothelial genes responsive to long-term (7 day) exposure to a unidirectional pulsatile shear stress of $19 \pm 12\,\text{dynes/cm}^2$. They also identified a limited panel of genes that were regulated by flow exposure but not inflammatory cytokines, notably among these the transcription factor KLF2. A follow-up study using the approach of Dai *et al.* demonstrated the prominent role that KLF2 plays in atheroprotective flow-mediated endothelial gene expression.[45] Genome-wide transcriptional profiling was used to determine transcriptional targets of KLF2 which was implicated in the orchestrated regulation of endothelial transcriptional programs controlling inflammation, thrombosis/hemostasis, vascular tone, and blood vessel development. Overexpression and knockdown studies in the context of flow revealed that the expression of ~15% of flow regulated genes was dependent on the flow-mediated KLF2 upregulation.

5.4. *In vivo Genomics Approaches*

More recently we have employed an *in vivo* approach to elucidating global endothelial gene expression and functional phenotype associated with sites of athero-susceptibility and athero-resistance in hemodynamically distinct regions of arteries. In the first study of its kind, we profiled gene expression in arterial EC freshly harvested from small ($\sim 1\,\text{cm}^2$) representative regions of athero-susceptibility and athero-resistance in the arteries of normal swine, using RNA amplification to overcome sampling limitations.[46]

Specifically, a region of disturbed flow (the inner and lateral curvature of the aortic arch) was compared to a region of relatively undisturbed flow (the descending thoracic aorta) on cDNA microarrays. Paired replicate analysis and a FDR based statistical approach were used to identify a set of ~2000 genes that were differentially expressed between these sites in the absence of any pathological changes. Analysis of biological pathways and gene networks revealed a pattern that was consistent with priming for enhanced inflammation under DF, evident as a disruption of the dynamic balance in expression of suites of genes known to drive pathology (Fig. 4). Specifically, though enhanced pro-inflammatory gene expression was observed under DF compared to UF, this coincided with enhanced anti-oxidative gene expression that is considered athero-protective. The redox sensitive transcription factor NFκB was found to be enhanced but inactive

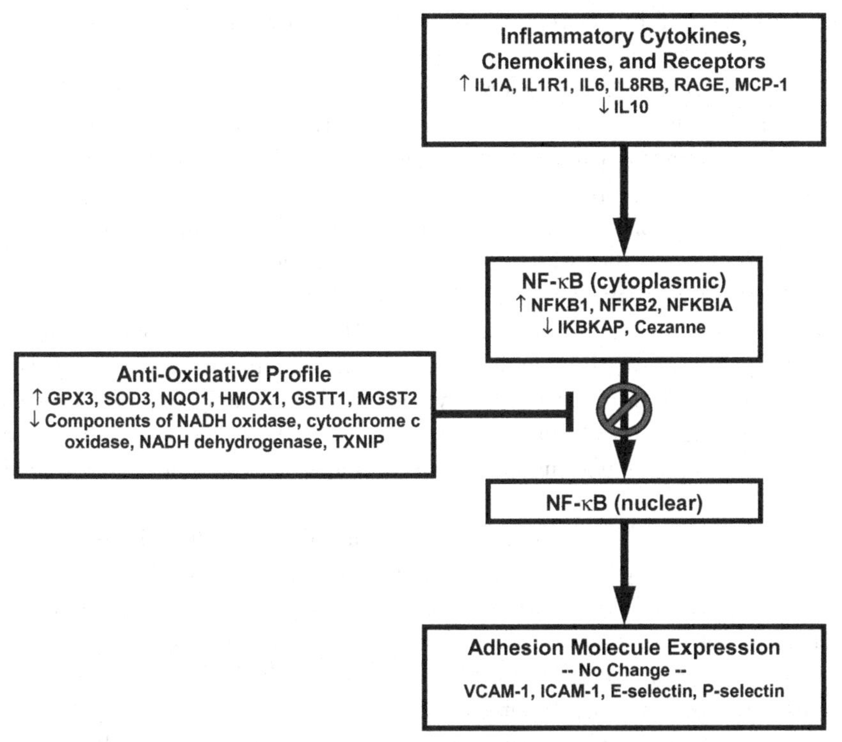

Fig. 4. Summary of observations from an *in vivo* microarray study profiling endothelial gene expression in hemodynamically-distinct sites of normal swine (from Passerini *et al.*, PNAS, 2004). Proinflammatory gene expression in disturbed flow regions is balanced by protective antioxidative mechanisms that prevent NFκB activation and subsequent transcription of vascular adhesion molecules.

in DF, and downstream vascular adhesion molecule expression functionally associated with monocyte recruitment to inflamed endothelium was not observed.[46]

This study provided the first *in vivo* evidence for a balanced steady state in endothelial gene expression at athero-susceptible regions of the normal artery, indicating that cells could be primed for inflammation but were physiologically stable in the absence of atherosclerotic risk factors. Hajra *et al.*[47] similarly noted priming of the NFκB pathway in normal mice at regions of high probability for atherosclerosis but preferential activation of this pathway at these sites in lipopolysaccharide-treated or hypercholesterolemic $LDLR^{-/-}$ mice. Though it may seem obvious in retrospect, this represents somewhat of a paradigm shift from the line of thinking that EC in regions of predisposition to atherosclerosis would display inherently pathological gene expression profiles. These results have led us to focus on risk factors for atherosclerosis (e.g. dyslipidemia, diabetes, aging) acting in the context of differential arterial hemodynamics to provide the tipping point for atherogenesis by shifting the balance of gene expression in atheroprone regions.

In a similar follow-up study comparing three distinct arterial regions in swine, gender and diet were also introduced as risk factors.[48] A relatively short-term (two week) hypercholesterolemic diet was compared to a normal one, and animals remained pre-lesional. Hierarchical clustering analysis showed preferential grouping of samples from the same arterial regions over gender and diet. Moreover, there were few differentially expressed genes within the same region based on gender or diet. Taken together, these studies implicate hemodynamics as a prominent determinant of endothelial phenotype *in vivo*.

Overall, the above studies suggest that disturbed flow is associated with a steady-state *in vivo* endothelial gene expression profile consistent with priming for inflammation at representative sites of susceptibility to atherosclerosis. A logical extension of these studies would be to identify some common molecular signature associated with athero-susceptibility across multiple comparable sites of flow disturbance.

In a recent follow-up study using the swine model, Civelek *et al.*[49] identified 133 genes to be commonly differentially expressed across four athero-susceptible (DF) and three athero-protected (UF) sites. Using the pathway mining approaches of EASE, GSEA and IPA, they identified endoplasmic reticulum (ER) stress-related protein biosynthesis as the common prevalent endothelial genomic signature in all of the athero-susceptible locations. They went on to show associated activation of 2 of 3 branches of the unfolded protein response (UPR) signaling pathway. They concluded that chronic ER stress and activated UPR characterizes the prepathological state of endothelium and prime the cells for pathological change at sites of spatial susceptibility to atherosclerosis.

In another follow-up study using the swine model, Fang *et al.*[50] aimed to elucidate the role of microRNAs (miRNAs) in mediating endothelial phenotypes that direct the susceptibility to atherosclerosis. These are conserved small non-coding RNAs which regulate cell phenotype through control of message RNA stability and/or translation of downstream targets. MicroRNA expression profiling using a multi-species miRNA microarray identified 7 down-regulated and 28 up-regulated endothelial miRNAs in the DF region of aortic arch compared to the UF region in the thoracic aorta, including miR-10a/b, which was among the most down-regulated. Whole-genome transcriptome analysis was then performed in HAEC over-expressed or suppressed in miR-10a. Suppression revealed increased upregulation of the NFκB pathway and ER stress consistent with the results of Civelek *et al.* and implicating miR-10a as potentially an important regulator of the athero-susceptible phenotype at sites of predisposition to disease.

The *in vivo* genomics approach to endothelial phenotyping is also being used to elucidate a role for regional hemodynamics underlying disease susceptibility beyond that in arteries. Simmons *et al.*[51] have applied the approach to the study of sclerotic disease of the aortic valve. Histological findings and shared risk factors with atherosclerotic disease of arteries suggest a common etiology involving chronic inflammatory processes potentiated by systemic factors. Furthermore, there is a recognized side-specific vulnerability to calcific lesions that correlates with complex fluid dynamics that are distinctly different on either side of the valve, analogous to regional susceptibility to atherosclerosis in arteries. They specifically isolated EC from the two sides of the aortic valve in normal swine and used cDNA microarrays to identify 584 genes differentially expressed at a FDR of 5% between the aortic and ventricular sides of the valve. Analysis of biological themes and pathways led the authors to conclude that the endothelium on the disease-prone aortic side of the valve is permissive to calcification but is protected in the normal valve against inflammation and lesion initiation by antioxidative mechanisms, analogous to the findings in arteries.

5.5. *Comparison of In vitro vs. In vivo Approaches:*

Both *in vitro* and *in vivo* studies have an important role to play in contributing to our understanding of endothelial heterogeneity, mechanobiology and disease, and the two approaches will ideally complement each other. A strength of the *in vitro* approach in the context of the current discussion is that it is reductionist by nature, allowing mechanistic studies in a precisely controlled environment that can also demonstrate cause and effect with respect to the role of applied fluid mechanics. Its limitations include the inability to observe the cells in the context of their normal physiological environment and an incomplete understanding of the impact of the cell culture environment on the native phenotype. The choice of cell type (e.g. HAEC vs. HUVEC), shear stress protocol, exposure time, and analysis techniques for genomics data can yield very different results between studies and a lack of concordance with *in vivo* findings. Therefore, careful consideration must be given to these factors in the design of experiments. The use of genomics approaches with *in vitro* flow models is now being extended to determine the effects of hemodynamically-induced endothelial phenotype on cocultures with smooth muscle cells.[52–53]

Though the *in vivo* approach provides the opportunity to make direct observations as to the state of the cells in their normal environment under conditions where they have been long adapted to their physiological flow regime, an important limitation associated with this approach is that the observations in response to differential hemodynamics are strictly correlative. They cannot be controlled for or separated from other systemic factors associated with the complex physiological milieu in the same way as for the *in vitro* reductionist approach. Establishing causality will be an important extension of the current studies. One way to accomplish this is through the use of models that manipulate the hemodynamic condition. For example, Cheng *et al.*[54] used a coarctation to induce flow disturbance in the carotid artery of mice and demonstrated altered eNOS expression.

An additional challenge to endothelial cell phenotyping *in vivo* is the choice of animal model. Analysis of human tissues must generally be done postmortem. Large animal models like the swine are more hemodynamically relevant and provide sufficient quantities of cells for analysis, but are expensive to maintain under a controlled environment and not subject to the same type of convenient genetic manipulation as are mice. Studies of the role of endothelium in more advanced stages of disease are further challenged by the need to isolate a pure endothelial cell population from a heterogenous plaque. Techniques such as laser capture microdissection (LCM) can help to overcome this obstacle. For example, Volger *et al.*[55] used LCM in the transcriptional profiling of endothelium from focal atherosclerotic lesions of postmortem human arteries, identifying common indicators of pathological change that distinguished advanced atherosclerotic plaques from early plaques or disease free regions. Studies such as these will be particularly insightful if they can be linked more directly to the hemodynamics through measurement or manipulation.

6. Summary

In summary, genomics approaches to endothelial phenotyping are providing insight into the role of hemodynamics and endothelial mechanobiology on normal cardiovascular physiology and susceptibility to disease. In this context, observations made in the course of these global studies provide a different perspective than that of the single gene approach and have given us a greater appreciation for endothelial heterogeneity and plasticity. The emerging picture is more complex than once thought. For example, endothelial cells normally are not inherently inflammatory in a sight of predisposition to disease, but rather exhibit differences consistent with their role as active and adaptive mediators of vascular physiology. These differences may be permissive in that they affect the balance of gene expression and activation of biological pathways, rendering EC more susceptible to inflammatory challenges or stresses induced, for example, by known risk factors. Future studies will focus on models to study the convergence of such factors with differential arterial hemodynamics in the modulation of cell signaling and gene expression affecting the mechanisms of atherosclerosis.

Acknowledgments

The author gratefully acknowledges Drs. Craig Simmons and Mete Civelek for their critical review of the manuscript; the UCD Expression Analysis Core and Bioinformatics Core for their contributions to array processing and data analysis and for seed grant funding which partially supported the studies; and the funding from the American Heart Association (BGIA 0765156Y) to AGP which supported the case study data presented in the chapter.

Web Resources

The following provide links to some common resources referred to in this chapter:

(i) Affymetrix homepage: http://www.affymetrix.com/index.affx
(ii) Illumina homepage: http://www.illumina.com/
(iii) Luminex homepage: http://www.luminexcorp.com/index.html
(iv) Patterns from Gene Expression (PaGE): http://www.cbil.upenn.edu/PaGE
(v) DAVID resources (including EASE): http://david.abcc.ncifcrf.gov/

(vi) Ingenuity Pathways Analysis (IPA): http://www.ingenuity.com/
(vii) Gene Set Enrichment Analysis (GSEA): http://www.broad.mit.edu/gsea
(viii) XCluster: http://genetics.stanford.edu/~sherlock/cluster.html
(ix) Microarray Gene Expression Data (MGED) Society (including MIAME): http://www.mged.org
(x) Bioconductor Project: http://www.bioconductor.org

References

1. Katagiri, F., and Glazebrook, J. (2009) Overview of mRNA expression profiling using DNA microarrays. *Curr Protoc Mol Biol* Chapter 22, Unit 22, 24.
2. Van Gelder, R. N., *et al.* (1990) Amplified RNA synthesized from limited quantities of heterogeneous cDNA. *Proc Natl Acad Sci U S A* **87**(5), 1663–1667.
3. Polacek, D. C., *et al.* (2003) Fidelity and enhanced sensitivity of differential transcription profiles following linear amplification of nanogram amounts of endothelial mRNA. *Physiol Genomics* **13**(2), 147–156.
4. Shendure, J., and Ji, H. (2008). Next-generation DNA sequencing. *Nat Biotechnol* **26**(10), 1135–1145.
5. Allison, D. B., Cui, X., Page, G. P., and Sabripour, M. (2006) Microarray data analysis: from disarray to consolidation and consensus. *Nat Rev Genet* **7**(1), 55–65.
6. Grant, G. R., Manduchi, E., and Stoeckert, C. J., Jr. (2007) Analysis and management of microarray gene expression data. *Curr Protoc Mol Biol* Chapter 19, Unit 19, 16.
7. Ball, C. A., *et al.* (2002) Standards for microarray data. *Science* **298**(5593), 539.
8. Brazma, A., *et al.* (2001) Minimum information about a microarray experiment (MIAME)-toward standards for microarray data. *Nat Genet* **29**(4), 365–371.
9. Benjamini, Y., and Hockberg, Y. (1995) Controlling the false discovery rate: a practical and powerful approach to multiple testing. *J R Statistical Soc Ser B — Methodological* **57**, 289–300.
10. Grant, G. R., Liu, J., and Stoeckert, C. J., Jr. (2005) A practical false discovery rate approach to identifying patterns of differential expression in microarray data. *Bioinformatics* **21**(11), 2684–2690.
11. Hosack, D. A., Dennis, G., Jr., Sherman, B. T., Lane, H. C., Lempicki, R. A. (2003) Identifying biological themes within lists of genes with EASE. *Genome Biol* **4**(10), R70.
12. Subramanian, A., *et al.* (2005) Gene set enrichment analysis: a knowledge-based approach for interpreting genome-wide expression profiles. *Proc Natl Acad Sci U S A* **102**(43), 15545–15550.

13. Eisen, M. B., Spellman, P. T., Brown, P. O., and Botstein, D. (1998) Cluster analysis and display of genome-wide expression patterns. *Proc Natl Acad Sci U S A* **95**(25), 14863–14868.
14. Collins, T., and Cybulsky, M. I. (2001) NF-kappaB: pivotal mediator or innocent bystander in atherogenesis? *J Clin Invest* **107**(3), 255–264.
15. Libby, P. (2002) Inflammation in atherosclerosis. *Nature* **420**(6917), 868–874.
16. Murakami, T., *et al.* (2000) The gene expression profile of human umbilical vein endothelial cells stimulated by tumor necrosis factor alpha using DNA microarray analysis. *J Atheroscler Thromb* **7**(1), 39–44.
17. Zhou, J., *et al.* (2002) Genomic-scale analysis of gene expression profiles in TNF-alpha treated human umbilical vein endothelial cells. *Inflamm Res* **51**(7), 332–341.
18. Viemann, D., *et al.* (2004) Transcriptional profiling of IKK2/NF-kappa B- and p38 MAP kinase-dependent gene expression in TNF-alpha-stimulated primary human endothelial cells. *Blood* **103**(9), 3365–3373.
19. Dunning, M. J., Smith, M. L., Ritchie, M. E., and Tavare, S. (2007) beadarray: R classes and methods for Illumina bead-based data. *Bioinformatics* **23**(16), 2183–2184.
20. Smyth, G. K. (2005) Limma: linear models for microarray data. *Bioinformatics and Computational Biology Solutions using R and Bioconductor*, (eds.) Gentleman, R., Carey, V., Dudoit, S., Irizarry, R., and Huber, W. (Springer, New York), pp. 397–420.
21. Smyth, G. K. (2004) Linear models and empirical bayes methods for assessing differential expression in microarray experiments. *Stat Appl Genet Mol Biol* **3**, Article3.
22. Yang, Y. H., *et al.* (2002) Normalization for cDNA microarray data: a robust composite method addressing single and multiple slide systematic variation. *Nucleic Acids Res* **30**(4), e15.
23. Aird, W. C. (2007) Phenotypic heterogeneity of the endothelium: II. Representative vascular beds. *Circ Res* **100**(2), 174–190.
24. Aird, W. C. (2007) Phenotypic heterogeneity of the endothelium: I. Structure, function, and mechanisms. *Circ Res* **100**(2), 158–173.
25. Gargalovic, P. S., *et al.* (2006) Identification of inflammatory gene modules based on variations of human endothelial cell responses to oxidized lipids. *Proc Natl Acad Sci U S A* **103**(34), 12741–12746.
26. Chi, J. T., *et al.* (2003) Endothelial cell diversity revealed by global expression profiling. *Proc Natl Acad Sci U S A* **100**(19), 10623–10628.
27. Davies, P. F., Polacek, D. C., Shi, C., Helmke, B. P. (2002) The convergence of haemodynamics, genomics, and endothelial structure in studies of the focal origin of atherosclerosis. *Biorheology* **39**(3–4), 299–306.
28. Thom, T., *et al.* (2006) Heart disease and stroke statistics–2006 update: a report from the American Heart Association Statistics Committee and Stroke Statistics Subcommittee. *Circulation* **113**(6), e85–151.
29. Steinberg, D. (2002) Atherogenesis in perspective: hypercholesterolemia and inflammation as partners in crime. *Nat Med* **8**(11), 1211–1217.

30. Lusis, A. J. (2000) Atherosclerosis. *Nature* **407**(6801), 233–241.
31. Glagov, S., Zarins, C., Giddens, D. P., and Ku, D. N. (1988) Hemodynamics and atherosclerosis. Insights and perspectives gained from studies of human arteries. *Arch Pathol Lab Med* **112**(10), 1018–1031.
32. Wissler, R. W. (1994) New insights into the pathogenesis of atherosclerosis as revealed by PDAY. Pathobiological Determinants of Atherosclerosis in Youth. *Atherosclerosis* **108** Suppl, S3–20.
33. Davies, P. F., Reidy, M. A., Goode, T. B., and Bowyer, D. E. (1976) Scanning electron microscopy in the evaluation of endothelial integrity of the fatty lesion in atherosclerosis. *Atherosclerosis* **25**(1), 125–130.
34. Li, Y. S., Haga, J. H., and Chien, S. (2005) Molecular basis of the effects of shear stress on vascular endothelial cells. *J Biomech* **38**(10), 1949–1971.
35. Gimbrone, M. A., Jr., *et al.* (1999) Special communication: the critical role of mechanical forces in blood vessel development, physiology and pathology. *J Vasc Surg* **29**(6), 1104–1151.
36. Li, A. C., and Glass, C. K. (2002) The macrophage foam cell as a target for therapeutic intervention. *Nat Med* **8**(11), 1235–1242.
37. Berk, B. C. (2008) Atheroprotective signaling mechanisms activated by steady laminar flow in endothelial cells. *Circulation* **117**(8), 1082–1089.
38. McCormick, S. M., *et al.* (2001) DNA microarray reveals changes in gene expression of shear stressed human umbilical vein endothelial cells. *Proc Natl Acad Sci U S A* **98**(16), 8955–8960.
39. Wasserman, S. M., *et al.* (2002) Gene expression profile of human endothelial cells exposed to sustained fluid shear stress. *Physiol Genomics* **12**(1), 13–23.
40. Chen, B. P., *et al.* (2001) DNA microarray analysis of gene expression in endothelial cells in response to 24-h shear stress. *Physiol Genomics* **7**(1), 55–63.
41. Garcia-Cardena, G., Comander, J., Anderson, K. R., Blackman, B. R., and Gimbrone, M. A., Jr. (2001) Biomechanical activation of vascular endothelium as a determinant of its functional phenotype. *Proc Natl Acad Sci U S A* **98**(8), 4478–4485.
42. Brooks, A. R., Lelkes, P. I., and Rubanyi, G. M. (2002) Gene expression profiling of human aortic endothelial cells exposed to disturbed flow and steady laminar flow. *Physiol Genomics* **9**(1), 27–41.
43. Dai G. *et al.* (2004) Distinct endothelial phenotypes evoked by arterial waveforms derived from atherosclerosis-susceptible and -resistant regions of human vasculature. *Proc Natl Acad Sci U S A* **101**(41), 14871–14876.
44. Dekker, R. J., *et al.* (2002) Prolonged fluid shear stress induces a distinct set of endothelial cell genes, most specifically lung Kruppel-like factor (KLF2). *Blood* **100**(5), 1689–1698.
45. Parmar, K. M., *et al.* (2006) Integration of flow-dependent endothelial phenotypes by Kruppel-like factor 2. *J Clin Invest* **116**(1), 49–58.
46. Passerini, A. G., *et al.* (2004) Coexisting proinflammatory and antioxidative endothelial transcription profiles in a disturbed flow region of the adult porcine aorta. *Proc Natl Acad Sci U S A* **101**(8), 2482–2487.

47. Hajra, L., *et al.* (2000) The NF-kappa B signal transduction pathway in aortic endothelial cells is primed for activation in regions predisposed to atherosclerotic lesion formation. *Proc Natl Acad Sci U S A* **97**(16), 9052–9057.
48. Passerini, A. G., *et al.* (2005) Regional determinants of arterial endothelial phenotype dominate the impact of gender or short-term exposure to a high-fat diet. *Biochem Biophys Res Commun* **332**(1), 142–148.
49. Civelek, M., Manduchi, E., Riley, R. J., Stoeckert, C. J., Jr., and Davies, P. F. (2009) Chronic endoplasmic reticulum stress activates unfolded protein response in arterial endothelium in regions of susceptibility to atherosclerosis. *Circ Res* **105**(5), 453–461.
50. Fang, Y., Civelek, M., Shi, C., Manduchi, E., Davies, P. F. (2009) MicroRNA-10a suppresses unfolded protein response and NF-kappa B pathway that mediate athero-prone endothelial phenotype. In *Biomedical Engineering Society Annual Meeting* (Pittsburgh, PA).
51. Simmons, C. A., Grant, G. R., Manduchi, E., and Davies, P. F. (2005) Spatial heterogeneity of endothelial phenotypes correlates with side-specific vulnerability to calcification in normal porcine aortic valves. *Circ Res* **96**(7), 792–799.
52. Chiu, J. J., *et al.* (2005) Shear stress inhibits smooth muscle cell-induced inflammatory gene expression in endothelial cells: role of NF-kappaB. *Arterioscler Thromb Vasc Biol* **25**(5), 963–969.
53. Hastings, N. E., Simmers, M. B., McDonald, O. G., Wamhoff, B. R., and Blackman, B. R. (2007) Atherosclerosis-prone hemodynamics differentially regulates endothelial and smooth muscle cell phenotypes and promotes pro-inflammatory priming. *Am J Physiol Cell Physiol* **293**(6), C1824–1833.
54. Cheng, C., *et al.* (2005) Shear stress affects the intracellular distribution of eNOS: direct demonstration by a novel in vivo technique. *Blood* **106**(12), 3691–3698.
55. Volger, O. L., *et al.* (2007) Distinctive expression of chemokines and transforming growth factor-beta signaling in human arterial endothelium during atherosclerosis. *Am J Pathol* **171**(1), 326–337.

Chapter 8

ENDOTHELIAL CELL PROLIFERATION AND DIFFERENTIATION IN RESPONSE TO SHEAR STRESS

LINGFANG ZENG, ANNA ZAMPETAKI and QINGBO XU*
Cardiovascular Division, The James Black Centre,
King's College London BHF Centre,
London, SE5 9NU, UK
**qingbo.xu@kcl.ac.uk*

Atherosclerotic lesions preferentially locate at branch or bifurcation areas along the vessel wall, indicating that mechanical forces created by local flow patterns may exert different effect on the lesion development. Since the integrity of endothelium plays a role in the lesion formation, endothelial cell (EC) growth, proliferation and apoptosis that may be followed by endothelial progenitor cell (EPC) repair could be key issues. Recent evidence indicates that laminar shear stress can stimulate multi-potent stem or progenitor cells from different sources to differentiate toward EC lineage, which provides a promising cell source for cell-based therapeutic application in cardiovascular diseases. However, the underlying mechanism is far from well-understood. This chapter will give an overview of the effect of local flow pattern on EC differentiation, proliferation, survival and apoptosis and the possible underlying mechanism.

1. Introduction

Endothelial cells (ECs) are the key cellular components of blood vessel wall, functioning as a selectively permeable barrier controlling materials transportation between blood and tissues. Besides this, ECs are also involved in the modulation of vessel tone through interaction with underneath smooth muscle cells (SMCs) and immunity through interaction with monocytes, lymphocytes, etc via inflammation reactions. Like all other cell types, ECs' cellular function can be regulated by environmental biological active molecules, like growth factors, cytokines, peptides, etc. and communication with other cells.

Similar to other cell types, mature ECs have their own life spans and undergo natural turnover, leading to local transient endothelium denudation and permeability change. The denuded endothelium will be quickly repaired via endothelial cell migration, proliferation and/or endothelial progenitor cell differentiation. It is well-known that the dysfunction/denudation of endothelium is the initial step of vascular diseases, such as atherosclerosis development. Factors that enhance EC turnover or reduce EC repair will increase the risk of atherosclerosis. In contrast, factors that reduce EC turnover or increase EC repair will be atheroprotective. Many pro-atherogenesis risk factors have been defined, such as modified low-density-lipoproteins (LDL), free radicals, genetic alterations, aging, infections, immune response and biomechanical stress, etc.[1–4]

Shear stress (τ) is the force per unit created when a tangential force (blood flow) acts on a surface (endothelium), which is directly proportional to the velocity of blood flow, and inversely proportional to the cube of the arterial radius (R), where Q is flow rate and μ is fluid viscosity.[5]

$$\tau = 4\mu Q/R^3 \tag{1.1}$$

Therefore, small changes in R will greatly influence τ, and vice versa. Along the arterial tree, the presence of branch point or arch curve, a plaque or surgical device may modify the local geometry, influencing the magnitude, directionality and spatiotemporal distribution of shear stress. It is well-established that blood flow in the straight part of arterial wall is considered unidirectional and high shear stress (laminar flow), while in the branch point or arch area or a plaque it is bidirectional disturbed flow and low shear stress (Fig. 1A and refer to reference[5] for review). Specifically, local flow patterns modulate the gene expression, signal transduction and cellular behaviour of ECs.[6]

Importantly, atherosclerosis is featured by its geographical distribution along the vessel wall, i.e. preferentially localizing in the branch points and curved regions but rarely in the straight part, indicating that local flow patterns play a significant role in the development of atherogenesis. Accumulating evidence indicates that different flow patterns trigger different signal pathways in ECs and exert regulatory roles in physiological or pathophysiological processes, such as cell proliferation, differentiation, survival and apoptosis. Detailed investigation on the effect of hemodynamic forces in EC cellular functions will provide new insight into the underlying mechanism involved in atherogenesis development and provide therapeutic tools to intervene vascular diseases.

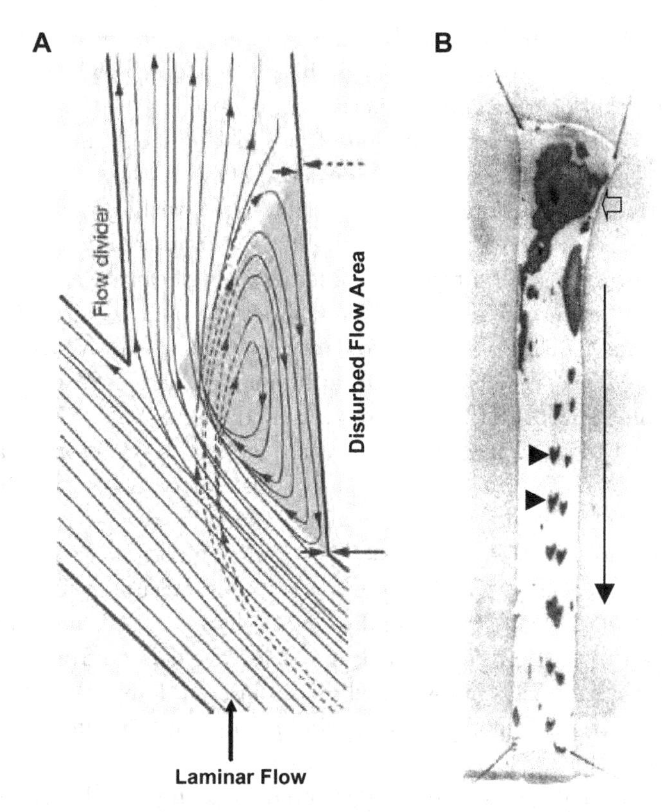

Fig. 1. Lipid generally accumulates in disturbed flow area along the arterial tree. (A) A schematic illustration of flow pattern in the branch point of an artery. In the straight part of the artery, the blood flow is unidirectional laminar flow; while in the branch point, there is a disturbed flow area where the flow is bidirectional. Adapted from Davies PF, *Nat Clin Pract Cardiovasc Med*, 2009.[5] (B) Sudan IV-stained thoracic aorta from rabbits fed 2% cholesterol for 4 months, showing the characteristic development of early fatty streak lesions in the aortic arch (open arrow) and branch orifices (arrow head). The arrow indicates the flow direction. Adapted from Schwenke DC *et al.*, Arteriosclerosis, 1989.[9]

2. Effect of Shear Stress on EC Turnover and Survival

2.1. *Disturbed Flow Increases EC Permeability*

A characteristic feature of atherosclerosis is focal LDL accumulation and fat streak formation proceeding lesion development. LDL transport from blood flow to arterial wall has local variation. By intravenously injecting horseradish peroxidase (HRP) and ^{125}I-labeled human LDL into normal rabbit, Stemerman *et al.*[7] found that the luminal surface of the aortas showed many small punctuate foci of brown reaction product to HRP, representing the focal heightened permeability to HRP. In the same HRP reacting foci, there was accumulation of ^{125}I-labeled LDL, indicating that the wall permeability to LDL has focal distribution pattern. These foci were confirmed to be branch disturbed flow area with low shear stress. Fed with 2% cholesterol for 16 days, LDL accumulated in the branch points of normal rabbit arteries proceeding fat streak formation. LDL accumulation patterned along the flow direction, and these areas were confirmed experiencing disturbed flow with low or zero shear stress, to be athero-prone areas (Fig. 1).[8–11] LDL accumulation derives from increased arterial wall transport of LDL and decreased degradation. The arterial wall transport of LDL can be mediated through LDL receptor uptake by ECs and increased permeability, in which the latter plays a main role. The increase of arterial wall permeability generally results from cell-to-cell junction loss between adjacent ECs and denudation of ECs in the endothelium, especially in artery injury conditions. Accumulating evidence show that de-endothelialization or EC damage causes LDL accumulation in arterial wall.[12–14] LDL accumulation can also be derived from increased lipid biosynthesis in ECs in disturbed area. Liu *et al.* found that disturbed flow activated sterol-response-element binding protein 1 and increased lipid biosynthesis in ECs.[15]

The accumulation of LDL in disturbed area implies that local flow pattern affects arterial wall permeability, which is mainly controlled by VE-cadherin-mediated adherens junction. VE-cadherin is a type II cadherin, specifically expressed in ECs. The extracellular domains of VE-cadherin form hexamers in which the VE-cadherin dimers from two adjacent cells interact in *trans* through extracellular domain 1 and VE-cadherin trimers from the same cell interact in *cis* via extracellular domain 4, mediating the adheren junction between two adjacent cells.[16] The intracellular domain of VE-cadherin interacts with cytoskeleton, α-catenin, β-catenin, vinculin and/or plakoglobin and crosstalks with vascular endothelial cell growth factor (VEGF) receptor, maintaining endothelium integrity.[17–19] Lack of VE-cadherin causes embryonic lethality due to defect in vascular remodelling.[20] VE-cadherin expression and its linkage to cytoskeleton are regulated by local flow patterns. Transient steady flow, which can be regarded as disturbed flow, down-regulates VE-cadherin proteins and decreased its pericellular location.[21] En face staining reveals that there is less amount of VE-cadherin in disturbed flow area as compared to adjacent athero-resistant area, especially in ApoE$^{-/-}$ mice.[22] On the other hand, long term laminar flow increases its interaction with cytoskeleton to form numerous stress fibre bundles distributed parallel to flow direction.[23] Disturbed flow-decrease of VE-cadherin may be through X-box binding protein 1 (XBP1). XBP1 is a basic leucine zip transcription factor, functioning as a key signal transducer in endoplasmic reticulum stress response.[24–26] Our recent findings[27] showed that laminar flow down-regulated while disturbed flow up-regulated XBP1 expression and splicing, and that high level of XBP1 proteins (especially the spliced isoform) were detected in the bifurcation or branch area of the arterial wall in aged ApoE$^{-/-}$ mice. Furthermore, the enhanced expression of spliced XBP1 down-regulated VE-cadherin protein level through transcriptional suppression and matrix metalloprotease (MMP)-mediated degradation, leading to endothelial dysfunction and atherosclerosis development in mice artery isograft model (Fig. 2).

Besides the effects of local flow, other atherosclerotic risk factors such as lipopolysaccharide (LPS) and oxidized LDL can also cause the shedding of VE-cadherin through MMPs.[28] Down-regulation of VE-cadherin will increase endothelium permeability to LDL, which accumulates beneath the endothelial layer and is oxidized by reactive oxygen species (ROS), and in turn further increases permeability, leading to atherosclerosis development.

2.2. *Disturbed Flow Promotes EC Proliferation and Apoptosis*

In addition to controlling pericellular permeability, VE-cadherin also regulates EC proliferation and apoptosis through interaction with Wnt/β-catenin and crosstalk with VEGF receptor signal pathways.[29] Ligand binding of VEGF to its receptor will interact with VE-cadherin and causes VE-cadherin shedding via endocytosis, releasing β-catenin translocation into nuclear and directing the transcription of genes responsible for cell proliferation. Disturbed flow down-regulating VE-cadherin may increase EC proliferation bypass the VEGF signal pathway. Indeed, disturbed flow increases EC proliferation *in vitro* and *in vivo*. In the *in vitro* culture system, disturbed flow is generally created by orbital, oscillatory and/or gradient shear stress. Exposed to orbital shear stress

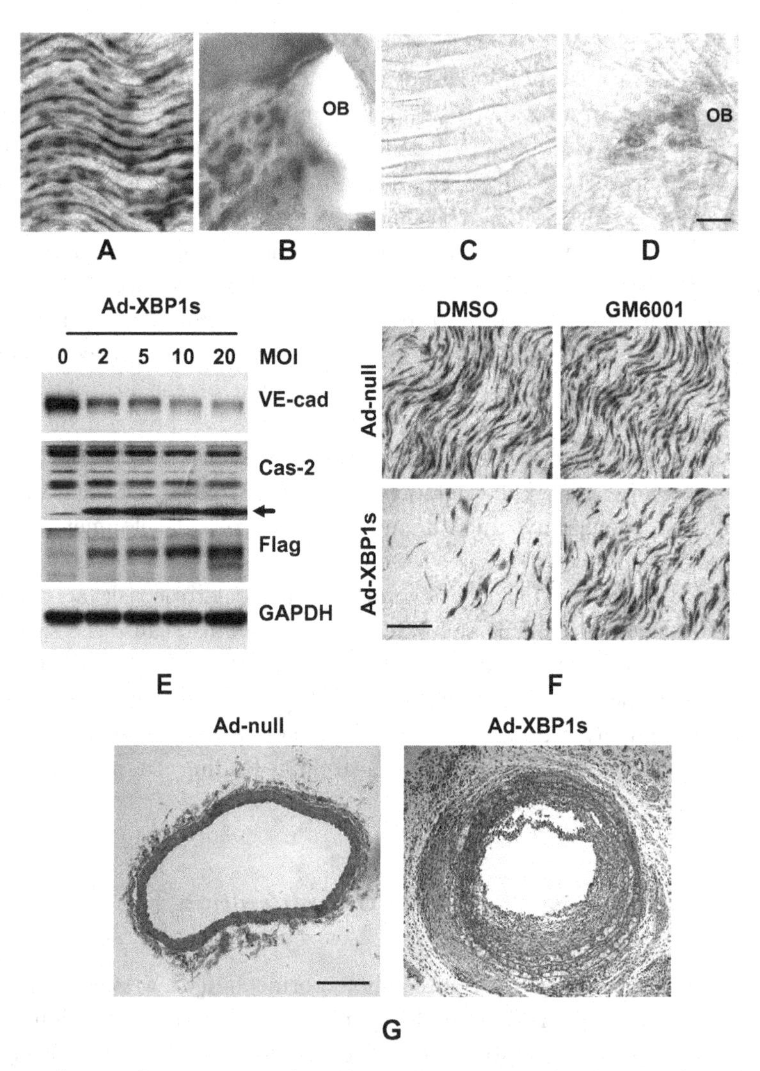

Fig. 2. Sustained activation of XBP1 splicing was related to atherosclerosis development. En face staining with X-gal showed ECs in the straight part (A) and branch area (B); En face staining with anti-XBP1 antibody showed XBP1 was highly expressed in branch area (D) but not in the straight part (C). (E) Sustained activation of XBP1 splicing via adenoviral gene transfer (Ad-XBP1s) induced VE-cadherin down-regulation and caspase activation. Arrow indicates the cleaved band of Caspase-2. Exogenous XBP1 was revealed by anti-Flag antibody. (F) MMP inhibitor GM6001 significantly rescued Ad-XBP1s-induced EC loss from vessel walls. (G) Over-expression of spliced XBP1 via Ad-XBP1s induced atherosclerosis development in artery allograft model in ApoE$^{-/-}$ mice. Control virus Ad-null was included in (F) and (G) as negative control. Bars: 100 μm.

created by an orbital shaker (210 rpm), EC proliferation was increased by 29% in cell number counting and 2 fold in ^{3}H-thymidine incorporation.[30] On the contrast, results from the same group showed that EC proliferation was decreased by 16% in cell counting and 38% in ^{3}H-thymidine incorporation when ECs were exposed to laminar flow created by a parallel plate.[30] As to gradient shear stress, it seems that temporal gradients shear stress but not spatial gradients shear stress increases EC proliferation. Sudden onset of flow stimulated EC proliferation by 105%, but ramped flow had no significant effect. Similarly, steady flow suppressed EC proliferation.[31] When human umbilical vein endothelial cells (HUVECs) were exposed to oscillatory flow at 12 dynes/cm^2, DNA synthesis was increased by about 2 fold as measured by ^{3}H-thymidine incorporation.[32] Similar to HUVECs' response to oscillatory flow, when porcine carotid arteries were exposed to oscillatory flow *ex vivo* for 3 days, the DNA synthesis in ECs was significantly increased as measured by Ki-67 staining.[33] *In vivo* EC proliferation in the intact endothelium along the arterial wall can be assessed by Br-dU incorporation and *en face* staining with anti-Br-dU immunostaining. Injected into the mice tail vein, Br-dU incorporation was observed in sites prone to lesion development, especially in ApoE$^{-/-}$ mice, but not in the straight parts resistant to lesion development.[22] Disturbed flow-induced DNA synthesis and proliferation is related to XBP1 splicing and p70/p85 S6 kinase (pp70(S6k)) activation.[27,32,34] Proliferating HUVECs shows higher level of XBP1 splicing as compared to quiescent cells, while both the XBP1 siRNA and Inositol requiring enzyme 1α (IRE1 α) siRNA knockdown suppresses Br-dU in proliferating HUVECs.[27] On the other hand, pp70(S6k) inhibitor, rapamycin, can block disturbed flow-induced DNA synthesis.[32]

Proliferation is usually linked to apoptosis while quiescence links to cell survival. That is to say ECs in disturbed flow area may have a higher apoptosis rate as compared to laminar flow.[6] Disturbed flow-induced EC apoptosis is related to up-regulation of reactive oxygen species (ROS), deficiency of nitric oxide (NO) and/or XBP1 splicing-induced VE-cadherin down-regulation.

Reactive oxygen species (ROS) plays a very important role in many cellular processes, including cell differentiation, proliferation and apoptosis. The excess production of ROS causes NF-κB and capases activation, leading to inflammation and cell apoptosis, which is very common in many diseases including atherosclerosis.[35] Low shear stress or disturbed flow-induced superoxide production seems to be mainly derived from vascular nicotinamide adenine dinucleotide phosphate (NADPH) oxidases (Nox).[36] Several groups have reported that oscillatory flow up-regulated Nox mRNA and activity, resulting in the increase of superoxide production.[37–40] Oscillatory flow-induced superoxide production seems to be regulated by bone morphogenic protein (BMP) 2/4 in an autocrine-like manner. Oscillatory flow increased BMP2/4 expression and secretion, while BMP4 siRNA can ablate oscillatory flow-induced superoxide production.[38,39] BMP 2 and 4 are TGF-β superfamily membrane cytokines that are expressed by both ECs and smooth muscle cells and regulate multiple cellular processes involved in atherogenesis.[41] Treatment with BMP4 in ECs increased Nox1 mRNA expression and H_2O_2 and O_2^- production.[38] BMP4 infusion by osmotic pumps in mice induced hypertension via surperoxide production, BMP4 antagonist noggin and Nox inhibitor apomycin can block BMP4-induced hypertension.[42]

Nitric oxide (NO) is an important vaso-reactive molecule, regulating blood vessel tone and other cellular processes. The homeostasis between NO and ROS determine the cellular re-dox status. NO is produced by nitric oxide synthase (NOS) from L-arginine with the coupling of BH4, flavins FAD and FMN, calmodulin and NADPH.[43] There are three isoforms of NOS, neuronal NOS (nNOS), inducible NOS (iNOS) and endothelial NOS (eNOS), encoded by three separate genes. Targeted deletion of eNOS in ECs increased lesion development in $ApoE^{-/-}$ due to the lack of NO production.[44,45] However, over-expression of eNOS in ECs will also increase lesion development due to the uncoupling of eNOS to cofactors, leading to increase of superoxide production and lack of NO production.[46] NO protect ECs from oxidative stress-induced apoptosis through scavenging ROS and/or direct inactivation of caspase via nitrosylation. It has been reported that disturbed flow down-regulated eNOS expression or decreased the coupling of eNOS to cofactors, leading to the deficiency of NO production.[47,48]

As described above, disturbed flow activates XBP1 splicing, leading to VE-cadherin transcriptional suppression and increase of degradation. Lack of VE-cadherin can trigger caspase activation in ECs, while caspase activation can also increase the shedding of VE-cadherin.[49,50] Sustained activation of XBP1 splicing will trigger activation of multiple capases and EC apoptosis, leading to EC loss from the vessel walls. MMP inhibitor GM6001 can partially rescue over-expression of spliced XBP1 (Ad-XBP1s) induced VE-cadherin degradation and EC loss from the vessel wall, while reconstitution of VE-cadherin via adenoviral gene transfer could significantly rescue Ad-XBP1s-induced EC apoptosis. Inhibition of capases could totally block Ad-XBP1s-induced EC loss from the vessel walls.[27]

Taken together, disturbed flow firstly activates XBP1 splicing, which in turn suppresses VE-cadherin transcription and increases its degradation. The down-regulation of VE-cadherin will increase EC proliferation and apoptosis. Secondly, disturbed flow activates BMP2/4, which in turn activates Nox mRNA expression and activity in an autocrine manner, leading to superoxide production. Thirdly, NO production is impaired by disturbed flow. The overall effect is to increase EC proliferation and apoptosis (Fig. 3).

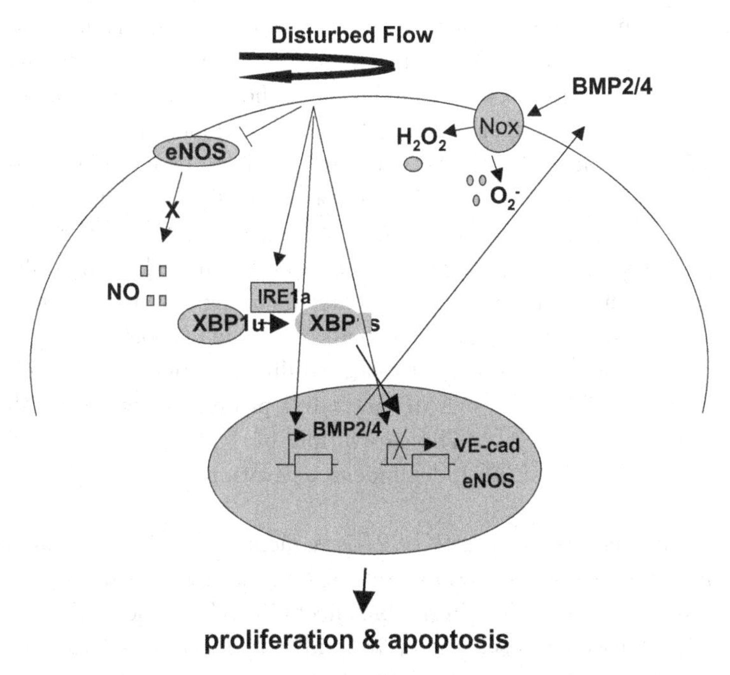

Fig. 3. Disturbed flow induces EC proliferation and apoptosis. Disturbed flow activates XBP1 splicing on one hand, which down-regulates VE-cadherin via transcriptional suppression and MMP-mediated degradation, leading to caspase activation. On the other hand, disturbed flow activates BMP2/4 expression and secretion, which in turn activates Nox to produce ROS in an autocrine manner. Thirdly, NO production was impaired under disturbed flow. The overall effect increases EC proliferation with concomitant increase of apoptosis.

2.3. *Laminar Flow Increase EC Quiescence and Survival*

In contrast to disturbed flow, steady or laminar flow increases EC quiescence and survival, partially due to NO production, KLF2 and p21 activation.

It is well established that laminar flow-induced NO production is a fundamental mechanism of regulation of vascular tone, peripheral resistance and tissue perfusion.[51] The NO production by flow is in a dose dependent manner *in vitro* and *in vivo*.[52–54] Laminar flow induces NO production through both the transcriptional up-regulation of eNOS gene expression and the post-translational modification of eNOS protein. Laminar flow-induced eNOS gene expression is a combined effect of transient transcription with a long-term mRNA stabilization. The transcription is calcium dependent process, involving c-Src/Mek1/2/ NFkappaB signal pathway activation and p50/p60 binding to a GAGACC sequence present in the eNOS promoter, in which the coactivator p300 is recruited.[55–58] The mRNA stabilization involves the elongation of polyadenylation of the 3' tail.[59] In sheared cells, eNOS mRNA has a longer 3' poly(A) tail with much longer half-life as compared to static cells. eNOS normally localizes in caveolae structure in the cell membrane associated with caveolin. The activation of eNOS involves the dissociation with caveolin, phosphorylation at different serine residues in response to different stimuli, association with calmodulin and translocation into cellular compartments including ER membrane, peri-nuclear and nuclear. Laminar flow induces rapid dissociation of eNOS with caveolin and association with calmodulin, phosphorylation at serine 635 and serine1179 sites by AMP-activated protein kinase or PI3K-Akt dependent activation.[60–65] The activation of PI3K-Akt was mediated by c-Src dependent VEGF-independent activation of VEGF receptor 2 (KDR).[66]

Lung krüppel-like factor (KLF2) is a member of the KLF family of zinc finger transcription factors, involved in murine vasculogenesis and anti-inflammatory and anti-thromobic effects in ECs. Knockdown of KLF2 by siRNA increased EC sensitivity to oxidized LDL-induced EC injury,[67] while hemozygous deficiency of KLF2 increased diet-induced atherosclerosis in $ApoE^{-/-}$ mice.[68] Endothelial loss of KLF2 caused dysfunction in hemodynamic regulation and defect in tunica media formation and vessel stabilization, leading to embryonic lethality.[69,70] The expression of KLF2 in ECs is flow pattern specific *in vitro* and *in vivo*. Laminar flow induced sustained activation of KLF2 expression, while oscillatory flow suppressed

KLF2 expression *in vitro*. High level of KLF2 was detected in straight part of vessel wall ECs, while low level in disturbed flow area.[67] The level of KLF2 in ECs is related to the expression of vascular tone-regulating genes.[71] Flow-induced activation of KLF2 expression is PI3K dependent nucleolin binding to the $-138 \sim -111$ sequence in the promoter from transcription start site.[72–74] KLF2 protect ECs from oxidative stress and inflammation through inhibition of vascular permeability factor/VEGF-induced EC proliferation,[75] up-regulation of eNOS,[71,76] thrombomodulin,[76,77] CD59[78] and Nrf2-dependent heme oxygenase 1 (HO-1) gene expression[79] and suppression of TGF-β signal pathway[80] and ATF2 expression.[81] A widely used vasoprotective medicine, statin, protect ECs through KLF2-dependent up-regulation of HO-1 gene expression.[82,83] Shear stress-upregulated KLF2 expression could lower the concentration of statin required to protect EC from H_2O_2-induced apoptosis.[84] KLF2 was reported to modulate $p21^{waf1/cip1}$ (p21) expression in Jurkat T leukaemia cell therefore inhibiting its growth.[85]

p21 is the founding member of the Cip/Kip family of cyclin-dependent kinase inhibitors that includes p27 and p57.[86,87] These molecules bind to cyclin/CDK complex and inhibit their activity, which is essential for cell cycle progression. p21 preferentially binds to cyclin/CDK2 complex, leading to cell cycle arrest at G1/S transition. The expression level of p21 in ECs relates to EC proliferation and survival to apoptotic stimuli. Lai *et al.*[88] reported that reduced expression of p21 and p27 led to an uncontrolled proliferation of immatured ECs in retinaldehyde dehydrogenase 2 deficient ($Raldh2^{-/-}$) mice. Similarly, increased proliferation of ECs was observed in p21 deficient mice ($p21^{-/-}$), which had much higher apoptotic rate for ECs as compared to hemizygous ($p21^{+/-}$) or wild type mice.[89] In *in vitro*-cultured ECs, the decreased expression of p21 by TGF β or increased cleavage of p21 by caspase 3 or neutrophil protease 3 (RP3) is associated with increased apoptosis.[90,91] On the contrast, elevated expression of p21 in ECs is associated with cell cycle arrest and increased survival to apoptotic stimuli. It has been well established that laminar shear stress induced EC cell cycle arrest at late G1 phase through up-regulation of p53-mediated p21 expression.[92,93] Zhang *et al.*[94] reported that anti-angiogenic agent TNP-470-induced cell cycle arrest was also mediated by p53 and p21. Mattiussi *et al.*[95] reported that both laminar shear stress and the NO donor, sodium nitroprusside (SNP), increased EC survival to hypoxia-induced apoptosis via up-regulation of p21. Over-expression of p21 by adenoviral gene transfer of AdCMV. p21 vector protected HUVEC from hypoxia-induced cell death. When such vector was directly injected *in vivo*, ischemia-induced EC death was significantly reduced. However, when p21 level was brought down by antisense vector AdCMV. ASp21 in HUVECs, the shear stress and SNP-induced protection was abolished. The expression of p21 in ECs can be mediated by p53 dependent and independent pathways. Our previous study[96] demonstrated that laminar shear stress-induced p21 expression is p53 dependent. The p21 level in p53-null HCT116 cells was increased by TSA in a Sp1 dependent manner[97] but not responded to laminar flow, while p21 level in wild type HCT116 cells ($p53^{+/+}$) was increase by both TSA and laminar flow. As to p53-dependent activation of p21, the relationship between the acetylation status of p53 and the expression of p21 is somewhat complicated. It was widely accepted that UV-irradiation induced p53 acetylation at multiple lysine sites in different cell types, which correlated with up-regulation of p21 (see Ref. 98 for review). However, p53 acetylation was a rapid event, occurring within 4hrs after UV-irradiation, while expression of p21 was up-regulated at least 8 hrs later.[96,99] Actually, UV-irradiation induced rapid degradation of p21 through proteasome pathway.[100] On the contrary, our study showed that laminar flow induced p53 deacetylation at lysine320 and lysine373 sites (Lys317 and Lys370 for murine p53, respectively) with concomitant up-regulation of p21 level in mature ECs[96] and differentiated ESCs.[101] The flow-induced p53 deacetylation and p21 up-regulation was blocked by the presence of HDAC inhibitor, trichostatin A (TSA) or HDAC siRNA, indicating that flow-induced p53 deacetylation is responsible for up-regulation of p21 expression and cell survival in ECs.

In summary, laminar flow protects EC from apoptosis through (1) up-regulation of eNOS transcription and mRNA stabilization via c-Src/Mek1/2/NFkappaB pathway and activation of eNOS protein phosphorylation in an Akt or PKA dependent pathways, leading to NO production increase; (2) activation of KLF2 expression in a PI3K dependent recruitment of nucleolin to KLF2 promoter, which in turn activates Nrf2-dependent activation of HO-1 expression and carbon monoxide production; (3) activation of HDACs and p53 deacetylation, causing p21 activation. KLF2 can induce eNOS and p21 gene expression, while NO can also regulate p21 expression. The concomitant activation of the net work among KLF2-eNOS-p21 contributes to the laminar flow-induced EC cell cycle arrest and survival from apoptotic stimuli (Fig. 4).

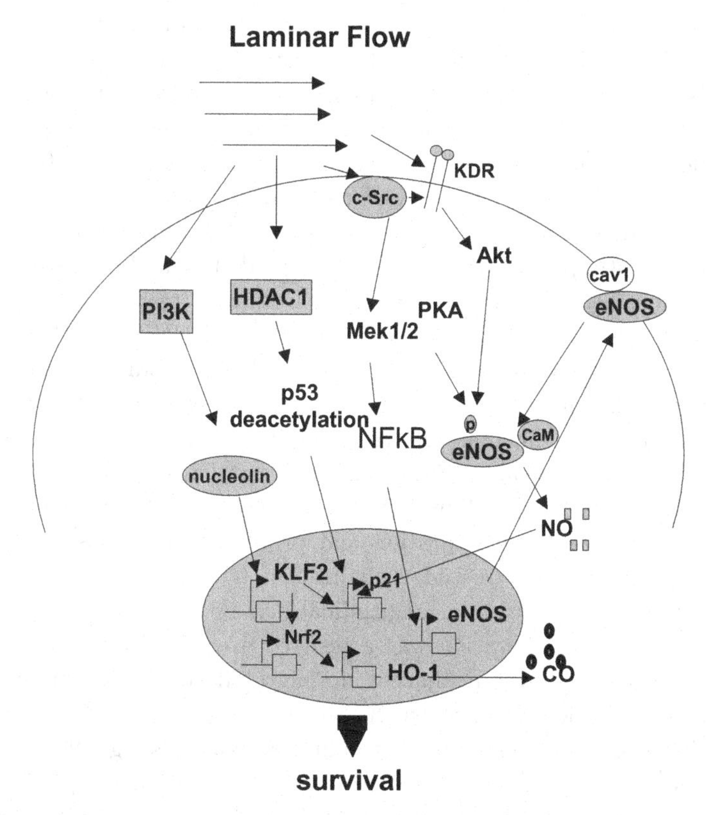

Fig. 4. Laminar flow induces EC cell cycle arrest and survival from apoptotic stimuli. Laminar flow activates eNOS via c-Src/Mek1/2/NFkB mediated transcription, dissociation with caveolin (cav1) and association with calmodulin (CaM), phosphorylation by Akt or PKA via ligand-independent KDR pathway, leading to NO production increase. Laminar flow activates KLF2 expression via PI3K/nucleolin, which in turn activates Nrf2-dependent transcription of HO-1, leading to CO production. Laminar flow also activates HDAC1, leading to p53 deacetylation-mediated p21 expression. KLF2 can activate both eNOS and p21 expression, while NO production can also induce p21 expression. The net-work among KLF2-NO-p21 leads to EC cell cycle arrest at late G1 phase and increase EC survival under oxidative stress.

3. Endothelium Repair

The integrity of the endothelial layer is crucial for the maintenance of normal vascular activity. However, as exposed to various endogenous stress conditions derived from shear stress, cyclic stretch, immune response and oxidative stress, etc and/or exogenous forces such as surgery and irradiation etc, endothelial cells will undergo natural turnover or damage, resulting in local denudation of the endothelium. This will cause the local disturbance to homeostasis, vascular wall tone, barrier function and leukocyte homing. Long term denudation of endothelium is the key factor to develop atherosclerosis. Therefore, the homeostasis of the arterial wall depends on the balance between vascular injury and repair.

The original concept for injury repair was that adjacent ECs migrate and subsequently proliferate to cover the denuded area. The first evidence for migration-mediated injury repair came from *in vitro* study.[102] Following a standardized "wound-healing" model in cultured HUVECs, cell migration from the edge area was observed consistently underway within 12 hrs after injury, and by 24 hr there was a considerable repopulation of the wound. A significant increase of ^{3}H-thymidine labelling was not observed until 36 hrs. Pre-treatment of the cells with irradiation abolished wound-induced ^{3}H-thymidine labelling but had no effect on cell migration. These results indicate that cell migration and proliferation are discrete events in wound healing. The re-endothelialization by adjacent EC migration was later observed *in vivo* in longitudinal denuded tracks in the thoracic aorta of rats.[103] Proliferation was a delayed event and only occurred in migrating cells but not in adjacent un-migrated cells. The migration of adjacent cells to denuded area starts with the orientation of centrosomes and redistribution of microfilaments bundles, which is signalled by FGF pathways.[104–109] As exposed to blood flow, the migration and proliferation of ECs to denuded area will be definitely affected by flow patterns. Laminar shear stress enhances EC migration to denuded area through activation of integrin/Rho signalling,[110,111] VE-cadherin expression and location[112] and VEGF signal pathways.[113] Disturbed flow can also enhance EC migration through tyrosine kinase activation, but less effectively compared to laminar flow.[110] It is believed that a small area of denudation can be re-endothelialized by adjacent cell migration, while a large area of denudation will involve in cell migration and subsequent proliferation.

Although mature ECs adjacent to the damaged cell can replace the lost cells, recent evidence indicates that endothelial progenitor cells (EPCs) are involved and play an important role in the re-endothelialization of denuded endothelium, especially in the areas with severe damage of endothelium. EPCs were first isolated by Asahara and colleagues[114] in 1997 from peripheral blood, characterized by the expression of surface marker CD34, CD133, and KDR, uptake of acetylated LDL and binding of *Ulex europeus* lectin.[115] Circulating EPCs are mainly derived from bone marrow via mobilization by vascular injury-released growth factors and cytokines.[116] The involvement of circulating EPCs in vascular injury repair was reported by various studies (reference[117] for review). In our study with vein graft mouse model, vena cava from *Tie2-LacZ* donor mice, in which ECs expressed β-gal and could be revealed by en face X-gal staining, was isografted to wild type recipient carotid arteries. Vice versa, wild type donor vena cava was isografted to *Tie2-LacZ* recipient mice carotid arteries. The disappearance in *Tie2-LacZ* to wild type and appearance in wild type to *Tie2-LacZ* grafts of the β-gal positive cells demonstrated the recipient origins of re-endothelialization in vascular injury repair. β-gal positive cell distribution pattern analysis indicated that regenerated ECs were possibly derived from circulating blood rather than anastomosed artery. Further experiments with vein graft in bone marrow chimeric mice, in which wild type mice received bone marrow from *Tie2-LacZ* mice while *Tie2-LacZ* mice receive bone marrow from wild type mice, demonstrated that both bone marrow-derived EPCs and non-bone marrow-derived EPCs participated in the re-endothelialization process. Bone marrow-derived EPCs took account for one third of the reendothelialization.[118] Our recent study demonstrated that bone marrow-derived EPCs were also involved in the repair of natural turnover of ECs caused by disturbed flow. Ten months after transplantation of bone marrow from $ApoE^{-/-}$/*Tie2-LacZ* mice to $ApoE^{-/-}$ mice, 3–4% of total ECs in atherosclerosis prone area were β-gal positive cells.[22] As described above, bone marrow-derived EPCs only took about one third of the reendothelialization of injured vessels, indicating that circulating EPCs should have other origins. Indeed, circulating EPCs has been demonstrated to be also derived from tissue resident progenitors including skeletal muscle,[119] spleen,[120] liver,[121] fat tissue[122] and adventitia of the arterial wall.[123] Besides the circulating EPCs, recent studies indicated that multipotent vascular stem cells exist in blood and vascular wall, involving in vascular injury repair (reference[124] for review). Despite its beneficial effect on re-endothelialization of denuded endothelium, EPCs also contribute to the development of vascular disease, such as atherosclerosis.[125]

4. Effect of Shear Stress on EC Differentiation

To investigate the effect of shear stress on EC differentiation, different groups used different cell sources and methods, but all achieved similar results, i.e. laminar flow enhanced-EC differentiation. The cell sources included embryonic stem cell (ESC),[101,126–128] ESC-derived Sca1$^+$ or Flk-1$^+$ cells,[129,130] mesenchymal stem cell (MSC)[131,132] or progenitor cell (MPC),[133,134] EPCs[135–141] isolated from bone marrow, peripheral blood and umbilical vein blood, multipotent stem cells isolated from adipose tissue[142] or placenta.[143] As to the methodology, the stem or progenitor cells were cultured on extracellular matrix (ECM)-coated media supplemented with/without growth factors prior to shear stress. Collagen type IV and fibronectin were the main ECMs used by most groups. Pulsatile/non-pulsatile laminar shear stress (6–15 dynes/cm^2) were generally applied to the pre-differentiated cells for different time duration. Comparing to static control, the sheared cells revealed much higher EC-like phenotype: expressing higher levels of EC marker proteins, such as CD31, CD144, eNOS and vWF, etc., forming capillary-like structures on matrigel surface *in vitro* and neo-vessels in matrigel plug implanted subcutaneously in mice, and repairing injured blood vessels in mouse model.

Mouse ESC cell line is a convenient cell source for differentiation studies. In our experiments,[101] ESCs were plated on collagen IV-coated glass slides in the absence of leukemia inhibitory factor (LIF) for 3 days, which allowed for ESCs to spontaneously differentiate into progenitors characterized by the occurrence of progenitor marker expression, such as Flk-1 and CD133. 12 dynes/cm^2 steady flow, created by growth medium flowing through cell surface in a rectangle chamber system, was then applied to the pre-differentiated cells, which promoted the progenitor cell proliferation and differentiation toward EC lineage. The sheared cells showed higher population of CD144 positive cells, forming nice tube-like structure on matrigel surface and blood vessels in matrigel plug in mice model. Most importantly, the differentiated ECs could incorporate into the injured femoral artery and reduced injury-induced neo-intima formation in ApoE$^{-/-}$ mice. Meanwhile, we found that laminar flow significantly decreased SMC marker gene expression like smooth muscle alpha actin (SMA), calponin and SM22, implying that laminar flow suppresses ESC differentiation toward SMC lineage. On the contrary, Illi *et al.*[127] found that both EC and SMC marker gene expression was up-regulated by shear when ESCs were cultured on fibronectin-coated media and under 10 dynes/cm^2 shear stress. Similarly, Huang *et al.*[126] reported that ESCs could synchronically differentiate into ECs and SMCs under the combination of a wall shear stress (WSS) from -0.98 to 2.2 dyn/cm^2

and a circumferential strain CS 4.6–9.6 $\times$ 10(4) dyn/cm^2 in a compliant microporous tube made of polyurethane. The luminal surface of the tube was fully covered with the cells by preincubation for two days in the presence of VEGF followed by additional 2 days shearing without VEGF. In the sheared group, cells in the superficial layer were regularly oriented in the direction of the pulsatile flow, exhibiting endothelial-like appearance; while the cells growing into the interstices in the deeper layer showed smooth muscle-like appearance. On the other hand, cells in static group only showed SMC-like appearance. The results from these different groups indicate that it is possible to direct ESCs differentiate into ECs or together with SMCs at the same time through modulation of the differentiation procedures. A recent study by Metallo *et al.*[128] showed that ESC-derived ECs possessed similar response to flow as primary ECs in morphology and gene expression profile.

Flk-1 and/or Sca-1 are EPC marker, usually used to isolate EPCs from ESC population after spontaneous differentiation in the absence of LIF and presence of VEGF for several days. Our study[129] demonstrated that Scal positive cells could differentiate into EC lineage under VEGF treatment or laminar shear stress with higher efficiency than ESC. At the same time, the SMC lineage differentiation was also suppressed by flow. A similar result was reported on isolated Flkl positive cells by Yamamoto *et al.*[130] Laminar flow increased Flkl proliferation and differentiation toward EC lineage, revealed by the increase of S and G2/M population and EC marker gene expression such as Flkl, Fltl, VE-cadherin and PECAM-1 at both mRNA and protein levels. EPCs isolated from other sources like human peripheral blood exhibited similar response to laminar flow *in vitro* as Flkl/Scal positive cells did. When cultured human blood-derived EPCs were subjected to laminar flow, the cell density was increased with higher G2/M subpopulation, EC specific markers such as eNOS, Flkl, Fltl, VE-cadherin were also increased at mRNA and protein levels as compare to EPCs kept under static conditions. The sheared EPCs showed an EC-like appearance with orientation along the flow direction, and could form tube-like structure on matrigel surface.[141] Whatever sources derived from, EPCs are at least bipotential progenitor cells, able to differentiate into EC and SMC lineages depending on differentiation procedures.[144,145] VEGF and laminar shear stress seem to favor EC differentiation, while PDGF and cyclic stretch favor SMC differentiation. Through modulating a specific procedure, it is possible to direct EPC differentiation toward specific lineage.

Other multipotent stem or progenitor cells are also widely used to study EC differentiation. These sources include bone marrow derived mesenchymal stem or progenitor cells, human placenta derived stem cells and adipose tissue resident stem cells. Wang *et al.*[133] reported that fluid shear stress created by a parallel plate system could enhance a murine embryonic mesenchymal progenitor cell line C3H/10T1/2 differentiate toward EC lineage, exhibiting EC marker expression, uptake of acetylated LDL and formation of capillary-like structures on matrigel. In addition, the expression of angiogenic factors was up-regulated while down-regulating growth factors associated with SMC differentiation. A recent report from Dong *et al.*[131] showed that canine bone marrow MSCs could be differentiated to ECs by laminar shear stress in a 3 dimensional tissue-engineered vascular grafts. Wu *et al.*[143] isolated multipotent stem cells, a subpopulation of $CD34^-CD133^-Flk1^-$ cells from human placenta and cultured in endothelial growth medium supplemented with VEGF, followed by laminar shear stress at 6 and 12 dynes/cm^2. VEGF treatment triggered the Flk1 expression, while high shear stress (12 dynes/cm^2) augmented EC differentiation with mature EC marker gene expression and capillary-like structure formation on matrigel. 6 dynes/$cm^2$was less effective than 12 dynes/cm^2 shear stress. This work indicates that VEGF and laminar shear stress can synergistically induce placenta derived-stem cell differentiation toward EC lineage. Similar synergistic effect between VEGF and shear stress can also be achieved on adipose-derived stem cell differentiation toward EC lineage.[142] Taken together, high shear stress laminar flow can enhance stem/progenitor cells differentiate toward EC lineage, while suppressing SMC commitment. VEGF can synergistically augment this process.

Cell differentiation is a multiple factor-involved multi-step process, the underlying mechanism of which is far from understood. VEGF is a well-known mitogenic growth factor for mature EC proliferation, and its role in EC differentiation has also established. Similar to mature ECs, laminar flow can activate VEGF receptor Flk1 in ESC-derived progenitor cells in a ligand-independent manner, which is essential for flow-induced EC differentiation. In our study,[101] inclusion of Flk1 inhibitor, SU1498, in the shear medium ablated flow-induced EC marker gene expression. Similar results were obtained on Flk1 positive progenitor cell differentiation by Yamammoto *et al.*[130] It was SU1498, not the neutralizing antibody against VEGF, which blocked shear stress-induced Flk1 positive progenitor cell differentiation toward ECs, indicating the ligand-independent activation of Flk1 is essential for EC differentiation under flow. Several down-stream signal pathways can be triggered by Flk1 activation. Our data[101] showed that PI3K /Akt inhibitor LY294002 not the MAP kinase inhibitor PD98059 blocked flow-induced ESC differentiation toward ECs. Similarly, Ye *et al.*[137] reported that laminar shear stress-induced EC differentiation from human cord blood EPCs was also dependent on Akt activation. HDACs seem to be Akt down stream effectors. The first indirect evidence for the involvement of HDACs in EC differentiation derived from HDACs inhibitor TSA blocking hypoxia-induced angiogenesis in tumor tissue.[146,147] Our data[101,129] and reports from Rossig *et al.*[139] demonstrated that laminar flow up-regulated HDAC activity in ESCs and EPCs, respectively. Inhibition of HDAC activity by TSA blocked flow-induced EC differentiation. Our study[101] further distinguished that HDAC1 and HDAC3 are the responsible HDACs, as HDAC1 and HDAC3 siRNAs could block flow-induced ESC differentiation toward ECs. Both HDAC1 and HDAC3 protein levels were up-regulated by laminar flow in ESCs, which was ablated by SU1498 and LY294002, indicating HDACs are the downstream of Flk1-PI3K/Akt pathway. HDACs not only modulate the epigenetic modification status of chromatin but also affect some transcription factor modification and its transcriptional activity, regulating gene expression. Our data[101] showed that laminar flow deacetylated p53, which in turn activated p21 expression, leading to EC differentiation. In the presence of HDAC3 siRNA or TSA, p53 acetylation was increased and flow could no longer deacetylate p53, resulting in p21 expression decrease. Both p53 siRNA and p21 siRNA ablated flow-induced EC marker expression in ESCs. The function of p21 might increase differentiated EC survival. Rossig *et al.*[139] reported that HDACs regulated HoxA9 expression, which was essential for flow induced EC differentiation. TSA blocked flow-induced HoxA9 expression, while HoxA9 siRNA abolished flow-induced EC marker gene expression. Except HDAC1 and HDAC3, HDAC5, HDAC7 and HDAC8 are also involved in vascular cell lineage determination. HDAC5 works together with Klf4 and Elk-1 suppressing SMC differentiation.[148] On the contrary, HDAC8 is restricted to SMC differentiation.[149] HDAC7 is essential for blood vessel formation but not necessary for EC differentiation.[150] Our data[151] indicated that HDAC7 expression and fully splicing coincided with SMC differentiation from ESCs. Laminar flow suppressed HDAC7 and HDAC8 expression and HDAC7 splicing with decrease of SMC marker expression.

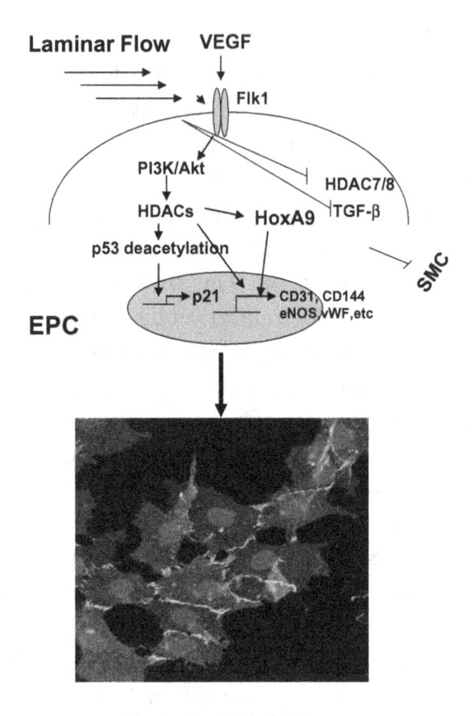

Fig. 5. Laminar flow induces EPC differentiation toward EC lineage. (A) A schematic illustration of the mechanism involved in EPC differentiation under laminar flow. Laminar flow activates Flk1 in a ligand-independent way, which leads to PI3K-Akt-HDACs cascade activation. The activation of HDACs causes p53 deaceetylation at Lys320/373 sites, which in turn activates p21 expression, resulting in differentiated EC survival. Alternatively, activation of HDACs leads to HoxA9 activation and down-stream target gene expression, which is involved in EC marker gene expression. HDACs may be directly involved in EC marker gene expression. On the other hand, laminar flow down-regulates HDAC7 and 8, and TGF-β signal pathway, suppressing SMC marker gene expression. The overall effect leads to EC differentiation.

TGF-β signal pathway is involved in SMC differentiation.[152] Wang *et al.*[134] reported that fluid shear stress induced mouse embryonic mesenchymal progenitor cell differentiation toward EC lineage through suppression of TGF-β receptor and Smads. Taken together, as illustrated in Fig. 5, we can postulate that laminar flow activates Flk1-PI3K-Akt-HDACs signal pathway, which in turn activates HoxA9, leading to EC marker gene expression and/or deacetylates p53 and therefore activates p21 expression, leading to differentiated EC survival. On the other hand, laminar flow turns down HDAC7, HDAC8 and TGF-β signal pathway, suppressing SMC differentiation. The overall effect primes the progenitor cells to differentiate into EC lineage, which contribute to the endothelium injury repair (Fig. 5).

5. Summary and Conclusion

Here we have endeavoured to summarize the recent results coming from studies on the effect of flow patterns on stem/progenitor cell differentiation and mature EC function *in vitro* and *in vivo.* Laminar shear stress can induce stem/progenitor cells differentiation toward EC lineage via Flk1-PI3K-Akt-HDACs signal pathway and suppress SMC differentiation through down-regulation HDAC7/8 and TGF-β pathway. On mature ECs, laminar shear stress induces cell cycle arrest and increase cell survival from apoptotic stimuli via KLF2-NO-p21 net work, it also increases EC migration. The overall of EC differentiation and migration is responsible for endothelium injury repair. In contrast, disturbed flow increases EC proliferation and apoptosis through activation of XBP1 splicing-induced VE-cadherin down-regulation, BMP2/4-mediated ROS production and deficiency of NO production via decreased eNOS expression. Different types of stem cells and progenitor cells can be primed to differentiate toward EC by laminar flow and/or VEGF. Different types of natural and synthetic polymer scaffolds have been made to support stem/progenitor cell differentiation toward all types of vascular cell lineages *in vitro* and *in vivo.* Extensive knowledge from research on both stem/progenitor cell differentiation and biodegradable materials will provide breakthrough on cell-based therapeutic vascular regenerative medicine.

One question we will ask is whether the disturbed flow areas serve as endothelial stem cell niche. The Br-dU incorporating or Ki-67 positive cells may actually be proliferating stem or progenitor cells in response to local or distal injury stimuli. Do these cells contribute to the circulating stem or progenitor cells in the peripheral blood? Does the trans-differentiation of these EC stem cells to other cell types contribute to the atherosclerosis development? In other words, atherosclerosis is a pathophysiological process involving in wrong differentiation direction of EC stem cells. The answer to these questions may enhance our knowledge on vascular biology and the mechanism involved in vascular disease development.

6. Disclosure

None of the authors has a conflict of interest.

Acknowledgement

This work is supported by grants from British Heart Foundation and Oak Foundation.

References

1. Libby, P. (2002) Inflammation in atherosclerosis. *Nature* **420**(6917), 868–874.
2. Li, C., and Xu, Q. (2007) Mechanical stress-initiated signal transduction in vascular smooth muscle cells *in vitro* and *in vivo*. *Cell Signal* **19**(5), 881–891.
3. Ross, R. (1999) Atherosclerosis — an inflammatory disease. *N Engl J Med* **340**(2), 115–126.
4. Steinberg, D. (1997) Low density lipoprotein oxidation and its pathobiological significance. *J Biol Chem* **272**(34), 20963–20966.
5. Davies, P. F. (2009) Hemodynamic shear stress and the endothelium in cardiovascular pathophysiology. *Nat Clin Pract Cardiovasc Med* **6**(1), 16–26.
6. Li, Y. S., Haga, J. H., and Chien, S. (2005) Molecular basis of the effects of shear stress on vascular endothelial cells. *J Biomech* **38**(10), 1949–1971.
7. Stemerman, M. B., Morrel, E. M., Burke, K. R., Colton, C. K., Smith, K. A., and Lees, R. S. (1986) Local variation in arterial wall permeability to low density lipoprotein in normal rabbit aorta. *Arteriosclerosis* **6**(1), 64–69.
8. Schwenke, D. C., and Carew, T. E. (1989) Initiation of atherosclerotic lesions in cholesterol-fed rabbits. II. Selective retention of LDL vs. selective increases in LDL permeability in susceptible sites of arteries. *Arteriosclerosis* **9**(6), 908–918.
9. Schwenke, D. C., and Carew, T. E. (1989) Initiation of atherosclerotic lesions in cholesterol-fed rabbits. I. Focal increases in arterial LDL concentration precede development of fatty streak lesions. *Arteriosclerosis* **9**(6), 895–907.
10. Wada, S., and Karino, T. (2002) Theoretical prediction of low-density lipoproteins concentration at the luminal surface of an artery with a multiple bend. *Ann Biomed Eng* **30**(6), 778–791.
11. Chien, S. (2003) Molecular and mechanical bases of focal lipid accumulation in arterial wall. *Prog Biophys Mol Biol* **83**(2), 131–151.
12. Minick, C. R., Stemerman, M. G., and Insull, W., Jr. (1977) Effect of regenerated endothelium on lipid accumulation in the arterial wall. *Proc Natl Acad Sci U S A* **74**(4), 1724–1728.

13. Falcone, D. J., Hajjar, D. P., and Minick, C. R. (1984) Lipoprotein and albumin accumulation in reendothelialized and deendothelialized aorta. *Am J Pathol* **114**(1), 112–120.
14. Roberts, A. B., Lees, A. M., Lees, R. S., Strauss, H. W., Fallon, J. T., Taveras, J., and Kopiwoda, S. (1983) Selective accumulation of low density lipoproteins in damaged arterial wall. *J Lipid Res* **24**(9), 1160–1167.
15. Liu, Y., Chen, B. P., Lu, M., Zhu, Y., Stemerman, M. B., Chien, S., and Shyy, J. Y. (2002) Shear stress activation of SREBP1 in endothelial cells is mediated by integrins. *Arterioscler Thromb Vasc Biol* **22**(1), 76–81.
16. Hewat, E. A., Durmort, C., Jacquamet, L., Concord, E., and Gulino-Debrac, D. (2007) Architecture of the VE-cadherin hexamer. *J Mol Biol* **365**(3), 744–751.
17. Bazzoni, G., and Dejana, E. (2004) Endothelial cell-to-cell junctions: molecular organization and role in vascular homeostasis. *Physiol Rev* **84**(3), 869–901.
18. Angst, B. D., Marcozzi, C., and Magee, A. I. (2001) The cadherin superfamily. *J Cell Sci* **114**(Pt 4), 625–626.
19. Ha, C. H., Bennett, A. M., and Jin, Z. G. (2008) A novel role of vascular endothelial cadherin in modulating c-Src activation and downstream signaling of vascular endothelial growth factor. *J Biol Chem* **283**(11), 7261–7270.
20. Carmeliet, P., Lampugnani, M. G., Moons, L., Breviario, F., Compernolle, V., Bono, F., Balconi, G., Spagnuolo, R., Oosthuyse, B., Dewerchin, M., Zanetti, A., Angellilo, A., Mattot, V., Nuyens, D., Lutgens, E., Clotman, F., de Ruiter, M. C., Gittenberger-de Groot, A., Poelmann, R., Lupu, F., Herbert, J. M., Collen, D., and Dejana, E. (1999) Targeted deficiency or cytosolic truncation of the VE-cadherin gene in mice impairs VEGF-mediated endothelial survival and angiogenesis. *Cell* **98**(2), 147–157.
21. Noria, S., Cowan, D. B., Gotlieb, A. I., and Langille, B. L. (1999) Transient and steady-state effects of shear stress on endothelial cell adherens junctions. *Circ Res* **85**(6), 504–514.
22. Foteinos, G., Hu, Y., Xiao, Q., Metzler, B., and Xu, Q. (2008) Rapid endothelial turnover in atherosclerosis-prone areas coincides with stem cell repair in apolipoprotein E-deficient mice. *Circulation* **117**(14), 1856–1863.
23. Ukropec, J. A., Hollinger, M. K., and Woolkalis, M. J. (2002) Regulation of VE-cadherin linkage to the cytoskeleton in endothelial cells exposed to fluid shear stress. *Exp Cell Res* **273**(2), 240–247.
24. Liou, H. C., Boothby, M. R., Finn, P. W., Davidon, R., Nabavi, N., Zeleznik-Le, N. J., Ting, J. P., and Glimcher, L. H. (1990) A new member of the leucine zipper class of proteins that binds to the HLA DR alpha promoter. *Science* **247**(4950), 1581–1584.
25. Calfon, M., Zeng, H., Urano, F., Till, J. H., Hubbard, S. R., Harding, H. P., Clark, S. G., and Ron, D. (2002) IRE1 couples endoplasmic reticulum load to secretory capacity by processing the XBP-1 mRNA. *Nature* **415**(6867), 92–96.

26. Yoshida, H., Matsui, T., Yamamoto, A., Okada, T., and Mori, K. (2001) XBP1 mRNA is induced by ATF6 and spliced by IRE1 in response to ER stress to produce a highly active transcription factor. *Cell* **107**(7), 881–891.
27. Zeng, L., Zampetaki, A., Margariti, A., Pepe, A. E., Alam, S., Martin, D., Xiao, Q., Wang, W., Jin, Z. G., Cockerill, G., Mori, K., Li, Y. S., Hu, Y., Chien, S., and Xu, Q. (2009) Sustained activation of XBP1 splicing leads to endothelial apoptosis and atherosclerosis development in response to disturbed flow. *Proc Natl Acad Sci U S A* **106**(20), 8326–8331.
28. Hashimoto, K., Kataoka, N., Nakamura, E., Tsujioka, K., and Kajiya, F. (2007) Oxidized LDL specifically promotes the initiation of monocyte invasion during transendothelial migration with upregulated PECAM-1 and downregulated VE-cadherin on endothelial junctions. *Atherosclerosis* **194**(2), e9–17.
29. Vestweber, D. (2008) VE-cadherin: the major endothelial adhesion molecule controlling cellular junctions and blood vessel formation. *Arterioscler Thromb Vasc Biol* **28**(2), 223–232.
30. Dardik, A., Chen, L., Frattini, J., Asada, H., Aziz, F., Kudo, F. A., and Sumpio, B. E. (2005) Differential effects of orbital and laminar shear stress on endothelial cells. *J Vasc Surg* **41**(5), 869–880.
31. White, C. R., Haidekker, M., Bao, X., and Frangos, J. A. (2001) Temporal gradients in shear, but not spatial gradients, stimulate endothelial cell proliferation. *Circulation* **103**(20), 2508–2513.
32. Kraiss, L. W., Ennis, T. M., and Alto, N. M. (2001) Flow-induced DNA synthesis requires signaling to a translational control pathway. *J Surg Res* **97**(1), 20–26.
33. Gambillara, V., Montorzi, G., Haziza-Pigeon, C., Stergiopulos, N., and Silacci, P. (2005) Arterial wall response to ex vivo exposure to oscillatory shear stress. *J Vasc Res* **42**(6), 535–544.
34. Kraiss, L. W., Weyrich, A. S., Alto, N. M., Dixon, D. A., Ennis, T. M., Modur, V., McIntyre, T. M., Prescott, S. M., and Zimmerman, G. A. (2000) Fluid flow activates a regulator of translation, p70/p85 S6 kinase, in human endothelial cells. *Am J Physiol Heart Circ Physiol* **278**(5), H1537–1544.
35. Orr, A. W., Hahn, C., Blackman, B. R., and Schwartz, M. A. (2008) p21-activated kinase signaling regulates oxidant-dependent NF-kappa B activation by flow. *Circ Res* **103**(6), 671–679.
36. Alexander, R. W. (2003) The Jeremiah Metzger Lecture. Pathogenesis of atherosclerosis: redox as a unifying mechanism. *Trans Am Clin Climatol Assoc* **114**, 273–304.
37. Silacci, P., Desgeorges, A., Mazzolai, L., Chambaz, C., and Hayoz, D. (2001) Flow pulsatility is a critical determinant of oxidative stress in endothelial cells. *Hypertension* **38**(5), 1162–1166.
38. Sorescu, G. P., Song, H., Tressel, S. L., Hwang, J., Dikalov, S., Smith, D. A., Boyd, N. L., Platt, M. O., Lassegue, B., Griendling, K. K., and Jo, H. (2004) Bone morphogenic protein 4 produced in endothelial cells by oscillatory

shear stress induces monocyte adhesion by stimulating reactive oxygen species production from a nox1-based NADPH oxidase. *Circ Res* **95**(8), 773–779.
39. Jo, H., Song, H., and Mowbray, A. (2006) Role of NADPH oxidases in disturbed flow- and BMP4-induced inflammation and atherosclerosis. *Antioxid Redox Signal* **8**(9–10), 1609–1619.
40. Zhang, H., Sunnarborg, S. W., McNaughton, K. K., Johns, T. G., Lee, D. C., and Faber, J. E. (2008) Heparin-binding epidermal growth factor-like growth factor signaling in flow-induced arterial remodeling. *Circ Res* **102**(10), 1275–1285.
41. Csiszar, A., Lehoux, S., and Ungvari, Z. (2009) Hemodynamic forces, vascular oxidative stress and regulation of BMP-2/4 expression. *Antioxid Redox Signal.*
42. Miriyala, S., Gongora Nieto, M. C., Mingone, C., Smith, D., Dikalov, S., Harrison, D. G., and Jo, H. (2006) Bone morphogenic protein-4 induces hypertension in mice: role of noggin, vascular NADPH oxidases, and impaired vasorelaxation. *Circulation* **113**(24), 2818–2825.
43. Schmidt, T. S., and Alp, N. J. (2007) Mechanisms for the role of tetrahydrobiopterin in endothelial function and vascular disease. *Clin Sci (Lond)* **113**(2), 47–63.
44. Kuhlencordt, P. J., Gyurko, R., Han, F., Scherrer-Crosbie, M., Aretz, T. H., Hajjar, R., Picard, M. H., and Huang, P. L. (2001) Accelerated atherosclerosis, aortic aneurysm formation, and ischemic heart disease in apolipoprotein E/endothelial nitric oxide synthase double-knockout mice. *Circulation* **104**(4), 448–454.
45. Mayr, U., Zou, Y., Zhang, Z., Dietrich, H., Hu, Y., and Xu, Q. (2006) Accelerated arteriosclerosis of vein grafts in inducible NO synthase(−/−) mice is related to decreased endothelial progenitor cell repair. *Circ Res* **98**(3), 412–420.
46. Ozaki, M., Kawashima, S., Yamashita, T., Hirase, T., Namiki, M., Inoue, N., Hirata, K., Yasui, H., Sakurai, H., Yoshida, Y., Masada, M., and Yokoyama, M. (2002) Overexpression of endothelial nitric oxide synthase accelerates atherosclerotic lesion formation in apoE-deficient mice. *J Clin Invest* **110**(3), 331–340.
47. Hastings, N. E., Simmers, M. B., McDonald, O. G., Wamhoff, B. R., and Blackman, B. R. (2007) Atherosclerosis-prone hemodynamics differentially regulates endothelial and smooth muscle cell phenotypes and promotes pro-inflammatory priming. *Am J Physiol Cell Physiol* **293**(6), C1824–1833.
48. Won, D., Zhu, S. N., Chen, M., Teichert, A. M., Fish, J. E., Matouk, C. C., Bonert, M., Ojha, M., Marsden, P. A., and Cybulsky, M. I. (2007) Relative reduction of endothelial nitric-oxide synthase expression and transcription in atherosclerosis-prone regions of the mouse aorta and in an *in vitro* model of disturbed flow. *Am J Pathol* **171**(5), 1691–1704.
49. Birdsey, G. M., Dryden, N. H., Amsellem, V., Gebhardt, F., Sahnan, K., Haskard, D. O., Dejana, E., Mason, J. C., and Randi, A. M. (2008)

Transcription factor Erg regulates angiogenesis and endothelial apoptosis through VE-cadherin. *Blood* **111**(7), 3498–3506.
50. Herren, B., Levkau, B., Raines, E. W., and Ross, R. (1998) Cleavage of beta-catenin and plakoglobin and shedding of VE-cadherin during endothelial apoptosis: evidence for a role for caspases and metalloproteinases. *Mol Biol Cell* **9**(6), 1589–1601.
51. Balligand, J. L., Feron, O., and Dessy, C. (2009) eNOS activation by physical forces: from short-term regulation of contraction to chronic remodeling of cardiovascular tissues. *Physiol Rev* **89**(2), 481–534.
52. Guo, X., and Kassab, G. S. (2009) Role of shear stress on nitrite and NOS protein content in different size conduit arteries of swine. *Acta Physiol (Oxf)*.
53. Yan, C., Huang, A., Kaley, G., and Sun, D. (2007) Chronic high blood flow potentiates shear stress-induced release of NO in arteries of aged rats. *Am J Physiol Heart Circ Physiol* **293**(5), H3105–3110.
54. Tao, J., Yang, Z., Wang, J. M., Tu, C., and Pan, S. R. (2006) Effects of fluid shear stress on eNOS mRNA expression and NO production in human endothelial progenitor cells. *Cardiology* **106**(2), 82–88.
55. Xiao, Z., Zhang, Z., Ranjan, V., and Diamond, S. L. (1997) Shear stress induction of the endothelial nitric oxide synthase gene is calcium-dependent but not calcium-activated. *J Cell Physiol* **171**(2), 205–211.
56. Davis, M. E., Grumbach, I. M., Fukai, T., Cutchins, A., and Harrison, D. G. (2004) Shear stress regulates endothelial nitric-oxide synthase promoter activity through nuclear factor kappaB binding. *J Biol Chem* **279**(1), 163–168.
57. Davis, M. E., Cai, H., Drummond, G. R., and Harrison, D. G. (2001) Shear stress regulates endothelial nitric oxide synthase expression through c-Src by divergent signaling pathways. *Circ Res* **89**(11), 1073–1080.
58. Chen, W., Bacanamwo, M., and Harrison, D. G. (2008) Activation of p300 histone acetyltransferase activity is an early endothelial response to laminar shear stress and is essential for stimulation of endothelial nitric-oxide synthase mRNA transcription. *J Biol Chem* **283**(24), 16293–16298.
59. Weber, M., Hagedorn, C. H., Harrison, D. G., and Searles, C. D. (2005) Laminar shear stress and 3' polyadenylation of eNOS mRNA. *Circ Res* **96**(11), 1161–1168.
60. Dimmeler, S., Fleming, I., Fisslthaler, B., Hermann, C., Busse, R., and Zeiher, A. M. (1999). Activation of nitric oxide synthase in endothelial cells by Akt-dependent phosphorylation. *Nature* **399**(6736), 601–605.
61. Rizzo, V., McIntosh, D. P., Oh, P., and Schnitzer, J. E. (1998) *In situ* flow activates endothelial nitric oxide synthase in luminal caveolae of endothelium with rapid caveolin dissociation and calmodulin association. *J Biol Chem* **273**(52), 34724–34729.
62. Chen, Z., Peng, I. C., Sun, W., Su, M. I., Hsu, P. H., Fu, Y., Zhu, Y., DeFea, K., Pan, S., Tsai, M. D., and Shyy, J. Y. (2009) AMP-activated protein kinase functionally phosphorylates endothelial nitric oxide synthase Ser633. *Circ Res* **104**(4), 496–505.

63. Zhang, Y., Lee, T. S., Kolb, E. M., Sun, K., Lu, X., Sladek, F. M., Kassab, G. S., Garland T, Jr., and Shyy, J. Y. (2006) AMP-activated protein kinase is involved in endothelial NO synthase activation in response to shear stress. *Arterioscler Thromb Vasc Biol* **26**(6), 1281–1287.
64. Dixit, M., Loot, A. E., Mohamed, A., Fisslthaler, B., Boulanger, C. M., Ceacareanu, B., Hassid, A., Busse, R., and Fleming, I. (2005) Gab1, SHP2, and protein kinase A are crucial for the activation of the endothelial NO synthase by fluid shear stress. *Circ Res* **97**(12), 1236–1244.
65. Gallis, B., Corthals, G. L., Goodlett, D. R., Ueba, H., Kim, F., Presnell, S. R., Figeys, D., Harrison, D. G., Berk, B. C., Aebersold, R., and Corson, M. A. (1999) Identification of flow-dependent endothelial nitric-oxide synthase phosphorylation sites by mass spectrometry and regulation of phosphorylation and nitric oxide production by the phosphatidylinositol 3-kinase inhibitor LY294002. *J Biol Chem* **274**(42), 30101–30108.
66. Jin, Z. G., Ueba, H., Tanimoto, T., Lungu, A. O., Frame, M. D., and Berk, B. C. (2003) Ligand-independent activation of vascular endothelial growth factor receptor 2 by fluid shear stress regulates activation of endothelial nitric oxide synthase. *Circ Res* **93**(4), 354–363.
67. Wang, N., Miao, H., Li, Y. S., Zhang, P., Haga, J. H., Hu, Y., Young, A., Yuan, S., Nguyen, P., Wu, C. C., and Chien, S. (2006) Shear stress regulation of Kruppel-like factor 2 expression is flow pattern-specific. *Biochem Biophys Res Commun* **341**(4), 1244–1251.
68. Atkins, G. B., Wang, Y., Mahabeleshwar, G. H., Shi, H., Gao, H., Kawanami, D., Natesan, V., Lin, Z., Simon, D. I., and Jain, M. K. (2008) Hemizygous deficiency of Kruppel-like factor 2 augments experimental atherosclerosis. *Circ Res* **103**(7), 690–693.
69. Lee, J. S., Yu, Q., Shin, J. T., Sebzda, E., Bertozzi, C., Chen, M., Mericko, P., Stadtfeld, M., Zhou, D., Cheng, L., Graf, T., MacRae, C. A., Lepore, J. J., Lo, C. W., and Kahn, M. L. (2006) KLF2 is an essential regulator of vascular hemodynamic forces *in vivo*. *Dev Cell* **11**(6), 845–857.
70. Kuo, C. T., Veselits, M. L., Barton, K. P., Lu, M. M., Clendenin, C., and Leiden, J. M. (1997) The LKLF transcription factor is required for normal tunica media formation and blood vessel stabilization during murine embryogenesis. *Genes Dev* **11**(22), 2996–3006.
71. Dekker, R. J., van Thienen, J. V., Rohlena, J., de Jager, S. C., Elderkamp, Y. W., Seppen, J., de Vries, C. J., Biessen, E. A., van Berkel, T. J., Pannekoek, H., and Horrevoets, A. J. (2005) Endothelial KLF2 links local arterial shear stress levels to the expression of vascular tone-regulating genes. *Am J Pathol* **167**(2), 609–618.
72. Huddleson, J. P., Ahmad, N., and Lingrel, J. B. (2006) Up-regulation of the KLF2 transcription factor by fluid shear stress requires nucleolin. *J Biol Chem* **281**(22), 15121–15128.
73. Ahmad, N., and Lingrel, J. B. (2005) Kruppel-like factor 2 transcriptional regulation involves heterogeneous nuclear ribonucleoproteins and acetyltransferases. *Biochemistry* **44**(16), 6276–6285.

74. Huddleson, J. P., Ahmad, N., Srinivasan, S., and Lingrel, J. B. (2005) Induction of KLF2 by fluid shear stress requires a novel promoter element activated by a phosphatidylinositol 3-kinase-dependent chromatin-remodeling pathway. *J Biol Chem* **280**(24), 23371–23379.
75. Bhattacharya, R., Senbanerjee, S., Lin, Z., Mir, S., Hamik, A., Wang, P., Mukherjee, P., Mukhopadhyay, D., and Jain, M. K. (2005) Inhibition of vascular permeability factor/vascular endothelial growth factor-mediated angiogenesis by the Kruppel-like factor KLF2. *J Biol Chem* **280**(32), 28848–28851.
76. Lin, Z., Kumar, A., SenBanerjee, S., Staniszewski, K., Parmar, K., Vaughan, D. E., Gimbrone, M. A., Jr., Balasubramanian, V., Garcia-Cardena, G., and Jain, M. K. (2005) Kruppel-like factor 2 (KLF2) regulates endothelial thrombotic function. *Circ Res* **96**(5), e48–57.
77. Lin, Z., Hamik, A., Jain, R., Kumar, A., and Jain, M. K. (2006) Kruppel-like factor 2 inhibits protease activated receptor-1 expression and thrombin-mediated endothelial activation. *Arterioscler Thromb Vasc Biol* **26**(5), 1185–1189.
78. Kinderlerer, A. R., Ali, F., Johns, M., Lidington, E. A., Leung, V., Boyle, J. J., Hamdulay, S. S., Evans, P. C., Haskard, D. O., and Mason, J. C. (2008) KLF2-dependent, shear stress-induced expression of CD59: a novel cytoprotective mechanism against complement-mediated injury in the vasculature. *J Biol Chem* **283**(21), 14636–14644.
79. Fledderus, J. O., Boon, R. A., Volger, O. L., Hurttila, H., Yla-Herttuala, S., Pannekoek, H., Levonen, A. L., and Horrevoets, A. J. (2008) KLF2 primes the antioxidant transcription factor Nrf2 for activation in endothelial cells. *Arterioscler Thromb Vasc Biol* **28**(7), 1339–1346.
80. Boon, R. A., Fledderus, J. O., Volger, O. L., van Wanrooij, E. J., Pardali, E., Weesie, F., Kuiper, J., Pannekoek, H., ten Dijke, P., and Horrevoets, A. J. (2007) KLF2 suppresses TGF-beta signaling in endothelium through induction of Smad7 and inhibition of AP-1. *Arterioscler Thromb Vasc Biol* **27**(3), 532–539.
81. Fledderus, J. O., van Thienen, J. V., Boon, R. A., Dekker, R. J., Rohlena, J., Volger, O. L., Bijnens, A. P., Daemen, M. J., Kuiper, J., van Berkel, T. J., Pannekoek, H., and Horrevoets, A. J. (2007) Prolonged shear stress and KLF2 suppress constitutive proinflammatory transcription through inhibition of ATF2. *Blood* **109**(10), 4249–4257.
82. Ali, F., Hamdulay, S. S., Kinderlerer, A. R., Boyle, J. J., Lidington, E. A., Yamaguchi, T., Soares, M. P., Haskard, D. O., Randi, A. M., and Mason, J. C. (2007) Statin-mediated cytoprotection of human vascular endothelial cells: a role for Kruppel-like factor 2-dependent induction of heme oxygenase-1. *J Thromb Haemost* **5**(12), 2537–2546.
83. Sen-Banerjee, S., Mir, S., Lin, Z., Hamik, A., Atkins, G. B., Das, H., Banerjee, P., Kumar, A., and Jain, M. K. (2005) Kruppel-like factor 2 as a novel mediator of statin effects in endothelial cells. *Circulation* **112**(5), 720–726.

84. Ali, F., Zakkar, M., Karu, K., Lidington, E. A., Hamdulay, S. S., Boyle, J. J., Zloh, M., Bauer, A., Haskard, D. O., Evans, P. C., and Mason, J. C. (2009) Induction of the cytoprotective enzyme heme oxygenase-1 by statins is enhanced in vascular endothelium exposed to laminar shear stress and impaired by disturbed flow. *J Biol Chem* **284**(28), 18882–18892.
85. Wu, J., and Lingrel, J. B. (2004) KLF2 inhibits Jurkat T leukemia cell growth via upregulation of cyclin-dependent kinase inhibitor p21WAF1/CIP1. *Oncogene* **23**(49), 8088–8096.
86. Gartel, A. L., and Tyner, A. L. (2002) The role of the cyclin-dependent kinase inhibitor p21 in apoptosis. *Mol Cancer Ther* **1**(8), 639–649.
87. Aoudjit, F., and Sevigny, J. (2004) P21(Waf1/Cip1) in endothelial cell survival. *Cardiovasc Res* **61**(4), 648–650.
88. Lai, L., Bohnsack, B. L., Niederreither, K., and Hirschi, K. K. (2003) Retinoic acid regulates endothelial cell proliferation during vasculogenesis. *Development* **130**(26), 6465–6474.
89. Bruhl, T., Heeschen, C., Aicher, A., Jadidi, A. S., Haendeler, J., Hoffmann, J., Schneider, M. D., Zeiher, A. M., Dimmeler, S., and Rossig, L. (2004) p21Cip1 levels differentially regulate turnover of mature endothelial cells, endothelial progenitor cells, and *in vivo* neovascularization. *Circ Res* **94**(5), 686–692.
90. Pendergraft, W. F. 3rd, Rudolph, E. H., Falk, R. J., Jahn, J. E., Grimmler, M., Hengst, L., Jennette, J. C., and Preston, G. A. (2004) Proteinase 3 sidesteps caspases and cleaves p21(Waf1/Cip1/Sdi1) to induce endothelial cell apoptosis. *Kidney Int* **65**(1), 75–84.
91. Yan, Q., and Sage, E. H. (1998) Transforming growth factor-beta1 induces apoptotic cell death in cultured retinal endothelial cells but not pericytes: association with decreased expression of p21waf1/cip1. *J Cell Biochem* **70**(1), 70–83.
92. Lin, K., Hsu, P. P., Chen, B. P., Yuan, S., Usami, S., Shyy, J. Y., Li, Y. S., and Chien, S. (2000) Molecular mechanism of endothelial growth arrest by laminar shear stress. *Proc Natl Acad Sci U S A* **97**(17), 9385–9389.
93. Akimoto, S., Mitsumata, M., Sasaguri, T., and Yoshida, Y. (2000) Laminar shear stress inhibits vascular endothelial cell proliferation by inducing cyclin-dependent kinase inhibitor p21(Sdi1/Cip1/Waf1). *Circ Res* **86**(2), 185–190.
94. Zhang, Y., Griffith, E. C., Sage, J., Jacks, T., and Liu, J. O. (2000) Cell cycle inhibition by the anti-angiogenic agent TNP-470 is mediated by p53 and p21WAF1/CIP1. *Proc Natl Acad Sci U S A* **97**(12), 6427–6432.
95. Mattiussi, S., Turrini, P., Testolin, L., Martelli, F., Zaccagnini, G., Mangoni, A., Barlucchi, L. M., Antonini, A., Illi, B., Cirielli, C., Padron, J., Nicolo, C., Testi, R., Osculati, F., Biglioli, P., Capogrossi, M. C., and Gaetano, C. (2004) p21(Waf1/Cip1/Sdi1) mediates shear stress-dependent antiapoptotic function. *Cardiovasc Res* **61**(4), 693–704.
96. Zeng, L., Zhang, Y., Chien, S., Liu, X., and Shyy, J. Y. (2003) The role of p53 deacetylation in p21Waf1 regulation by laminar flow. *J Biol Chem* **278**(27), 24594–24599.

97. Sowa, Y., Orita, T., Hiranabe-Minamikawa, S., Nakano, K., Mizuno, T., Nomura, H., and Sakai, T. (1999) Histone deacetylase inhibitor activates the p21/WAF1/Cip1 gene promoter through the Sp1 sites. *Ann N Y Acad Sci* **886**, 195–199.
98. Prives, C., and Manley, J. L. (2001) Why is p53 acetylated? *Cell* **107**(7), 815–818.
99. Medrano, E. E., Im, S., Yang, F., and Abdel-Malek, Z. A. (1995) Ultraviolet B light induces G1 arrest in human melanocytes by prolonged inhibition of retinoblastoma protein phosphorylation associated with long-term expression of the p21Waf-1/SDI-1/Cip-1 protein. *Cancer Res* **55**(18), 4047–4052.
100. Bendjennat, M., Boulaire, J., Jascur, T., Brickner, H., Barbier, V., Sarasin, A., Fotedar, A., and Fotedar, R. (2003) UV irradiation triggers ubiquitin-dependent degradation of p21(WAF1) to promote DNA repair. *Cell* **114**(5), 599–610.
101. Zeng, L., Xiao, Q., Margariti, A., Zhang, Z., Zampetaki, A., Patel, S., Capogrossi, M. C., Hu, Y., and Xu, Q. (2006) HDAC3 is crucial in shear- and VEGF-induced stem cell differentiation toward endothelial cells. *J Cell Biol* **174**(7), 1059–1069.
102. Sholley, M. M., Gimbrone, M. A., Jr., and Cotran, R. S. (1977) Cellular migration and replication in endothelial regeneration: a study using irradiated endothelial cultures. *Lab Invest* **36**(1), 18–25.
103. Hirsch, E. Z., Chisolm, G. M. 3rd, and White, H. M. (1983) Reendothelialization and maintenance of endothelial integrity in longitudinal denuded tracks in the thoracic aorta of rats. *Atherosclerosis* **46**(3), 287–307.
104. Schubert, H. D., and Trokel, S. (1984) Endothelial repair following Nd:YAG laser injury. *Invest Ophthalmol Vis Sci* **25**(8), 971–976.
105. Rogers, K. A., Sandig, M., McKee, N. H., and Kalnins, V. I. (1989) The distribution of microfilament bundles in rabbit endothelial cells in the intact aorta and during wound healing *in situ*. *Biochem Cell Biol* **67**(9), 553–562.
106. Rogers, K. A., Sandig, M., McKee, N. H., and Kalnins, V. I. (1992) The distribution of centrosomes in migrating endothelial cells during wound healing *in situ*. *Biochem Cell Biol* **70**(10–11), 1135–1141.
107. Bjornsson, T. D., Dryjski, M., Tluczek, J., Mennie, R., Ronan, J., Mellin, T. N., and Thomas, K. A. (1991) Acidic fibroblast growth factor promotes vascular repair. *Proc Natl Acad Sci U S A* **88**(19), 8651–8655.
108. Coomber, B. L. (1993) Centrosome reorientation in regenerating endothelial monolayers requires bFGF. *J Cell Biochem* **52**(3), 289–296.
109. Ettenson, D. S., and Gotlieb, A. I. (1995) Basic fibroblast growth factor is a signal for the initiation of centrosome redistribution to the front of migrating endothelial cells at the edge of an *in vitro* wound. *Arterioscler Thromb Vasc Biol* **15**(4), 515–521.
110. Hsu, P. P., Li, S., Li, Y. S., Usami, S., Ratcliffe, A., Wang, X., and Chien, S. (2001) Effects of flow patterns on endothelial cell migration into a zone of mechanical denudation. *Biochem Biophys Res Commun* **285**(3), 751–759.

111. Urbich, C., Dernbach, E., Reissner, A., Vasa, M., Zeiher, A. M., and Dimmeler, S. (2002) Shear stress-induced endothelial cell migration involves integrin signaling via the fibronectin receptor subunits alpha(5) and beta(1). *Arterioscler Thromb Vasc Biol* **22**(1), 69–75.
112. Albuquerque, M. L., and Flozak, A. S. (2002) Wound closure in sheared endothelial cells is enhanced by modulation of vascular endothelial-cadherin expression and localization. *Exp Biol Med (Maywood)* **227**(11), 1006–1016.
113. Hughes, S. K., Wacker, B. K., Kaneda, M. M., and Elbert, D. L. (2005) Fluid shear stress modulates cell migration induced by sphingosine 1-phosphate and vascular endothelial growth factor. *Ann Biomed Eng* **33**(8), 1003–1014.
114. Asahara, T., Murohara, T., Sullivan, A., Silver, M., van der Zee, R., Li, T., Witzenbichler, B., Schatteman, G., and Isner, J. M. (1997) Isolation of putative progenitor endothelial cells for angiogenesis. *Science* **275**(5302), 964–967.
115. Aicher, A., Zeiher, A. M., and Dimmeler, S. (2005) Mobilizing endothelial progenitor cells. *Hypertension* **45**(3), 321–325.
116. Shi, Q., Rafii, S., Wu, M. H., Wijelath, E. S., Yu, C., Ishida, A., Fujita, Y., Kothari, S., Mohle, R., Sauvage, L. R., Moore, M. A., Storb, R. F., and Hammond, W. P. (1998) Evidence for circulating bone marrow-derived endothelial cells. *Blood* **92**(2), 362–367.
117. Xu, Q. (2007) Progenitor cells in vascular repair. *Curr Opin Lipidol* **18**(5), 534–539.
118. Xu, Q., Zhang, Z., Davison, F., and Hu, Y. (2003) Circulating progenitor cells regenerate endothelium of vein graft atherosclerosis, which is diminished in ApoE-deficient mice. *Circ Res* **93**(8), e76–86.
119. Majka, S. M., Jackson, K. A., Kienstra, K. A., Majesky, M. W., Goodell, M. A., and Hirschi, K. K. (2003) Distinct progenitor populations in skeletal muscle are bone marrow derived and exhibit different cell fates during vascular regeneration. *J Clin Invest* **111**(1), 71–79.
120. Wassmann, S., Werner, N., Czech, T., and Nickenig, G. (2006) Improvement of endothelial function by systemic transfusion of vascular progenitor cells. *Circ Res* **99**(8), e74–83.
121. Aicher, A., Rentsch, M., Sasaki, K., Ellwart, J. W., Fandrich, F., Siebert, R., Cooke, J. P., Dimmeler, S., and Heeschen, C. (2007) Nonbone marrow-derived circulating progenitor cells contribute to postnatal neovascularization following tissue ischemia. *Circ Res* **100**(4), 581–589.
122. Planat-Benard, V., Silvestre, J. S., Cousin, B., Andre, M., Nibbelink, M., Tamarat, R., Clergue, M., Manneville, C., Saillan-Barreau, C., Duriez, M., Tedgui, A., Levy, B., Penicaud, L., and Casteilla, L. (2004) Plasticity of human adipose lineage cells toward endothelial cells: physiological and therapeutic perspectives. *Circulation* **109**(5), 656–663.
123. Hu, Y., Zhang, Z., Torsney, E., Afzal, A. R., Davison, F., Metzler, B., and Xu, Q. (2004) Abundant progenitor cells in the adventitia contribute to atherosclerosis of vein grafts in ApoE-deficient mice. *J Clin Invest* **113**(9), 1258–1265.

124. Pacilli, A., and Pasquinelli, G. (2009) Vascular wall resident progenitor cells: a review. *Exp Cell Res* **315**(6), 901–914.
125. Zampetaki, A., Kirton, J. P., and Xu, Q. (2008) Vascular repair by endothelial progenitor cells. *Cardiovasc Res* **78**(3), 413–421.
126. Huang, H., Nakayama, Y., Qin, K., Yamamoto, K., Ando, J., Yamashita, J., Itoh, H., Kanda, K., Yaku, H., Okamoto, Y., and Nemoto, Y. (2005) Differentiation from embryonic stem cells to vascular wall cells under *in vitro* pulsatile flow loading. *J Artif Organs* **8**(2), 110–118.
127. Illi, B., Scopece, A., Nanni, S., Farsetti, A., Morgante, L., Biglioli, P., Capogrossi, M. C., and Gaetano, C. (2005) Epigenetic histone modification and cardiovascular lineage programming in mouse embryonic stem cells exposed to laminar shear stress. *Circ Res* **96**(5), 501–508.
128. Metallo, C. M., Vodyanik, M. A., de Pablo, J. J., Slukvin, I. I., and Palecek, S. P. (2008) The response of human embryonic stem cell-derived endothelial cells to shear stress. *Biotechnol Bioeng* **100**(4), 830–837.
129. Xiao, Q., Zeng, L., Zhang, Z., Margariti, A., Ali, Z. A., Channon, K. M., Xu, Q., and Hu, Y. (2006) Sca-1+ progenitors derived from embryonic stem cells differentiate into endothelial cells capable of vascular repair after arterial injury. *Arterioscler Thromb Vasc Biol* **26**(10), 2244–2251.
130. Yamamoto, K., Sokabe, T., Watabe, T., Miyazono, K., Yamashita, J. K., Obi, S., Ohura, N., Matsushita, A., Kamiya, A., and Ando, J. (2005) Fluid shear stress induces differentiation of Flk-1-positive embryonic stem cells into vascular endothelial cells *in vitro*. *Am J Physiol Heart Circ Physiol* **288**(4), H1915–1924.
131. Dong, J. D., Gu, Y. Q., Li, C. M., Wang, C. R., Feng, Z. G., Qiu, R. X., Chen, B., Li, J. X., Zhang, S. W., Wang, Z. G., and Zhang, J. (2009) Response of mesenchymal stem cells to shear stress in tissue-engineered vascular grafts. *Acta Pharmacol Sin* **30**(5), 530–536.
132. Kreke, M. R., Sharp, L. A., Lee, Y. W., and Goldstein, A. S. (2008) Effect of intermittent shear stress on mechanotransductive signaling and osteoblastic differentiation of bone marrow stromal cells. *Tissue Eng Part A* **14**(4), 529–537.
133. Wang, H., Riha, G. M., Yan, S., Li, M., Chai, H., Yang, H., Yao, Q., and Chen, C. (2005) Shear stress induces endothelial differentiation from a murine embryonic mesenchymal progenitor cell line. *Arterioscler Thromb Vasc Biol* **25**(9), 1817–1823.
134. Wang, H., Li, M., Lin, P. H., Yao, Q., and Chen, C. (2008) Fluid shear stress regulates the expression of TGF-beta1 and its signaling molecules in mouse embryo mesenchymal progenitor cells. *J Surg Res* **150**(2), 266–270.
135. Obi, S., Yamamoto, K., Shimizu, N., Kumagaya, S., Masumura, T., Sokabe, T., Asahara, T., and Ando, J. (2009) Fluid shear stress induces arterial differentiation of endothelial progenitor cells. *J Appl Physiol* **106**(1), 203–211.
136. Daculsi, R., Grellier, M., Remy, M., Bareille, R., Pierron, D., Fernandez, P., and Bordenave, L. (2008) Unusual transduction response of

progenitor-derived and mature endothelial cells exposed to laminar pulsatile shear stress. *J Biomech* **41**(12), 2781–2785.

137. Ye, C., Bai, L., Yan, Z. Q., Wang, Y. H., and Jiang, Z. L. (2008) Shear stress and vascular smooth muscle cells promote endothelial differentiation of endothelial progenitor cells via activation of Akt. *Clin Biomech (Bristol, Avon)* **23** Suppl 1, S118–124.
138. Sreerekha, P. R., and Krishnan, L. K. (2006) Cultivation of endothelial progenitor cells on fibrin matrix and layering on dacron/ polytetrafluoroethylene vascular grafts. *Artif Organs* **30**(4), 242–249.
139. Rossig, L., Urbich, C., Bruhl, T., Dernbach, E., Heeschen, C., Chavakis, E., Sasaki, K., Aicher, D., Diehl, F., Seeger, F., Potente, M., Aicher, A., Zanetta, L., Dejana, E., Zeiher, A. M., and Dimmeler, S. (2005) Histone deacetylase activity is essential for the expression of HoxA9 and for endothelial commitment of progenitor cells. *J Exp Med* **201**(11), 1825–1835.
140. Sho, E., Sho, M., Nanjo, H., Kawamura, K., Masuda, H., and Dalman, R. L. (2004) Hemodynamic regulation of CD34+ cell localization and differentiation in experimental aneurysms. *Arterioscler Thromb Vasc Biol* **24**(10), 1916–1921.
141. Yamamoto, K., Takahashi, T., Asahara, T., Ohura, N., Sokabe, T., Kamiya, A., and Ando, J. (2003) Proliferation, differentiation, and tube formation by endothelial progenitor cells in response to shear stress. *J Appl Physiol* **95**(5), 2081–2088.
142. DiMuzio, P., and Tulenko, T. (2007) Tissue engineering applications to vascular bypass graft development: the use of adipose-derived stem cells. *J Vasc Surg* **45** Suppl A, A99–103.
143. Wu, C. C., Chao, Y. C., Chen, C. N., Chien, S., Chen, Y. C., Chien, C. C., Chiu, J. J., and Linju Yen, B. (2008) Synergism of biochemical and mechanical stimuli in the differentiation of human placenta-derived multipotent cells into endothelial cells. *J Biomech* **41**(4), 813–821.
144. Yamashita, J., Itoh, H., Hirashima, M., Ogawa, M., Nishikawa, S., Yurugi, T., Naito, M., and Nakao, K. (2000) Flk1-positive cells derived from embryonic stem cells serve as vascular progenitors. *Nature* **408**(6808), 92–96.
145. Gerecht-Nir, S., Ziskind, A., Cohen, S., and Itskovitz-Eldor, J. (2003) Human embryonic stem cells as an *in vitro* model for human vascular development and the induction of vascular differentiation. *Lab Invest* **83**(12), 1811–1820.
146. Liu, L. T., Chang, H. C., Chiang, L. C., and Hung, W. C. (2003) Histone deacetylase inhibitor up-regulates RECK to inhibit MMP-2 activation and cancer cell invasion. *Cancer Res* **63**(12), 3069–3072.
147. Sawa, H., Murakami, H., Ohshima, Y., Murakami, M., Yamazaki, I., Tamura, Y., Mima, T., Satone, A., Ide, W., Hashimoto, I., and Kamada, H. (2002) Histone deacetylase inhibitors such as sodium butyrate and trichostatin A inhibit vascular endothelial growth factor (VEGF) secretion from human glioblastoma cells. *Brain Tumor Pathol* **19**(2), 77–81.

148. Yoshida, T., Gan, Q., and Owens, G. K. (2008) Kruppel-like factor 4, Elk-1, and histone deacetylases cooperatively suppress smooth muscle cell differentiation markers in response to oxidized phospholipids. *Am J Physiol Cell Physiol* **295**(5), C1175–1182.
149. Waltregny, D., De Leval, L., Glenisson, W., Ly Tran, S., North, B. J., Bellahcene, A., Weidle, U., Verdin, E., and Castronovo, V. (2004) Expression of histone deacetylase 8, a class I histone deacetylase, is restricted to cells showing smooth muscle differentiation in normal human tissues. *Am J Pathol* **165**(2), 553–564.
150. Chang, S., Young, B. D., Li, S., Qi, X., Richardson, J. A., and Olson, E. N. (2006) Histone deacetylase 7 maintains vascular integrity by repressing matrix metalloproteinase 10. *Cell* **126**(2), 321–334.
151. Margariti, A., Xiao, Q., Zampetaki, A., Zhang, Z., Li, H., Martin, D., Hu, Y., Zeng, L., and Xu, Q. (2009) Splicing of HDAC7 modulates the SRF-myocardin complex during stem-cell differentiation towards smooth muscle cells. *J Cell Sci* **122**(Pt 4), 460–470.
152. Xiao, Q., Zeng, L., Zhang, Z., Hu, Y., and Xu, Q. (2007) Stem cell-derived Sca-1+ progenitors differentiate into smooth muscle cells, which is mediated by collagen IV-integrin alpha1/beta1/alphav and PDGF receptor pathways. *Am J Physiol Cell Physiol* **292**(1), C342–352.

Chapter 9

VASCULAR DIFFERENTIATION OF STEM CELLS BY MECHANICAL FORCES

TIMOTHY M. MAUL[*,‡,§,¶], ALEJANDRO NIEPONICE[†,‡,§,||] and DAVID A VORP[*,†,‡,§,**]

*Departments of *Bioengineering and †Surgery,*
‡Center for Vascular Remodeling and Regeneration and
§McGowan Institute for Regenerative Medicine,
University of Pittsburgh, Pittsburgh, PA
¶maultm@upmc.edu
||nieponicea@upmc.edu
***vorpda@upmc.edu*

Current challenges in vascular medicine such as bypass grafting, stenting, and angioplasty have driven the field of vascular regenerative medicine and tissue engineering. Stem cells have shown promise as important components to these applications. Stem cells from multiple tissue sources have demonstrated the capability to differentiate into smooth muscle and endothelial cells in both laboratory and animal models. While early research focused on the biochemical mechanisms behind this phenomenon, more recent data demonstrated that mechanical stimulation can provide important signals to guide the differentiation of stem cells towards vascular phenotypes. The three mechanical stimuli relevant to the vascular system (stretch, shear, and pressure) have been applied in isolation or in combination to stem cells in two- and three-dimensional systems. This chapter provides a review of such work to date, including the magnitude, frequency, and timing of mechanical stimuli used in guiding stem cell differentiation. Experiments utilizing concurrent biochemical stimulation are also discussed, highlighting the importance of a synergistic effort between the biochemical and biomechanical environments. Ultimately, a more complete understanding of these interactions will be necessary to yield important breakthroughs for the future of vascular regenerative medicine.

It is well established that vascular SMCs and ECs, and indeed many other cell types, are sensitive to biomechanical and/or biochemical stimulation,[1–10] and data is continuously emerging to suggest that bone marrow derived mesenchymal stem cells (MSCs) are no different. Primary cultures of MSCs have consistently demonstrated multiple differentiation capacities.[12–19] Specifically, *in vitro* biochemical and biomechanical conditions have been identified which stimulate the differentiation of these stem cells towards adipocytes,[19,21] osteoblasts,[19,21,23,24] stroma,[24,25] chondrocytes,[19,25,26] cardiomyocytes,[27–32] SMCs,[20,34–39] and ECs.[27,40–45]

Although the effects of mechanical stimuli on fully differentiated SMCs and ECs has been extensively studied and demonstrated to be important for the normal physiologic function of these cells,[46–48] the use of physiologically-relevant biomechanical stimuli have only recently begun to be employed, not only for MSC differentiation, but other stem cell sources as well. Therefore, the potential of biomechanical forces on their own, or in combination with biological factors, has not been fully elucidated and has gone underutilized in the field of vascular regenerative medicine. The primary vascular-related forces studied to date are cyclic stretch (both uniaxial and equiaxial), shear stress (laminar, pulsatile, and oscillatory), and to a lesser extent hydrostatic pressure. Each of these forces will be reviewed in this chapter.

1. Stretch

Hamilton *et al.*,[20] were among the first to demonstrate that cyclic uniaxial stretch was sufficient to promote SMC protein production in MSCs (Fig. 1) while inhibiting division. These results were confirmed in a three dimensional model showing that MSCs to produce SMC-specific proteins under static tension or cyclic stretch, and decreased proliferation (as measured by MTT) under cyclic stretch.[49] These results may be related to the redirection of the cells towards differentiation instead of proliferation, a concept that has previously been proposed for differentiated SMCs.[50] Concurrent with the results published by Hamilton *et al.*, Park *et al.*[34] made the important distinction related to the type of cyclic stretch: uniaxial or equiaxial. Their results demonstrated that uniaxial stretch, but not equiaxial stretch, is necessary for the increase in SMC gene transcription and protein production. They also noted that the increase in SMC gene transcription was transient, which they attributed to the re-orientation of MSCs perpendicular to the direction of strain. This re-orientation is common among most cell types exposed to cyclic stretch and was also demonstrated by Hamilton *et al.*[20] However, 3-D cultures tended to show alignment in the direction of the static stress lines established by the organizing matrix. These stress fields themselves are capable of inducing differentiation.[49] This concept is reinforced by Kurpinski *et al.*,[33] who

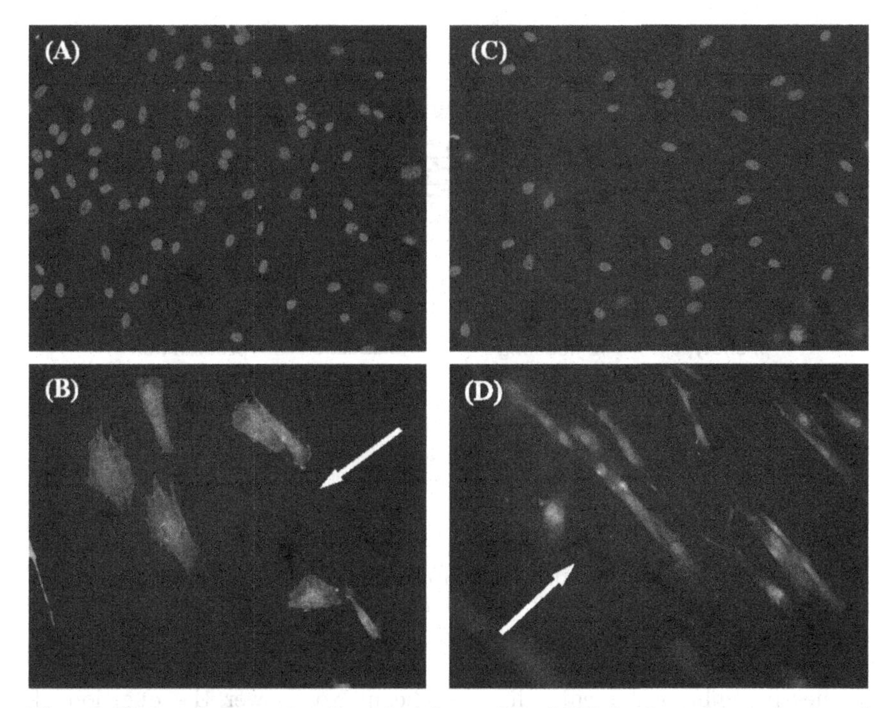

Fig. 1. The application of cyclic uniaxial stretch to MSCs leads to the production of smooth muscle proteins (A) SMA and (B) h1-calponin. Control cultures (C-D) were negative for (C) SMA and (D) h1-calponin.[20]

showed a stronger and more consistent increase in the expression of SMC markers by forcing the alignment of the MSCs in the direction of stretch (Fig. 2). In recent work by our group, we have further determined that 5% uniaxial stretch appears to be a threshold for the increased expression of more mature SMC proteins such as calponin and MHC.[51] While these studies were conducted at the normal cardiovascular frequency of 1 Hz, others have looked at the effects of lower frequency stimulation. Choi *et al.*[52] showed that low frequency (0.03 Hz) equiaxial stretch between 5% and 15% for up to 14 days did not affect surface expression of the stem cell markers CD90 and CD105, but did increase the production of collagen at 5–10% cyclic stretch. Contrasted with this, we found that low magnitude (1%) high frequency (2.5 Hz) uniaxial stretch had a local effect on a subpopulation of MSCs, causing expression of SMA, calponin, and myosin heavy chain.[51] Thus, it appears that magnitude and frequency have important roles to play in MSC differentiation. Although the studies performed to date have focused on determining thresholds and basic descriptions of behavior,

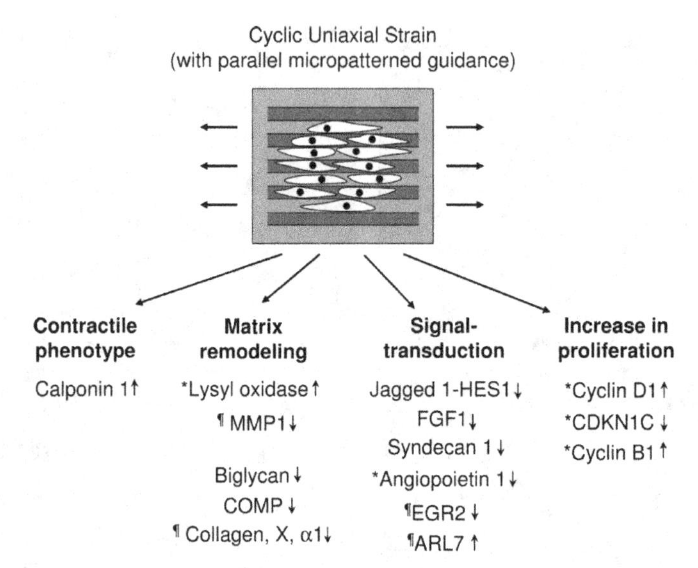

Fig. 2. Forcing alignment in the direction of strain increases contractile phenotype and proliferation markers in MSCs in addition to other changes in matrix and signal transduction.[33]

studies in embryonic stem cells have begun to answer the question of mechanism. Shimizu *et al.*,[53] using flk-1$^+$ mouse embryonic stem cells (ESCs) exposed to 4–12% uniaxial strain at 1 Hz for 24 hours showed a dose-dependent increase in SMC markers at the gene and protein level along with a decrease in the expression of flk-1. More importantly PDGFRβ kinase inhibitors showed a complete blockage of the expression of SMC markers. Such inhibition of differentiation was not found with neutralizing antibodies against PDGF, thus suggesting that the PDGFRβ is directly activated by the mechanical motion imparted upon the cell in a ligand-independent fashion.

In addition to changes in differentiation resulting from cyclic stretch, several reports have demonstrated differing effects on proliferation as a result of cyclic stretch. The 10%, 1 Hz uniaxial cyclic stretch from Hamilton *et al.*[20], which allowed the cells to re-orient and align perpendicular to the direction of strain, showed a stark inhibition of proliferation in the absence apoptosis. However, in the uniaxial stretch experiments (5%, 1 Hz) from Kurpinski *et al.*,[33] which forced the cells to align parallel to the direction of strain, proliferation was increased. Song *et al.*[54] have also reported increased proliferation under uniaxial stretch at low magnitude (2–8%, 1 Hz) over short periods of time (up to 60 minutes) by the MTT assay. Choi *et al.*[52] have expanded upon this to demonstrate that low frequency (0.03 Hz) cyclic equiaxial strain between 5% and 15% increases proliferation (by MTT assay) in the early stages of culture (<3 days). However, longer exposure (14 days) to strain did not show any increased proliferation over controls. We have also found that 1% uniaxial cyclic stretch at 1Hz increased cell number relative to higher magnitudes of stimulation or control cultures.[51] Taken together with the previous studies, it would appear that low levels of cyclic stretch (either low magnitude and/or low frequency) are capable of increasing MSC proliferation with apparently minimal effect on cellular differentiation.

There have also been several studies investigating the influence of stretch on MSC differentiation to other cell types.[9,55–60] Altman *et al.*[9] demonstrated that appropriately applied mechanical forces (stretch and torsion), without biochemical stimulation, induced MSC differentiation to a ligament cell lineage. The results of that study — particularly the increase in ECM production as a result of cyclic stretch — are consistent with others[56,61] that have shown MSCs exposed to cyclic stretch increased collagen I and III synthesis in similar manner to valve interstitial cells.

Thomas and El-Haj[55] determined the dose-response of a cyclic stretch applied to 10-day-old cultures in osteo-inductive culture medium, with an emphasis in understanding osteoblast differentiation. They demonstrated that increasing stretch magnitude resulted in elevated alkaline phosphatase levels, characteristic of early osteoblast differentiation. Similarly, MSCs treated with osteo-inductive media and exposed to intermittent (30 minutes-2 hours per day) cyclic stretching at both 1 Hz and 0.5 Hz have demonstrated osteoblast differentiation through increases in alkaline phosphatase, Runx2, and osteocalcin, collagen I, and collagen III production.[57–60] In the short-term, this intermittent cyclic stretching with media containing dexamethasone was found to be more osteo-inductive than dexamethasone alone.[59] In addition to the rise in osteoblast proteins expression, adipogenic proteins such as PPAR-γ were decreased by intermittent stretch, leading to the conclusion that cyclic stretching modulates adipogenesis in favor of osteoblastogenesis.[57]

2. Shear

Although shear stress is another important biomechanical force in the cardiovascular system, there have only been a few reports on the effects of shear stress on MSC as well as ESC differentiation. Kobayashi *et al.*[38] determined that pressure-dominated shear stress (120/60 mmHg, 1 dyne/cm^2) as well as combined pressure and pulsatile shear forces (120/60 mmHg, 7–14 dyne/scm^2, 90° phase shifted) were responsible for increasing SM-MHC (SM-1 isoform) and SMA protein expression in MSCs. Theirs was the first study suggesting that MSCs are capable of differentiating toward SMC lineages as a result of fluid flow. Yamamoto *et al.*[62] and Wang *et al.*[63] each demonstrated that flk-1$^+$ ESCs and C3H/10T1/2 embryonic MSCs (eMSC), respectively, exposed to physiologic levels of shear stress will express the EC proteins CD31, flk-1, flt-1, vWF, and VE-cadherin at both the protein and mRNA levels. In addition, the embryonic eMSCs also expressed higher levels of VEGF and lower levels of TGF-β and PDGF-B and lower levels of the PDGF receptor. In follow-up studies, Wang *et al.*[64] showed that the applied shear stress suppresses TGF-β signaling through downregulation of TGFβ1, its receptor, and the TGF-β signaling molecules SMAD2, 4, and 5. In addition, the negative TGF-β signaling molecule SMAD7 was upregulated by the shear stress; thus demonstrating that the complete inhibition of TGF-β signaling may play an important role in the EC differentiation of embryonic derived MSCs. The importance of TGF-β signaling in SMC differentiation of this particular cell population has been previously established.[65,66] Further mechanistic studies in bone marrow derived MSCs by Glossop *et al.*[67] have shown that MSCs respond to shear stress with IL-1β expression through a MAPK-related pathway. The MAPK pathway, among others, has been well-established in other, more differentiated cell types, as a dominant pathway in mechanotransduction,[68] and it would appear that such pathways are likely utilized for differentiation of stem cells.

The synergistic combination of growth factors and shear stress has recently been shown in placenta derived MSCs.[69] Combination of endothelial growth media (which contains VEGF, FGF, IGF and heparin) and shear stresses greater than 6 dynes/cm^2 promoted more significant increases in PECAM-1, vWF, flt-1 and flk-1 expression than either stimulus alone. EC-like behavior (LDL uptake and sprouting) was also increased on Matrigel following pre-conditioning with growth factors and shear stress. Recently, we have looked at the gene expression of MSCs under 20 dynes/cm^2 steady shear stress and found that several EC markers, including vWF, PECAM, and VEGF-A are increased and remain elevated with the application of shear. In addition, ECM molecules such as collagen

I and III and elastin are also increased by the application of 20 dynes/cm^2, while SMC related genes show some transient increases but approach baseline levels by day 3.[51]

In addition to increases in differentiation markers, shear stress also has a thrombo-protective effect in endothelial progenitor cells. Exposure to 5–25 dynes/cm^2 laminar shear stress increased endothelial nitric oxide synthase (eNOS) mRNA and nitric oxide production in a dose-dependent manner within 4 hours of exposure.[70] Other studies have shown that similar levels of laminar shear stress inhibit PAI-1 and increase prostaglandin production, both of which are anti-thrombogenic molecules.[71] Similar properties have been well-demonstrated in fully differentiated ECs upon exposure to shear stress,[72,73] and may potentially be exploited with the use of stem and progenitor cells in tissue engineered vascular grafts. Recent data from Nieponice *et al.*[22] has shown that small diameter grafts will acutely thrombose *in vivo* without the addition of stem cells. Although the mechanism for such anti-thrombotic activity was not explored in their experiments, the data from Tao *et al.*[70] seems to suggest that shear stress may be the mechanism that should be explored further. However, one must also consider that the timing of the application of these forces may be critical to the functionality of the ECs upon differentiation. Previous work has shown that ECs derived from embryonic stem cells through chemical differentiation do not functionally respond to shear stress like terminally differentiated ECs (Fig. 3),[11] yet show the same consistent marker expression (Flk-1, Flt-1, VE-cadherin, and CD31) as mature ECs.[74]

In addition to cardiovascular differentiation, other studies involving shear stress and stem cells have focused on osteoblast differentiation. Oscillatory fluid shear stress was found to increase the expression of bone-related genes such as osteopontin and osteocalcin as well as increase proliferation when applied to MSCs grown in osteo-inductive culture medium.[75] Similar effects have been demonstrated using steady shear stress, but without any increases in proliferation as reported in the oscillatory shear study.[76–78] It is important to note that the shear stresses employed in musculoskeletal studies are on the order of about 2 dynes/cm^2, which is much lower than the shear stresses employed in cardiovascular studies. Also, the differentiation of osteo-progenitors appears to be strongly dependant upon the timing of the shear stress application following osteo-induction and is related to PGI_2 and prostaglandin production.[77]

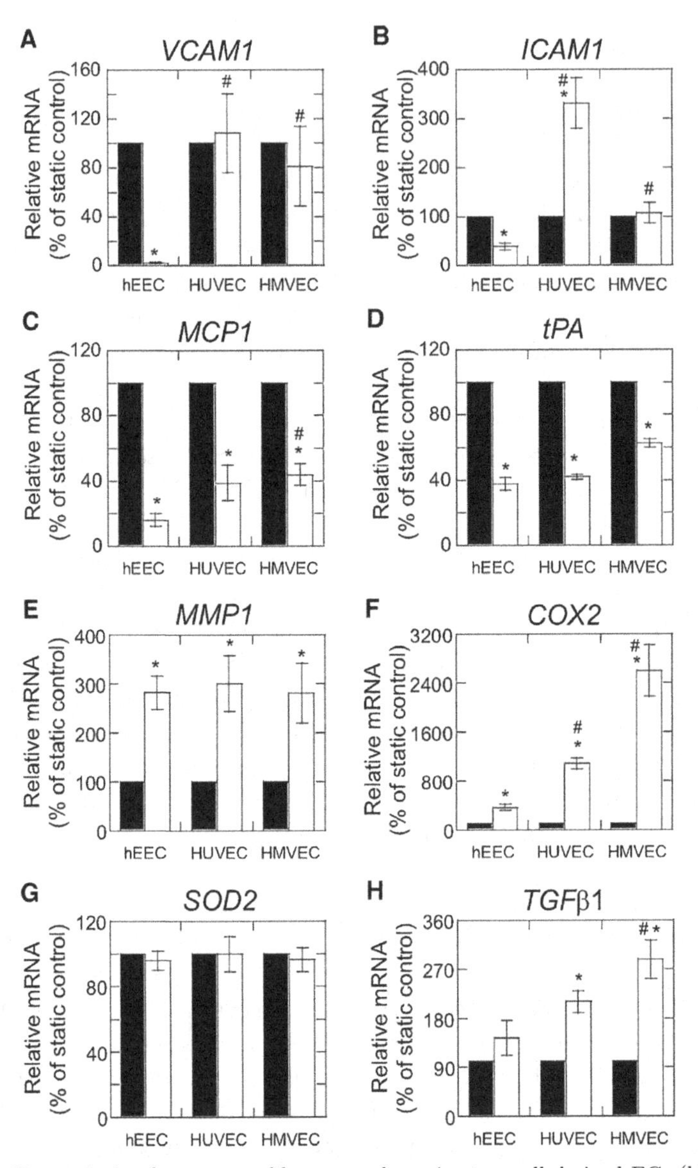

Fig. 3. Transcriptional response of human embryonic stem cell derived ECs (hEECs), human umbilical vein ECs (HUVECs), and human microvascular ECs (HMVECs) cultured under 15 dyn/cm^2 shear stress for 24 h (white bars) or control conditions (black bars) demonstrate the response to shear is not as robust in hEECs, which may have important consequences for the inflammatory repsonse. ($^*p < 0.05$ for shear vs. static culture; $\#p < 0.05$ for comparing response to hEECs). Figure reproduced from[11] with permission from John Wiley & Sons, Inc.

3. Hydrostatic Pressure

As for adult SMCs and ECs, hydrostatic pressure has also been an understudied stimulus for stem cells. Although Kobayashi *et al.*[38] reported a pressure-dominated vascular differentiation response by MSCs, their study was not able to decouple the effects of pressure from shear stress. This was the first study that attempted to elucidate the effects of pressure (despite still being coupled with shear forces) to cardiovascular cell differentiation in stem cells. The majority of studies on the effects of simple hydrostatic pressure (both cyclic and static) on stem cells have centered on musculoskeletal precursors, namely osteoblast-, osteoclast- and chondrocyte-precursors derived from MSCs.

Hydrostatic pressure appears to increase differentiation potential of osteoblast-induced MSCs and osteo-progenitors into osteoblasts[79,80] and inhibit the differentiation potential of osteoclast-induced MSCs.[81,82] A similar effect has been demonstrated for chondrocyte-induced MSCs, with pressure increasing chondrocyte-specific matrix production and driving the chondrogenic phenotype.[83–87] The frequency and magnitude of pressure stimulation in chondrocyte-precursors appears to affect differentiation[87] more than osteoblast-[79,80] and osteoclast-precursors.[81,82] Although these studies indicate that MSCs are indeed sensitive to hydrostatic pressure, they do not decouple the pressure stimulus from other stimuli such as a chemical inductor or other mechanical stimuli, and therefore may be masking the true nature of the pressure effect. Also, in a similar manner to the effects of shear stress on osteo-progenitors, pressure-induced differentiation appears to depend upon the timing of application following induction.[81,84] We have recently attempted to isolate the effects of cyclic pressure alone using physiologically-relevant pressure stimuli. Using several magnitudes and frequencies of stimulation, we found that cyclic pressure is a potent inductor of proliferation, but does not seem to alter protein production in subconfluent MSCs. However, application of cyclic pressure does increase the gene expression of several EC related genes including PECAM and E-selectin.[51]

4. Combined Forces

Realizing that the vascular environment is not simply a single force acting on each cell type, Huang *et al.*[88] were among the first to look at combined stretch, pressure and shear in ESCs. Their study demonstrated both EC

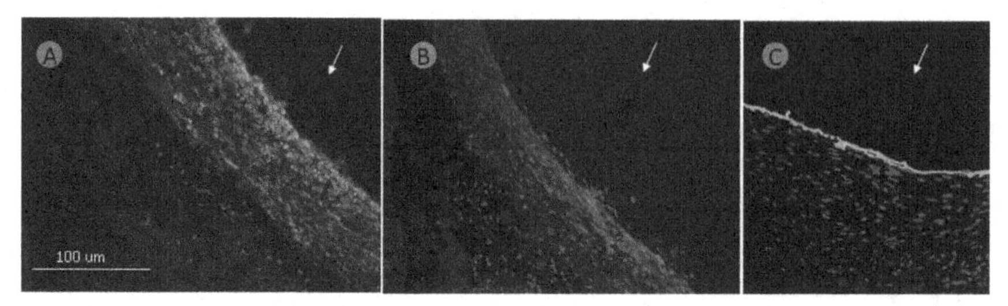

Fig. 4. Immunohistochemistry of a stem cell seeded biodegradable scaffold stains positive for smooth muscle α-actin (A), calponin (B), and von Willebrand factor (C) after *in vivo* implantation in the arterial circulation. Arrows denote the lumen.[22]

and SMC organization and differentiation as a result of pulsatile flow through a compliant tube seeded with ESCs. However, for MSCs, such combined forces appear to predominantly cause SMC differentiation, as described by O'Cearbhaill, *et al.*[89] This type of work has been previously established with *in vivo* models where there MSCs were seeded into a vascular graft and implanted.[90–92] However, in these studies, the fate of the MSCs was uncertain since the cells were not tracked. Recent work by Nieponice *et al.*[22] has shown that muscle derived stem cells seeded in their undifferentiated state and implanted as an aortic interposition graft participate in the remodeling of the graft and remain within the wall after several weeks *in vivo*. They also found that the wall was populated with SMC cells expressing SMA and calponin, while the lumen was lined with ECs expressing vWF (Fig. 4).

5. Summary

Although the mechanical environment is important for maintaining the phenotype and functionality of terminally differentiated cells,[46,93–101] only recently has attention been given to the role that mechanical forces play in the differentiation of MSCs. The previous studies described in this review demonstrate the important potential of using mechanical stimulation to guide MSC (and ESC) differentiation. Summary tables are provided for the varied studies for cyclic stretch (Table 1) and shear stress (Table 2). From the tables, it is readily apparent that mechanical stimulation of stem cells will increase the production of genes and/or proteins that are consistent with EC and SMC differentiation. More consistent results are

Table 1. Summary of the markers relevant to vascular cells and vascular tissue engineering for stimulation of stem cells with cyclic stretch. Double arrows indicate signal sustainability as up, down, or returning to baseline. rMSC = rat mesnchymal stem cell; hMSC = human mesenchymal stem cell; mESC = Flk1^{+} mouse embryonic stem cell; UN = uniaxial; EQ = equiaxial; OI = osteo-inductive medium; BME = β mercaptoethanol.

Marker	Change	Cell Type	Magnitude	Frequency	Duration	Chemical Supplement	Direction	Reference
SMC								
SMA	↑	rMSC	10%	1 Hz	7 d	N	UN	(Hamilton *et al.*, 2004)
	↑	mESC	2–12%	1 Hz	24 h	BME	UN	(Shimizu *et al.*, 2008)
	↑ ⇔	hMSC	10%	1 Hz	1–3 d	N	UN	(Park *et al.*, 2004)
	↓ ⇓	hMSC	10%	1 Hz	1–3 d	N	EQ	(Park *et al.*, 2004)
Calponin	↑	rMSC	5–10%	1 Hz	7 d	N	UN	(Hamilton *et al.*, 2004)
	↑	hMSC	5%	1 Hz	2–4 d	N	UN	(Kurpinski *et al.*, 2006)
SM22α	↑ ⇔	hMSC	10%	1 Hz	1–3 d	N	UN	(Park *et al.*, 2004)
	↑ ⇑	rMSC	10%	1 Hz	1–3 d	N	UN	(Maul, 2007)
	↑	mESC	2–12%	1 Hz	24 h	BME	UN	(Shimizu *et al.*, 2008)
	↓ ⇓	hMSC	10%	1 Hz	1–3 d	N	EQ	(Park *et al.*, 2004)
Caldesmon	↔	rMSC	10%	1 Hz	7 d	N	UN	(Hamilton *et al.*, 2004)
	↔	rMSC	10%	1 Hz	1–3 d	N	UN	(Maul, 2007)
SM-MMHC	↑	mESC	2–12%	1 Hz	24 h	BME	UN	(Shimizu *et al.*, 2008)
	↑	rMSC	10%	1 Hz	5 d	N	UN	(Maul, 2007)
	↑	rMSC	1%	2.75 Hz	5 d	N	UN	
EC								
Flk-1	↓	mESC	8%	1 Hz	24 h	BME	UN	(Shimizu *et al.*, 2008)
	↔ ⇑	rMSC	10%	1 Hz	1–3 d	N	UN	(Maul, 2007)
PECAM	↔ ⇔	rMSC	10%	1 Hz	1–3 d	N	UN	(Maul, 2007)
VE-cadherin	↔	hMSC	10%	1 Hz	1–3 d	N	UN	(Park *et al.*, 2004)

(*Continued*)

Table 1. (*Continued*)

Marker	Change	Cell Type	Magnitude	Frequency	Duration	Chemical Supplement	Direction	Reference
ECM								
Collagen I	↑	hMSC	8%	1 Hz IM	7 d	OI	UN	(Jagodzinski *et al.*, 2004)
	↑ ⇑	hMSC	10%	0.0167 Hz	14 d	OI	UN 3D	(Altman *et al.*, 2002)
	↑ ⇑	hMSC	10%	1 Hz	1–3 d	N	UN	(Park *et al.*, 2004)
	↔	hMSC	10%	1 Hz	1–3 d	N	EQ	(Park *et al.*, 2004)
	↔ ⇔	rMSC	10%	1 Hz	1–3 d	N	UN	(Maul, 2007)
Collagen II	↔	hMSC	10%	1 Hz	1–3 d	N	UN	(Park *et al.*, 2004)
	↑ ⇔	rMSC	10%	1 Hz	1–3 d	N	UN	(Maul, 2007)
Collagen III	↑ ⇑	hMSC	2,8%	1 Hz IM	7 d	OI	UN	(Jagodzinski *et al.*)
	↑ ⇑	hMSC	10%	0.0167 Hz	14 d	OI	UN3D	(Altman *et al.*, 2002)
	↔	hMSC	10%	1 Hz	1–3 d	N	UN	(Park *et al.*, 2004)
	↑ ⇑	rMSC	10%	1 Hz	1–3 d	N	UN	(Maul, 2007)
Proliferation								
MTT, DNA, or Cell Count	↑ ⇑	rMSC	0.3%	0.5 Hz	1–8 d IM	OI	EQ	(Yoshikawa *et al.*, 1997)
	↑	hMSC	10%	0.0167 Hz	21 d	OI	UN 3D	(Altman *et al.*, 2002)
	↑	rMSC	2–8%	1 Hz	15–60 min	N	UN	(Song *et al.*, 2007)
	↑	mESC	4–8%	1 Hz	24 h	BME	UN	(Shimizu *et al.*, 2008)
	↑ ⇔	hMSC	5,8%	0.033 Hz	3–14 d	N	EQ	(Choi *et al.*, 2007)
	↔	hMSC	10,15%	0.033 Hz	3–14 d	N	EQ	
	↓	rMSC	10%	1 Hz	7 d	N	UN	(Hamilton *et al.*, 2004)
	↓	rMSC	10%	1 Hz	6 d	N	UN 3D	(Nieponice *et al.*, 2006)

Table 2. Summary of the markers relevant to vascular cells and vascular tissue engineering for stimulation of stem cells with shear stress. Double arrows indicate signal sustainability as up, down, or returning to baseline. rMSC = rat mesenchymal stem cell; hMSC = human mesenchymal stem cell; mESC = Flk1$^+$ mouse embryonic stem cell; eMSC = embryonic mesenchymal stem cell line C3H/10T1/2, pSC = placenta derived stem cell. OFF = oscillitory fluid flow; OI = osteo-inductive medium; BME = β mercaptoethanol.

Marker	Change	Cell Type	Magnitude	Frequency	Duration	Chemical Supplement	Reference
SMC							
SMA	↑ ⇑	rMSC	7–14 dynes/cm^2	1 Hz	7–21 d	SMC Growth Medium	(Kobayashi *et al.*, 2004)
	↑ ⇑	rMSC	7–14 dynes/cm^2	1 Hz	7–21 d	SMC Growth Medium	(Kobayashi *et al.*, 2004)
	↑ ⇔	mESC	1.5–5 dynes/cm^2	Steady	24–72 h	BME	(Yamamoto *et al.*, 2005)
	↓ ⇓	pSC	12 dynes/cm^2	Steady	12–24 h	EC Growth Medium	(Wu *et al.*, 2008)
SM22α	↑ ⇔	mESC	1.5–5 dynes/cm^2	Steady	24 h	BME	(Yamamoto *et al.*, 2005)
	↔ ⇔	rMSC	20 dynes/cm^{2+}	Steady	1–3 d	N	(Maul, 2007)
SM-MMHC	↑	rMSC	7–14 dynes/cm^2	1 Hz	7–21 d	SMC Growth Medium	(Kobayashi *et al.*, 2004)
Caldesmon	↑ ⇓	rMSC	20 dynes/cm^{2+}	Steady	1–3 d	N	(Maul, 2007)
TGF-β	↓	eMSC	15 dynes/cm^2	Steady	12 h	N	(Wang *et al.*, 2005)
PDGF-B	↓	eMSC	15 dynes/cm^2	Steady	12 h	N	(Wang *et al.*, 2005)
PDGFR	↓	eMSC	15 dynes/cm^2	Steady	12 h	N	(Wang *et al.*, 2005)
EC							
VE-cadherin	↑ ⇑	mESC	1.5–5 dynes/cm^2	Steady	24–72 h	BME	(Yamamoto *et al.*, 2005)
Flk-1	↑ ⇑	mESC	1.5–5 dynes/cm^2	Steady	24–72 h	BME	(Yamamoto *et al.*, 2005)
	↑ ⇑	pSC	6–12 dynes/cm^2	Steady	3–24 h	EC Growth Medium	(Wu *et al.*, 2008)
PECAM	↑ ⇑	mESC	1.5–5 dynes/cm^2	Steady	24–72 h	BME	(Yamamoto *et al.*, 2005)
	↑	eMSC	15 dynes/cm^2	Steady	12 h	N	(Wang *et al.*, 2005)
	↑ ⇑	pSC	6–12 dynes/cm^2	Steady	3–24 h	EC Growth Medium	(Wu *et al.*, 2008)

(*Continued*)

Table 2. (*Continued*)

Marker	Change	Cell Type	Magnitude	Frequency	Duration	Chemical Supplement	Reference
vWF	↑	eMSC	15 dynes/cm^2	Steady	12 h	N	(Wang *et al.*, 2005)
	↑ ⇑	rMSC	20 dynes/cm^{2+}	Steady	1–3 d	N	(Maul, 2007)
	↑ ⇑	pSC	6–12 dynes/cm^2	Steady	3–24 h	EC Growth Medium	(Wu *et al.*, 2008)
VEGF	↑	eMSC	15 dynes/cm^2	Steady	12 h	N	(Wang *et al.*, 2005)
	↑⇑	rMSC	20 dynes/cm^{2+}	Steady	1–3 d	N	(Maul, 2007)
	↔ ⇔	pSC	6–12 dynes/cm^2	Steady	3–24 h	EC Growth Medium	(Wu *et al.*, 2008)
NOS	↑ ⇑	rMSC	20 dynes/cm^{2+}	Steady	1–3 d	N	(Maul, 2007)
	↑	pSC	6–12 dynes/cm^2	Steady	24 h	EC Growth Medium	(Wu *et al.*, 2008)
ECM							
Collagen I	↔	hMSC	20 dynes/cm^2	1 Hz OFF	24 h	OI	(Li *et al.*, 2004)
	↑ ⇑	rMSC	20 dynes/cm^{2+}	Steady	1–3 d	N	(Maul, 2007)
Collagen III	↑ ⇑	rMSC	20 dynes/cm^{2+}	Steady	1–3 d	N	(Maul, 2007)
Elastin	↑ ⇑	rMSC	20 dynes/cm^{2+}	Steady	1–3 d	N	(Maul, 2007)
Proliferation							
Propidium Iodide,	↑	mESC	0–20 dynes/cm^2	Steady	24 h	BME	(Yamamoto *et al.*, 2005)
BrDU, Cell Count	↑	hMSC	20 dynes/cm^2	1 Hz OFF	24 h	OI	(Li *et al.*, 2004)
	↔	rMSC	0.36–2.7 dynes/cm^2	Steady	30 min IM	OI	(Kreke and Goldstein, 2004)

usually obtained with a synergistic effect of biochemical and mechanical stimulation, but several studies do indicate that mechanical stimulation alone is sufficient to induce differentiation.

Although limited in scope, the cardiovascular-related studies to date have clearly demonstrated the ability of cyclic stretch and shear stress to generate SMC and EC differentiation in MSCs and ESCs The motivation to study the role of mechanical stimulation towards cardiovascular cells has be generated, in part, by recent *in vivo* data suggesting that MSCs have the ability to home to sites of vascular injury, and in this mechanically dynamic environment generate vascular SMCs and ECs.[102–106] While the data seems to indicate that cyclic stretch predominantly guides MSCs towards SMCs, and shear stress guides MSCs and ESCs towards ECs, combined stimulation — cyclic shear stress with pressure or cyclic shear with pressure and stretch — appears to be able to drive both SMC and EC differentiation. In addition, there is very little data utilizing cyclic pressure that is physiologically relevant to the cardiovascular system, even though there is clear evidence that pressure is an important stimulus for both ECs and SMCs.[46–48] The few cardiovascular-related studies have also utilized a limited range of magnitudes and paid no attention to the effects of frequency despite the wide range of both that are present from early development to maturity throughout the vasculature. These factors may ultimately be important in determining the lineage to which the stem cells differentiate but without coordinated study, we can only speculate as to their role in MSC differentiation.

References

1. Akhouayri, O., Lafage-Proust, M. H., Rattner, A., Laroche, N., Caillot-Augusseau, A., Alexandre, C., and Vico, L. (1999) Effects of static or dynamic mechanical stresses on osteoblast phenotype expression in three-dimensional contractile collagen gels. *J Cell Biochem* **76**(2), 217–230.
2. Kanda, K., Matsuda, T. (1994) Mechanical stress-induced orientation and ultrastructural change of smooth muscle cells cultured in three-dimensional collagen lattices. *Cell Transplant* **3**(6), 481–492.
3. Kanda, K., Matsuda, T., and Oka, T. (1993) Mechanical stress induced cellular orientation and phenotypic modulation of 3-D cultured smooth muscle cells. *ASAIO J* **39**, M686–M690.
4. Nomura, S., and Takano-Yamamoto, T. (2000) Molecular events caused by mechanical stress in bone. *Matrix Biol* **19**(2), 91–96.

5. Okano, T., Satoh, S., Oka, T., and Matsuda, T. (1997) Tissue engineering of skeletal muscle. Highly dense, highly oriented hybrid muscular tissues biomimicking native tissues. *ASAIO J* **43**(5), M749–753.
6. Smith, R. L., Rusk, S. F., Ellison, B. E., Wessells, P., Tsuchiya, K., Carter, D. R., Caler, W. E., Sandell, L. J., and Schurman, D. J. (1996) *In vitro* stimulation of articular chondrocyte mRNA and extracellular matrix synthesis by hydrostatic pressure. *J Orthop Res* **14**(1), 53–60.
7. Zeichen, J., van Griensven, M., and Bosch, U. (2000) The proliferative response of isolated human tendon fibroblasts to cyclic biaxial mechanical strain. *Am J Sports Med* **28**(6), 888–892.
8. Smith, P. G., Moreno, R., and Ikebe, M. (1997) Strain increases airway smooth muscle contractile and cytoskeletal proteins *in vitro*. *Am J Physiol* **272**(1 Pt 1), L20–27.
9. Altman, G. H., Horan, R. L., Martin, I., Farhadi, J., Stark, P. R., Volloch, V., Richmond, J. C., Vunjak Novakovic, G., and Kaplan, D. L. (2002) Cell differentiation by mechanical stress. *The FASEB Journal* **16**(2), 270–272.
10. Gomes, M. E., Bossano, C. M., Johnston, C. M., Reis, R. L., and Mikos, A. G. (2006) *In vitro* localization of bone growth factors in constructs of biodegradable scaffolds seeded with marrow stromal cells and cultured in a flow perfusion bioreactor. *Tissue Eng.*
11. Metallo, C. M., Vodyanik, M. A., de Pablo, J. J., Slukvin, II, and Palecek, S. P. (2008) The response of human embryonic stem cell-derived endothelial cells to shear stress. *Biotechnol Bioeng* **100**(4), 830–837.
12. Huss, R. (2000) Isolation of primary and immortalized CD34-hematopoietic and mesenchymal stem cells from various sources. *Stem Cells* **18**(1), 1–9.
13. Huss, R. (2000) Perspectives on the morphology and biology of CD34-negative stem cells. *J Hematother. Stem Cell Res* **9**(6), 783–793.
14. Friedenstein, A. J. (1995) Marrow stromal fibroblasts. *Calcif Tissue Int* **56**(Suppl 1), S17.
15. Caplan, A. I. (1991) Mesenchymal stem cells. *J Orthop Res* **9**(5), 641–650.
16. Conget, P. A., and Minguell, J. J. (1999) Phenotypical and functional properties of human bone marrow mesenchymal progenitor cells. *J Cell Physiol* **181**(1), 67–73.
17. Bruder, S. P., Fink, D. J., and Caplan, A. I. (1994) Mesenchymal stem cells in bone development, bone repair, and skeletal regeneration therapy. *J Cell Biochem* **56**(3), 283–294.
18. Prockop, D. J. (1997) Marrow stromal cells as stem cells for nonhematopoietic tissues. *Science* **276**(5309), 71–74.
19. Pittenger, M. F., Mackay, A. M., Beck, S. C., Jaiswal, R. K., Douglas, R., Mosca, J. D., Moorman, M. A., Simonetti, D. W., Craig, S., and Marshak, D. R. (1999) Multilineage potential of adult human mesenchymal stem cells. *Science* **284**(5411), 143–147.
20. Hamilton, D. W., Maul, T. M., and Vorp, D. A. (2004) Characterization of the response of bone marrow derived progenitor cells to cyclic strain: Implications for vascular tissue engineering applications. *Tissue Eng* **10**(3/4), 361–370.

21. Lanotte, M., Scott, D., Dexter, T. M., and Allen, T. D. (1982) Clonal preadipocyte cell lines with different phenotypes derived from murine marrow stroma: factors influencing growth and adipogenesis *in vitro*. *J Cell Physiol* **111**(2), 177–186.
22. Nieponice, A., Soletti, L., Guan, J., Hong, Y., Gharaibeh, B. M., Maul, T. M., Huard, J., Wagner, W. R., and Vorp, D. A. (2009) *In-vivo* assessment of a tissue-engineered vascular graft combining a biodegradable elastomeric scaffold and muscle-derived stem cells in a rat model. *Tissue Eng* (submitted).
23. Friedenstein, A. J., Precursor cells of mechanocytes. Int. Rev. Cytol. 1976;47:327–359.
24. Friedenstein, A. J., Chailakhyan, R. K., and Gerasimov, U. V. (1987) Bone marrow osteogenic stem cells: *in vitro* cultivation and transplantation in diffusion chambers. *Cell Tissue Kinet* **20**(3), 263–272.
25. Caplan, A. I. (2005) Review: mesenchymal stem cells: cell-based reconstructive therapy in orthopedics. *Tissue Eng* **11**(7–8), 1198–1211.
26. Solchaga, L. A., Welter, J. F., Lennon, D. P., and Caplan, A. I. (2004) Generation of pluripotent stem cells and their differentiation to the chondrocytic phenotype. *Methods Mol Med* **100**, 53–68.
27. Goodell, M. A., Jackson, K. A., Majka, S. M., Mi, T., Wang, H., Pocius, J., Hartley, C. J., Majesky, M. W., Entman, M. L., Michael, L. H., and Hirschi, K. K. (2001) Stem cell plasticity in muscle and bone marrow. *Ann N Y Acad Sci* **938**, 208–218. discussion 218–220.
28. Grounds, M. D., White, J. D., Rosenthal, N., and Bogoyevitch, M. A. (2002) The role of stem cells in skeletal and cardiac muscle repair. *The Journal of Histochemistry and Cytochemistry* **50**(5), 589–610.
29. Bayes-Genis, A., Roura, S., Soler-Botija, C., Farre, J., Hove-Madsen, L., Llach, A., and Cinca, J. (2005) Identification of cardiomyogenic lineage markers in untreated human bone marrow-derived mesenchymal stem cells. *Transplant Proc* **37**(9), 4077–4079.
30. Zhang, S., Jia, Z., Ge, J., Gong, L., Ma, Y., Li, T., Guo, J., Chen, P., Hu, Q., Zhang, P., Liu, Y., Li, Z., Ma, K., Li, L., and Zhou, C. (2005) Purified human bone marrow multipotent mesenchymal stem cells regenerate infarcted myocardium in experimental rats. *Cell Transplant* **14**(10), 787–798.
31. Shim, W. S., Jiang, S., Wong, P., Tan, J., Chua, Y. L., Tan, Y. S., Sin, Y. K., Lim, C. H., Chua, T., Teh, M., Liu, T. C., and Sim, E. (2004) *Ex vivo* differentiation of human adult bone marrow stem cells into cardiomyocyte-like cells. *Biochem Biophys Res Commun* **324**(2), 481–488.
32. Makino, S., Fukuda, K., Miyoshi, S., Konishi, F., Kodama, H., Pan, J., Sano, M., Takahashi, T., Hori, S., Abe, H., Hata, J., Umezawa, A., and Ogawa, S. (1999) Cardiomyocytes can be generated from marrow stromal cells *in vitro*. *J Clin Invest* **103**(5), 697–705.
33. Kurpinski, K., Chu, J., Hashi, C., and Li, S. (2006) Anisotropic mechanosensing by mesenchymal stem cells. *Proc Natl Acad Sci U S A* **103**(44), 16095–16100.

34. Park, J. S., Chu, J. S., Cheng, C., Chen, F., Chen, D., and Li, S. (2004) Differential effects of equiaxial and uniaxial strain on mesenchymal stem cells. *Biotechnol Bioeng* **88**(3), 359–368.
35. Galmiche, M. C., Koteliansky, V. E., Briere, J., Herve, P., and Charbord, P. (1993) Stromal cells from human long-term marrow cultures are mesenchymal cells that differentiate following a vascular smooth muscle differentiation pathway. *Blood* **82**(1), 66–76.
36. Ross, J. J., Hong, Z., Willenbring, B., Zeng, L., Isenberg, B., Lee, E. H., Reyes, M., Keirstead, S. A., Weir, E. K., Tranquillo, R. T., and Verfaillie, C. M. (2006) Cytokine-induced differentiation of multipotent adult progenitor cells into functional smooth muscle cells. *J Clin Invest.*
37. Arakawa, E., Hasegawa, K., Yanai, N., Obinata, M., and Matsuda, Y. (2000) A mouse bone marrow stromal cell line, TBR-B, shows inducible expression of smooth muscle-specific genes. *FEBS Lett* **481**(2), 193–196.
38. Kobayashi, N., Yasu, T., Ueba, H., Sata, M., Hashimoto, S., Kuroki, M., Saito, M., and Kawakami, M. (2004) Mechanical stress promotes the expression of smooth muscle-like properties in marrow stromal cells. *Exp Hematol* **32**(12), 1238–1245.
39. Kinner, B., Zaleskas, J. M., and Spector, M. (2002) Regulation of smooth muscle actin expression and contraction in adult human mesenchymal stem cells. *Exp Cell Res* **278**(1), 72–83.
40. Gehling, U. M., Ergun, S., Schumacher, U., Wagener, C., Pantel, K., Otte, M., Schuch, G., Schafhausen, P., Mende, T., Kilic, N., Kluge, K., Schafer, B., Hossfeld, D. K., and Fiedler, W. (2000) *In vitro* differentiation of endothelial cells from AC133-positive progenitor cells. *Blood* **95**(10), 3106–3112.
41. Reyes, M., Dudek, A., Jahagirdar, B., Koodie, L., Marker, P. H., and Verfaillie, C. M. (2002) Origin of endothelial progenitors in human postnatal bone marrow. *J Clin Invest* **109**(3), 337–346.
42. Takahashi, T., Kalka, C., Masuda, H., Chen, D., Silver, M., Kearney, M., Magner, M., Isner, J. M., and Asahara, T. (1999) Ischemia- and cytokine-induced mobilization of bone marrow-derived endothelial progenitor cells for neovascularization. *Nat Med* **5**(4), 434–438.
43. Oswald, J., Boxberger, S., Jorgensen, B., Feldmann, S., Ehninger, G., Bornhauser, M., and Werner, C. (2004) Mesenchymal stem cells can be differentiated into endothelial cells *in vitro*. *Stem Cells* **22**(3), 377–384.
44. Rafii, S., Meeus, S., Dias, S., Hattori, K., Heissig, B., Shmelkov, S., Rafii, D., and Lyden, D. (2002) Contribution of marrow-derived progenitors to vascular and cardiac regeneration. *Semin Cell Dev Biol* **13**(1), 61–67.
45. Fujiyama, S., Amano, K., Uehira, K., Yoshida, M., Nishiwaki, Y., Nozawa, Y., Jin, D., Takai, S., Miyazaki, M., Egashira, K., Imada, T., Iwasaka, T., and Matsubara, H. (2003) Bone marrow monocyte lineage cells adhere on injured endothelium in a monocyte chemoattractant protein-1-dependent manner and accelerate reendothelialization as endothelial progenitor cells. *Circulation Research (Online)* **93**(10), 980–989.

46. Chien, S. (2007) Mechanotransduction and endothelial cell homeostasis: the wisdom of the cell. *Am J Physiol Heart Circ Physiol* **292**(3), H1209–1224.
47. Williams, B. (1998) Mechanical influences on vascular smooth muscle cell function. *J Hypertens* **16**(12 Pt 2), 1921–1929.
48. Wang J. H. C., Thampatty, B. P., and Kwang, W. J. (2008) Mechanobiology of Adult and Stem Cells. *International Review of Cell and Molecular Biology*. Vol. 271: Academic Press; 301–346.
49. Nieponice, A., Maul, T. M., Cumer, J. M., Soletti, L., and Vorp, D. A. (2006) Mechanical stimulation induces morphological and phenotypic changes in bone marrow-derived progenitor cells within a three-dimensional fibrin matrix. *J Biomed Mater Res A*.
50. Chamley-Campbell, J., Campbell, G. R., and Ross, R. (1979) The smooth muscle cell in culture. *Physiol Rev* **59**(1), 1–61.
51. Maul, T. M. (2007) Mechanobiology of Stem Cells: Implications for Vascular Tissue Engineering. Pittsburgh, PA: Bioengineering, University of Pittsburgh.
52. Choi, K.-M., Seo, Y.-K., Yoon, H.-H., Song, K.-Y., Kwon, S.-Y., Lee, H.-S., and Park, J.-K. (2007) Effects of mechanical stimulation on the proliferation of bone marrow-derived human mesenchymal stem cells. *Biotechnol Bioprocess Eng* **12**(6), 601–609.
53. Shimizu, N., Yamamoto, K., Obi, S., Kumagaya, S., Masumura, T., Shimano, Y., Naruse, K., Yamashita, J. K., Igarashi, T., and Ando, J. (2008) Cyclic strain induces mouse embryonic stem cell differentiation into vascular smooth muscle cells by activating PDGF receptor {beta}. *J Appl Physiol* **104**(3), 766–772.
54. Song, G., Ju, Y., Shen, X., Luo, Q., Shi, Y., and Qin, J. (2007) Mechanical stretch promotes proliferation of rat bone marrow mesenchymal stem cells. *Colloids Surf B Biointerfaces* **58**(2), 271–277.
55. Thomas, G. P., and el-Haj, A. J. (1996) Bone marrow stromal cells are load responsive *in vitro*. *Calcif Tissue Int* **58**(2), 101–108.
56. Ku, C. H., Johnson, P. H., Batten, P., Sarathchandra, P., Chambers, R. C., Taylor, P. M., Yacoub, M. H., and Chester, A. H. (2006) Collagen synthesis by mesenchymal stem cells and aortic valve interstitial cells in response to mechanical stretch. *Cardiovasc Res* **71**(3), 548–556.
57. David, V., Martin, A., Lafage-Proust, M.-H., Malaval, L., Peyroche, S., Jones, D. B., Vico, L., and Guignandon, A. (2007) Mechanical loading down-regulates peroxisome proliferator-activated receptor {gamma} in bone marrow stromal cells and favors osteoblastogenesis at the expense of adipogenesis. *Endocrinology* **148**(5), 2553–2562.
58. Yoshikawa, T., Peel, S. A., Gladstone, J. R., and Davies, J. E. (1997) Biochemical analysis of the response in rat bone marrow cell cultures to mechanical stimulation. *Biomed Mater Eng* **7**(6), 369–377.
59. Jagodzinski, M., Drescher, M., Zeichen, J., Hankemeier, S., Krettek, C., Bosch, U., and van Griensven, M. (2004) Effects of cyclic longitudinal

mechanical strain and dexamethasone on osteogenic differentiation of human bone marrow stromal cells. *Eur Cell Mater* **7**, 35–41. discussion 41.

60. Jing, Y., Li, L., Li, Y., Chen, M., Wu, W., Chen, H., and Liu, X. (2006) The effect of mechanical strain on proliferation and osteogenic differentiation of bone marrow mesenchymal stem cells from rats. *Sheng Wu Yi Xue Gong Cheng Xue Za Zhi* **23**(3), 542–545.
61. Engelmayr, G. C. Jr., Sales, V. L., Mayer, J. E. Jr., and Sacks, M. S. (2006) Cyclic flexure and laminar flow synergistically accelerate mesenchymal stem cell-mediated engineered tissue formation: Implications for engineered heart valve tissues. *Biomaterials* **27**(36), 6083–6095.
62. Yamamoto, K., Sokabe, T., Watabe, T., Miyazono, K., Yamashita, J. K., Obi, S., Ohura, N., Matsushita, A., Kamiya, A., and Ando, J. (2005) Fluid shear stress induces differentiation of Flk-1-positive embryonic stem cells into vascular endothelial cells *in vitro*. *Am J Physiol Heart Circ Physiol* **288**(4), H1915–1924.
63. Wang, H., Riha, G. M., Yan, S., Li, M., Chai, H., Yang, H., Yao, Q., and Chen, C. (2005) Shear stress induces endothelial differentiation from a murine embryonic mesenchymal progenitor cell line. *Arterioscler Thromb Vasc Biol* **25**(9), 1817–1823.
64. Wang, H., Li, M., Lin, P. H., Yao, Q., and Chen, C. (2008) Fluid shear stress regulates the expression of TGF-beta1 and its signaling molecules in mouse embryo mesenchymal progenitor cells. *J Surg Res* **150**(2), 266–270.
65. Hirschi, K. K., Rohovsky, S. A., and D'Amore, P. A. (1998) PDGF, TGF-beta, and heterotypic cell-cell interactions mediate endothelial cell-induced recruitment of 10T1/2 cells and their differentiation to a smooth muscle fate. [erratum appears in *J Cell Biol* 1998 Jun (1) **141**(5), 1287]. *J Cell Biol* **141**(3), 805–814.
66. Chen, S., Kulik, M., and Lechleider, R. J. (2003) Smad proteins regulate transcriptional induction of the SM22alpha gene by TGF-beta. *Nucleic Acids Res* **31**(4), 1302–1310.
67. Glossop, J. R., and Cartmell, S. H. (2009) Effect of fluid flow-induced shear stress on human mesenchymal stem cells: Differential gene expression of IL1B and MAP3K8 in MAPK signaling. *Gene Expr Patterns*, In Press, Corrected Proof.
68. Banes, A. J., Lee, G., Graff, R., Otey, C., Archambault, J., Tsuzaki, M., Elfervig, M., and Qi, J. (2001) Mechanical forces and signaling in connective tissue cells: cellular mechanisms of detection, transduction, and responses to mechanical deformation. *Current Opinion in Orthopedics* **12**(5), 389–396.
69. Wu, C. C., Chao, Y. C., Chen, C. N., Chien, S., Chen, Y. C., Chien, C. C., Chiu, J. J., and Linju Yen, B. (2008) Synergism of biochemical and mechanical stimuli in the differentiation of human placenta-derived multipotent cells into endothelial cells. *J Biomech* **41**(4), 813–821.
70. Tao, J., Yang, Z., Wang, J. M., Tu, C., and Pan, S. R. (2006) Effects of fluid shear stress on eNOS mRNA expression and NO production in human endothelial progenitor cells. *Cardiology* **106**(2), 82–88.

71. Yang, Z., Wang, J. M., Wang, L. C., Chen, L., Tu, C., Luo, C. F., Tang, A. L., Wang, S. M., and Tao, J. (2007) *In vitro* shear stress modulates antithrombogenic potentials of human endothelial progenitor cells. *J Thromb Thrombolysis* **23**(2), 121–127.
72. Chien, S., Li, S., and Shyy, Y. J. (1998) Effects of mechanical forces on signal transduction and gene expression in endothelial cells. *Hypertension (Online)* **31**(1 Pt 2), 162–169.
73. Topper, J. N., Cai, J., Falb, D., and Gimbrone, M. A. (1996) Identification of vascular endothelial genes differentially responsive to fluid mechanical stimuli: cyclooxygenase-2, manganese superoxide dismutase, and endothelial cell nitric oxide synthase are selectively up-regulated by steady laminar shear stress. *Proc Natl Acad Sci U S A* **93**(19), 10417–10422.
74. McCloskey, K. E., Smith, D. A., Jo, H., and Nerem, R. M. (2006) Embryonic stem cell-derived endothelial cells may lack complete functional maturation *in vitro*. *J Vasc Res* **43**(5), 411–421.
75. Li, Y. J., Batra, N. N., You, L., Meier, S. C., Coe, I. A., Yellowley, C. E., and Jacobs, C. R. (2004) Oscillatory fluid flow affects human marrow stromal cell proliferation and differentiation. *J Orthop Res* **22**(6), 1283–1289.
76. Kreke, M. R., and Goldstein, A. S. (2004) Hydrodynamic shear stimulates osteocalcin expression but not proliferation of bone marrow stromal cells. *Tissue Eng* **10**(5–6), 780–788.
77. Kreke, M. R., Huckle, W. R., and Goldstein, A. S. (2005) Fluid flow stimulates expression of osteopontin and bone sialoprotein by bone marrow stromal cells in a temporally dependent manner. *Bone* **36**(6), 1047–1055.
78. Holtorf, H. L., Jansen, J. A., and Mikos, A. G. (2005) Flow perfusion culture induces the osteoblastic differentiation of marrow stroma cell-scaffold constructs in the absence of dexamethasone. *J Biomed Mater Res A* **72**(3), 326–334.
79. Roelofsen, J., Klein Nulend, J., and Burger, E. H. (1995) Mechanical stimulation by intermittent hydrostatic compression promotes bone-specific gene expression *in vitro*. *J Biomech* **28**(12), 1493–1503.
80. Kim, S. H., Choi, Y. R., Park, M. S., Shin, J. W., Park, K. D., Kim, S. J., and Lee, J. W. (2007) ERK 1/2 activation in enhanced osteogenesis of human mesenchymal stem cells in poly(lactic-glycolic acid) by cyclic hydrostatic pressure. *J Biomed Mater Res A* **80**(4), 826–836.
81. Nagatomi, J., Arulanandam, B. P., Metzger, D. W., Meunier, A., and Bizios, R. (2002) Effects of cyclic pressure on bone marrow cell cultures. *J Biomech Eng* **124**(3), 308–314.
82. Rubin, J., Biskobing, D., Fan, X., Rubin, C., McLeod, K., and Taylor, W. R. (1997) Pressure regulates osteoclast formation and MCSF expression in marrow culture. *J Cell Physiol* **170**(1), 81–87.
83. Angele, P., Yoo, J. U., Smith, C., Mansour, J., Jepsen, K. J., Nerlich, M., and Johnstone, B. (2003) Cyclic hydrostatic pressure enhances the chondrogenic phenotype of human mesenchymal progenitor cells differentiated *in vitro*. *J Orthop Res* **21**(3), 451–457.

84. Elder, S. H., Fulzele, K. S., and McCulley, W. R. (2005) Cyclic hydrostatic compression stimulates chondroinduction of C3H/10T1/2 cells. *Biomech Model Mechanobiol* **3**(3), 141–146.
85. Miyanishi, K., Trindade, M. C., Lindsey, D. P., Beaupre, G. S., Carter, D. R., Goodman, S. B., Schurman, D. J., and Smith, R. L. (2006) Effects of hydrostatic pressure and transforming growth factor-beta 3 on adult human mesenchymal stem cell chondrogenesis *in vitro*. *Tissue Eng* **12**(6), 1419–1428.
86. Finger, A. R., Sargent, C. Y., Dulaney, K. O., Bernacki, S. H., and Loboa, E. G. (2007) Differential effects on messenger ribonucleic acid expression by bone marrow-derived human mesenchymal stem cells seeded in agarose constructs due to ramped and steady applications of cyclic hydrostatic pressure. *Tissue Eng* **13**(6), 1151–1158.
87. Elder, S. H., Goldstein, S. A., Kimura, J. H., Soslowsky, L. J., and Spengler, D. M. (2001) Chondrocyte differentiation is modulated by frequency and duration of cyclic compressive loading. *Ann Biomed Eng* **29**(6), 476–482.
88. Huang, H., Nakayama, Y., Qin, K., Yamamoto, K., Ando, J., Yamashita, J., Itoh, H., Kanda, K., Yaku, H., Okamoto, Y., and Nemoto, Y. (2005) Differentiation from embryonic stem cells to vascular wall cells under *in vitro* pulsatile flow loading. *J Artif Organs* **8**(2), 110–118.
89. O'Cearbhaill, E. D., Punchard, M. A., Murphy, M., Barry, F. P., McHugh, P. E., and Barron, V. (2008) Response of mesenchymal stem cells to the biomechanical environment of the endothelium on a flexible tubular silicone substrate. *Biomaterials*.
90. Noishiki, Y., Yamane, Y., Tomizawa, Y., and Matsumoto, A. (1995) Transplantation of autologous tissue fragments into an e-PTFE graft with long fibrils. *Artif Organs* **19**(1), 17–26.
91. Shin'oka, T., Imai, Y., and Ikada, Y. (2001) Transplantation of a tissue-engineered pulmonary artery. *N Engl J Med* **344**(7), 532–533.
92. Shin'oka, T., Matsumura, K., Hibino, N., Naito, Y., Murata, A., Kosaka, Y., and Kurosawa, H. (2003) Clinical practice of transplantation of regenerated blood vessels using bone marrow cells. *Nippon Naika Gakkai Zasshi* **92**(9), 1776–1780.
93. Abbott, B. L. (2003) ABCG2 (BCRP) expression in normal and malignant hematopoietic cells. *Hematol Oncol* **21**(3), 115–130.
94. Azuma, N., Duzgun, S. A., Ikeda, M., Kito, H., Akasaka, N., Sasajima, T., and Sumpio, B. E. (2000) Endothelial cell response to different mechanical forces. *J Vasc Surg* **32**(4), 789–794.
95. Chien, S. (2006) Molecular basis of rheological modulation of endothelial functions: importance of stress direction. *Biorheology* **43**(2), 95–116.
96. Cowan, D. B., and Langille, B. L. (1996) Cellular and molecular biology of vascular remodeling. *Curr Opin Lipidol* **7**(2), 94–100.
97. Garcia-Cardena, G., Comander, J., Anderson, K. R., Blackman, B. R., and Gimbrone, M. A. (2001) Biomechanical activation of vascular endothelium

as a determinant of its functional phenotype. *Proc Natl Acad Sci U S A* **98**(8), 4478–4485.

98. Joe, P., Wallen, L. D., Chapin, C. J., Lee, C. H., Allen, L., Han, V. K., Dobbs, L. G., Hawgood, S., and Kitterman, J. A. (1997) Effects of mechanical factors on growth and maturation of the lung in fetal sheep. *The American Journal of Physiology* **272**(1 Pt 1), L95–105.
99. Resnick, N., and Gimbrone, M. A. (1995) Hemodynamic forces are complex regulators of endothelial gene expression. *The FASEB Journal* **9**(10), 874–882.
100. Skalak, T. C., Price, R. J., and Zeller, P. J. (1998) Where do new arterioles come from? Mechanical forces and microvessel adaptation. *Microcirculation* **5**(2–3), 91–94.
101. Zhao, S., Suciu, A., Ziegler, T., Moore, J. E., Burki, E., Meister, J. J., and Brunner, H. R. (1995) Synergistic effects of fluid shear stress and cyclic circumferential stretch on vascular endothelial cell morphology and cytoskeleton. *Arteriosclerosis, Thrombosis, and Vascular Biology (Online)* **15**(10), 1781–1786.
102. Han, C. I., Campbell, G. R., and Campbell, J. H. (2001) Circulating bone marrow cells can contribute to neointimal formation. *J Vasc Res* **38**(2), 113–119.
103. Hirschi, K. K., and Goodell, M. A. (2002) Hematopoietic, vascular and cardiac fates of bone marrow-derived stem cells. *Gene Ther* **9**(10), 648–652.
104. Hirschi, K., and Goodell, M. (2001) Common origins of blood and blood vessels in adults? *Differentiation; Research in Biological Diversity.* **68**(4–5), 186–192.
105. Asahara, T., and Kawamoto, A. (2004) Endothelial progenitor cells for postnatal vasculogenesis. *Am J Physiol Cell Physiol* **287**(3), C572–579.
106. Asahara, T., Murohara, T., Sullivan, A., Silver, M., van der Zee, R., Li, T., Witzenbichler, B., Schatteman, G., and Isner, J. M. (1997) Isolation of putative progenitor endothelial cells for angiogenesis. *Science* **275**(5302), 964–967.

Chapter 10

TISSUE ENGINEERED BLOOD VESSELS: FROM THE BENCH TO THE BEDSIDE AND BACK AGAIN (DEVELOPMENT OF A VASCULAR CONDUIT FOR USE IN CONGENITAL HEART SURGERY)

BERNARD S. SALAMEH*, TAMAR L. MIRENSKY, TOSHIHARU SHINOKA and CHRISTOPHER K. BREUER†

Yale University School of Medicine, New Haven, CT

**Pediatric Surgery, 333 Cedar Street FMB 132*
PO Box 208062, New Haven, CT 06520-8062
Bernard.salameh@yale.edu
† christoper.breuer@yale.edu

Recent advancements in congenital heart surgery have enabled children born with congenital cardiac anomalies to have longer and better quality lives. Most congenital heart operations require the use of either autologous or bioprosthetic materials to reconstruct the heart and great vessels; hence the need to develop an ideal vascular graft. The development of tissue-engineered vascular conduits and grafts hold great promise in further advancing the fields of pediatric cardiothoracic and vascular surgery. To date, implantation of such grafts in human patients has also been successful and has presented us with an exciting, rapidly advancing field.

1. Introduction

Over the past three decades, advancements have been made in congenital heart surgery that have enabled children born with congenital cardiac anomalies to have longer and better quality lives. Most congenital heart operations require the use of either autologous or bioprosthetic materials to reconstruct the heart and great vessels.[1] Synthetic materials remain a significant source of post-operative morbidity and mortality. Currently available replacement vascular conduits include those made from autologous tissues such as pericardium, prosthetic grafts such as those made of polytetrafluoroethylene (Gore-tex®), and bioprosthetic grafts such as homografts. Use of autologous venous grafts is restricted because of limited availability. In patients undergoing congenital heart surgery, prosthetic grafts are widely available and "off the shelf"; however, they are associated with increased risks of infection, thrombosis and a lack of growth potential. Bioprosthetic grafts such as homografts have improved biocompatibility compared to synthetic grafts but are associated with a lack of growth potential as well as a poor durability due to high rates of ectopic calcification.

The development of an improved vascular conduit for use in congenital heart surgery is an area of active investigation. An ideal vascular graft would be durable and ready "off the shelf".[2] Additionally, an ideal vascular graft would be biocompatible and non-thrombogenic with a low incidence of hemolysis or infectious complications. Finally, an ideal vascular graft would be a biologic conduit that has the ability to remodel and grow with the patient.

Perhaps nowhere will the effect of the development of a tissue engineered vascular graft (TEVG) be greater than in congenital heart surgery. A graft with growth potential has the ability to transform the field and dramatically improve our capabilities for correcting congenital cardiac anomalies. The development of an autologous vascular graft with the ability to grow, repair, and remodel would not only improve the durability of these grafts, but also preclude the need for graft replacement due to somatic overgrowth and relative stenosis of the graft due to patients outgrowing their grafts.[1] The development of a vascular graft with growth potential would preclude the need for delaying surgery until patients are more fully grown and prevent the use of oversized vascular grafts, which have been shown to increase the morbidity and mortality associated with repair of congenital heart defects. In order to meet these needs, we developed the first TEVG for use in congenital cardiac surgery.

A serendipitous benefit of developing a vascular graft for use in congenital cardiac surgery is that this is one of the few areas in surgery in which vascular conduits are used in low-pressure, high-flow circuits. Such circuits are less prone to thrombosis or aneurysm formation making vascular grafts for use in these circulations an ideal clinical target for the first tissue engineered vascular graft.

1.1. *Pre-clinical Studies*

Weinberg and Bell were the first to attempt the creation of a complete vascular structure by seeding a bovine collagen matrix scaffold with autologous cells.[3] Thus, they were instrumental in developing the classical tissue-engineering paradigm for tissue-engineered conduits. Bovine aortic endothelial cells, smooth muscle cells, and adventitial fibroblasts were isolated. The middle layer of the blood vessel model, corresponding to the media of an artery, was prepared by casting culture medium, collagen, and smooth muscle cells together in an annular mold. The mixture jelled at 37°C and contracted within a few days to produce a tubular lattice around a central mandril. After one week, an open Dacron® mesh sleeve was slipped over the lattice to provide additional mechanical support. The outer layer, corresponding to the adventitia, was cast around the first lattice with adventitial fibroblasts rather than smooth muscle cells. Two weeks later, when the outer layer was fully contracted, the tube was carefully slipped off the mandrel with jeweler's forceps and either used for mechanical testing or lined with endothelial cells. For the latter, the model was cannulated, a suspension of endothelial cells was injected into the lumen, and the vessel was rotated around the longitudinal axis at 1 rev/min for one week to distribute endothelial cells uniformly on the luminal surface. The model grossly and microscopically resembled a muscular artery. The endothelial lining of the blood vessel model functioned like a normal endothelium. Weinberg and Bell were able to demonstrate that using the classical tissue-engineering paradigm, they could create neovessels *in vitro* with characteristics similar to mammalian muscular arteries. Unfortunately, these tissue engineered vascular grafts lacked the requisite biomechanical properties to behave as blood vessels due to a low burst pressure thus precluding their implantation and evaluation *in vivo* without the addition of a Dacron® sheet for reinforcement.

During the past 15 years we have attempted to use tissue-engineering methodology to develop an improved vascular graft. Tissue engineering is an interdisciplinary field that applies the principles of engineering and life sciences toward the development of biological substitutes that restore, maintain, or improve tissue function.[4] Our work has focused on the use of the classical tissue-engineering paradigm in which autologous cells are seeded onto a biodegradable scaffold. The scaffold provides sites for cell attachment and space for neotissue formation. As the scaffold degrades, neotissue forms ultimately creating a purely autologous biological scaffold without any synthetic components. Our lab along with others has focused on creating a living vascular conduit with growth potential for use in congenital heart surgery.

In the mid 1990's we designed a pilot study to assess the feasibility of a tissue engineering approach to construct tissue-engineered pulmonary artery conduits.[5] Bovine artery (Group A, $n = 4$) and vein (Group V, $n = 3$) segments were harvested, separated into individual cells, expanded *in vitro*, and seeded onto synthetic biodegradable (polyglactin/polyglycolic acid) tubular scaffolds (20 mm long × 15 mm diameter). After 7 days of *in vitro* culture, the autologous cell/polymer vascular constructs were used to replace a 2 cm segment of pulmonary artery in lambs Control animals received an acellular polymer tube sealed with fibrin glue. Animals were sacrificed at intervals from 11 to 24 weeks (mean follow-up 130.3 ± 30.8 days) after echocardiographic and angiographic studies. Explanted tissue-engineered conduits were assayed for collagen (4-hydroxyproline) and calcium content, and a tissue deoxyribonucleic acid assay (bis-benzimide dye) was used to estimate the number of cell nuclei as an index of tissue maturity. The acellular control graft developed progressive obstruction and thrombosis. All seven tissue-engineered grafts remained patent and demonstrated a non-aneurysmal increase in diameter (group A 18.3 ± 1.3 mm, 95.3% of native pulmonary artery; group V 17.1 ± 1.2 mm, 86.8% of native pulmonary artery). Histologically, none of the biodegradable polymer composing the scaffold remained in any tissue engineered grafts by 11 weeks. Collagen content in tissue-engineered grafts was $73.9\% \pm 8.0\%$ of adjacent native pulmonary artery. Elastic fibers were present in the media layer of tissue-engineered vessel wall and endothelial specific factor VIII was identified on the luminal surface. Deoxyribonucleic acid assay demonstrated a progressive decrease in the numbers of cell nuclei over 11 and 24 weeks, suggesting ongoing tissue remodeling. Calcium content of tissue-engineered grafts was elevated (group A = 7.95 ± 5.09; group V = 13.2 ± 5.48; native pulmonary artery = $1.2 = /-0.8$ mg/gm dry weight), but no macroscopic calcification was found. This study proved the feasibility of using tissue-engineering methodology to construct a neovessel for use as a vascular conduit in congenital heart surgery. TEVGs developed an endothelial lining and a vessel wall with robust extracellular matrix (ECM) formation, including collagen, without evidence of ectopic calcification.

In our following study, the focus shifted to scaffold design and fabrication.[6] The initial scaffold was constructed from biodegradable polymers originally designed for other biomedical applications. While creating a tissue engineered vascular graft with this scaffold was feasible, the design of the polyglycolic acid (PGA) scaffold was not optimal due to the relatively stiff nature of the PGA fibers, which resulted in poor compliance match and poor surgical handling. The hybrid polymeric scaffold fabricated from either PGA or polylactic acid (PLA) fiber-based mesh coated with a 50:50 copolymer of L-lactide and ε-caprolactone (PCLA/PGA or PCLA/PLA) was specifically designed for use as a biodegradable scaffold in the fabrication of a TEVG. The hybrid scaffolds are more elastic than the PGA scaffold, resulting in improved compliance match between the vessel and the conduit and possess better surgical handling characteristics. The PCLA/PGA scaffold was specifically designed for use as a vascular graft in congenital heart surgery. TEVGs were fabricated by seeding 5×10^6 cells (obtained from femoral veins of mongrel dogs) onto tube-shaped biodegradable polymer scaffolds composed of PGA nonwoven fabric sheets and a copolymer of poly-L-lactide and caprolactone (PCLA) ($n = 4$). After 7 days, the inferior vena cavas (IVCs) of the same dogs were replaced with these TEVGs. After 3, 4, 5, and 6 months, angiography was performed, and the dogs were sacrificed. The implanted TEVGs were examined both grossly and immunohistologically. The TEVGs showed no evidence of stenosis or dilatation. No thrombus was found inside the TEVGs, even without any anticoagulation therapy. Remnants of the polymer scaffolds were not observed in any of the 6 months specimens, demonstrating complete scaffold degradation prior to this period. The gross appearance was similar to that of the native IVCs. Immunohistological staining revealed the presence of factor VIII positive nucleated cells at the luminal surface of the TEVGs. In addition, lesions were observed where alpha-smooth muscle actin and desmin positive cells existed. The TEVG developed an endothelial lining and vessel wall with smooth muscle cells (SMCs) and robust ECM formation containing collagen and elastin. Therefore, we concluded that functional TEVGs can be made by seeding autologous cells onto a (PCLA/PGA) scaffold, thereby creating a TEVG that resembles native vessels morphologically and possesses excellent surgical handling characteristics.

We then explored alternative autologous cell sources. In our initial experiments, autologous vascular cells were isolated from vessel biopsies. This methodology was problematic in several respects. First it required an invasive procedure (biopsy) in addition to expansion of cells in culture prior to the definitive operation thereby increasing the risk of contamination and infection. Additionally, obtaining healthy autologous cells from diseased donors can be quite technically challenging. In an attempt to identify an alternative autologous cell source that could be obtained with minimal manipulation and without the use of cell culture, autologous cells obtained from bone marrow aspirates were explored. A study was designed to seed bone marrow cells (BMCs) onto a biodegradable scaffold in an attempt to construct a graft that would address the problems posed earlier.[7]

To demonstrate the contribution of BMCs to histiogenesis, cells were labeled with Alexa-594 conjugated anti-fluorescence/-Oregon Green, and seeded onto scaffolds that were implanted as IVC interposition grafts. Implanted grafts were analyzed immunohistochemically at 3 hours, and subsequently at 2, 4, and 8 weeks after implantation using antibodies against endothelial cell lineage markers, endothelium, and smooth muscle cells. Seeded BMCs expressing endothelial cell lineage markers, such as CD34, CD31, Flk-1 and Tie-2, adhered to the scaffold. This was followed by proliferation and differentiation, resulting in expression of endothelial cells markers, such as CD146, factor VIII and CD31, and smooth muscle cell markers, such as alpha-smooth muscle cell actin, SMemb, SM1 and SM2. Cells in TEVGs also produced vascular endothelial growth factor and angiopoietin-1. These results provided direct evidence that BMCs may be utilized in the construction of TEVGs. Seeded BMCs attached to the scaffold and became incorporated into the vascular neotissue immediately after graft implantation. TEVGs resembled native vessels morphologically, structurally and functionally.

In order to study the effect of cell source on the structure and function of TEVGs, we evaluated the endothelial function and mechanical properties of tissue-engineered conduits constructed with autologous mononuclear bone marrow cells (MN-BMCs) and a biodegradable scaffold using a canine IVC model.[8] Autologous MN-BMCs were obtained from a dog and seeded onto a biodegradable tubular scaffold consisting of PCLA/PGA sponge. This graft was implanted into the IVC of the same host dog on the day of surgery. TEVGs were analyzed biochemically, biomechanically, and histologically after implantation. When the TEVGs were explanted after one month and stimulated with acetylcholine, they produced nitrates and nitrites in a dose dependent manner. N^G-nitro-L-arginine methylester significantly inhibited these reactions. With stimulation by acetylcholine, factor VIII-positive cells of TEVGs produced endothelial nitric oxide synthase proteins, and the ratio of endothelial nitric oxide synthase/s17 mRNA was similar between native IVC and TEVGs at 1 and 3 months after implantation.

TEVGs had biochemical properties and wall thicknesses similar to those of the native IVC 6 months after implantation, and tolerated venous pressures well without any problems. The number of inflammatory cells in TEVGs and the ratio of CD4/s17 mRNA decreased significantly with time. We concluded that TEVGs constructed with MN-BMCs and biodegradable scaffolds have functional endothelium with nitric oxide production, durable mechanical properties, and the potential to remodel without significant ectopic calcification. Additionally, since TEVGs endothelialize within 1 month, only limited anticoagulation may be necessary post-operatively.

Constructing a tissue-engineered vascular graft by using bone marrow cells, which can be obtained easily and used immediately without cell culture, overcame many of the problems associated with the use of cultured cells. The method was further refined in order to remove red blood cells by performing density centrifugation and isolating the mononuclear fraction of the bone marrow. This technique had the added benefit of providing a source of autologous serum that could be used instead of media to bathe the seeded scaffold while preparing the graft for implantation.

Next, we compared neovessels created using a variety of cell sources in order to determine if the cell source affected neovessel formation.[9] Biodegradable polymers seeded with different types of cells (group V, cultured venous cells; group B, bone marrow cells without culture; and group C, non-cell-seeded graft as control) were implanted into the IVCs of dogs. The grafts were explanted at 4 weeks and assessed both histologically and biochemically. Upon histologic examination, a layer of Masson positive stained collagen, a layer of factor VIII positive endothelial cells and anti-alpha-smooth muscle antigen-immunoreactive cells were noted in groups V and B similar to that seen in native vascular tissue. A 4-hydroxyproline assay in group C showed significantly lower levels than in groups V and B or native tissue ($P < 0.05$). Additionally, the DNA content of the tissue-engineered vascular graft tended to be higher in group C than in groups V and B or in native tissue. To evaluate the growth potential of the TEVGs, we turned our attention to a juvenile animal model and magnetic resonance imaging.[10]

PGA nonwoven mesh tubes (3-cm length, 1.3-cm internal diameter) coated with a 10% copolymer solution of PCLA and statically seeded with autologous bone marrow derived mononuclear cells (1×10^6 cells/cm^2). Eight TEVGs (7 seeded, 1 unseeded control) were implanted as IVC

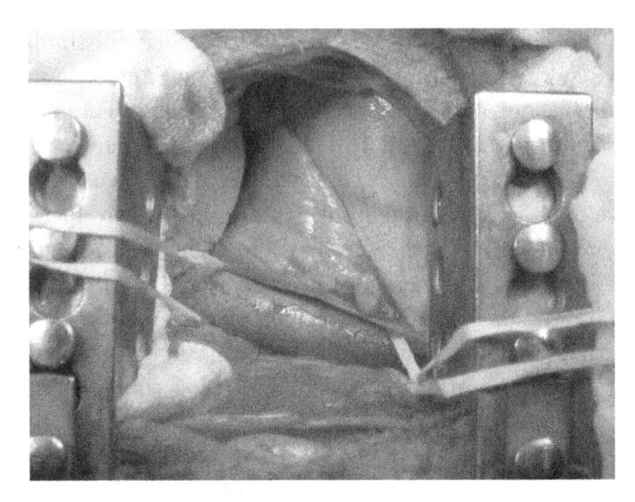

Fig. 1. Operative field. IVC interposition graft in juvenile lamb model.[10]

interposition grafts in juvenile lambs (Fig. 1). Subjects underwent bimonthly magnetic resonance angiography (Siemens 1.5 T) with vascular image analysis. One of 7-seeded grafts was explanted after 1 month and all others were explanted 6 months after implantation. Neotissue was characterized using qualitative histologic and immunohistochemical staining and quantitative biochemical analysis. All grafts explanted at 6 months were patent and increased in volume as measured by difference in pixel summation in magnetic resonance angiography at 1 month and 6 months. The volume of seeded TEVGs at explant averaged 126.9% $\pm$ 9.9% of their volume at 1 month. There was no evidence of aneurysmal dilation. TEVGs resembled the native IVC histologically and had comparable collagen (157.9 $\pm$ 26.4 ug/mg), elastin (186.9 $\pm$ 16.7 ug/mg), and glycosaminoglycan (9.7 $\pm$ 0.8 ug/mg) content. Immunohistochemical staining and Western blot analysis showed that Ephrin-B4, a determinant of normal venous development, was demonstarted in the seeded grafts 6 months after implantation. We concluded that the TEVGs not only resembled native vessels morphologically and histologically but also functionally, as they possessed a smooth muscle layer that was responsive to pharmacological stimulation and a functional endothelium that inhibited thrombosis. Therefore, tissue-engineering technology offers the ability to create vascular grafts that are living structures capable of growth, repair, and remodeling in response to their local environment milieu.

1.2. *Clinical Studies*

Based on our preclinical studies, coupled with the great need for an improved vascular conduit for use in congenital heart surgery, we proceeded with human trials at Tokyo Women's Medical University (Tokyo, Japan). The first patient was a four-year-old girl who had been diagnosed with a single right ventricle and pulmonary atresia and had undergone pulmonary-artery angioplasty and the Fontan procedure at the age of three years.[11] Angiography seven months later revealed total occlusion of the right intermediate pulmonary artery. Following ethics committee approval and informed consent, the patient underwent implantation of a TEVG in April 1999. An approximately 2-cm segment of peripheral vein was explanted and cells from its walls were isolated. The cells were cultured and expanded as previously described. The cell count in the culture increased substantially to approximately 12×10^6 cells by eight weeks. A tube that served as a scaffold for these cells was constructed from a polycaprolactone–polylactic acid copolymer (weight ratio, 1:1) reinforced with woven PGA. The biodegradable polymer conduit (10 mm in diameter, 20 mm in length, and 1 mm in thickness) was designed to degrade within eight weeks. Ten days after seeding, the graft was transplanted. The occluded pulmonary artery was reconstructed with the TEVG. No postoperative complications occurred. On follow-up angiography, the transplanted vessel was noted to be completely patent. Seven months after implantation, the patient was doing well with no evidence of graft occlusion or aneurysmal changes on chest radiography.

Dr. Shinoka received approval from the ethics committee at the Tokyo Women's University to continue his work and was allowed to begin a clinical investigation of the use of TEVGs in the surgical repair of congenital cardiac anomalies. The study was limited to children older than one year of age and restricted to repairs exposed to venous or pulmonary arterial pressures. Dr. Shinoka performed the first operation in May 2000, when he replaced a portion of a thrombosed pulmonary artery with an autologous tissue-engineered construct. Between May 2000 and December 2004, he performed a total of 48 operations using either autologous tissue engineered patches or conduits in the repair of complex congenital cardiac anomalies. He evaluated the use of two different types of tissue engineering scaffolds: (1) PCLA/PGA and (2) PCLA/PLA. In addition, he evaluated three different autologous cell sources including: (1) mature vascular cells (endothelial cells, smooth muscle cells and fibroblasts), (2) bone marrow cells and (3) bone marrow-derived mononuclear cells. Included as a subset in this clinical investigation were 25 patients with single ventricle cardiac anomalies who underwent modified Fontan procedures using an autologous, extra-anatomic tissue-engineered conduit from the inferior vena cava to the pulmonary artery. All 25 TEVGs were seeded with autologous bone marrow-derived mononuclear cells.

A total of 42 consecutive patients received tissue-engineered vascular autografts seeded with BMCs (1). Informed consent was obtained directly from patients older than 20 years and from the parents of younger patients. Twenty-three patients had a tube graft as an extracardiac total cavopulmonary connection (TCPC) graft (Fig. 2).

In 19 patients, a sheet-type patch was used. The mean age at operation was 7.3 years (range 1–24 years), and the mean body weight was 21.7 kg (range 7.5–64 kg). Inclusion criteria for patients for this procedure were as follows: elective surgery, age younger than 30 years, patients or familial full

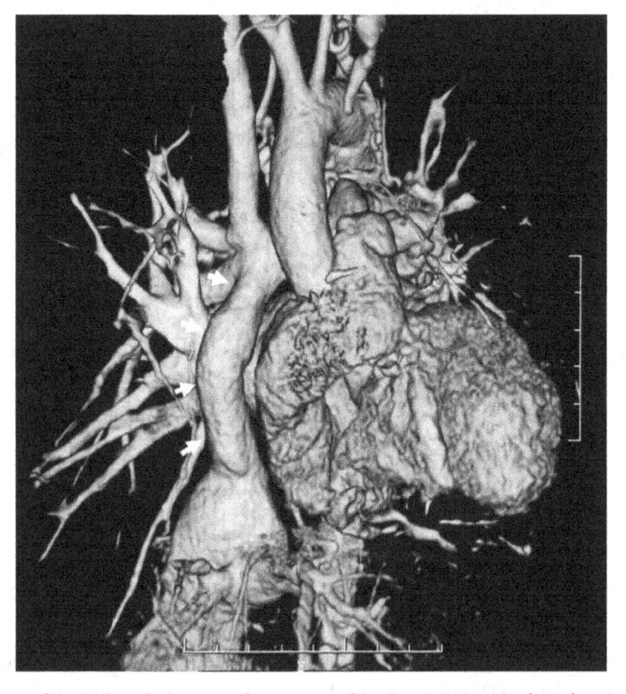

Fig. 2. Three-dimensional computed tomographic image 12 months after implantation of TCPC graft in a pediatric patient (patient 20). *White arrows* indicate location of tissue-engineered conduit.[1]

understanding of the procedure, and good quality of other organ function. Eighteen patients were male, and 24 were female. Thirty-six patients had undergone one or more previous operations. To examine the inflammatory reaction early after surgery, 20 patients who underwent TCPC at the same times (mean age 6.3 ± 3.1 years) with foreign materials served as a control group. White blood cell counts and the maximum postoperative C-reactive protein level were compared between groups.

Patient follow-up was scheduled at 6 to 12 months postoperatively and yearly thereafter. During follow-up visits, transthoracic echocardiography and multislice computed tomography, cineangiography, or magnetic resonance imaging angiogram were performed. Anticoagulation therapy with warfarin sodium and aspirin was continued until 3 to 6 months after the operation. International normalized ratio was kept from 1.5 to 2.0. Thereafter, anticoagulation therapy with aspirin alone was continued for an additional 12 months. At follow-up visits, additional clinical evaluations such as physical examination, chest roentgenography and electrocardiography were performed.

One year after implantation, computed tomography or magnetic resonance imaging was performed. Because the transectional shapes often appeared elliptic, the changes in maximal transectional area were calculated and compared with the area of the implanted tube. Calculation was performed according to the following formula: % Area change = [(Major axis $\times$ Major axis of graft) − (Implanted tube diameter)^2]/(implanted tube diameter)$^2 \times 100\%$. Results from 7 of 23 patients who underwent TCPC were included in this calculation. The PGA fibers were degraded by hydrolysis in approximately 2 months, the PLA fibers in 2 years. The remaining tensile strengths of the PLA fiber were 98.2% at 13 weeks, 88.1% at 26 weeks, 61.3% at 52 weeks, and 23.1% at 78 weeks; those of the PGA fiber were 81.3% at 1 week, 48.8% at 2 weeks, 7.6% at 3 weeks, and 4.6% at 4 weeks. Mean cell number seeded onto the scaffold was $320{,}000 \pm 29{,}900\,\text{cells/cm}^2$. Scanning electromicrography revealed seeded cells attached to the polymer surface. Giemsa staining demonstrated a sufficient number of seeded monolayer cells in the inner space of the scaffold wall. Immunohistochemical staining for anti-CD34 and fluorescence-activated cell sorter analysis demonstrated approximately 3% anti-CD34-positive cells.

Mean follow-up was 16.3 months (range 1.3–31.6 months, median 16.7 months). There were no in-hospital deaths after surgery. One patient with hypoplastic left heart syndrome died 3 months after the TCPC operation because of progressive tricuspid regurgitation and congestive heart failure. This late death was not related to the implanted tissue-engineered graft. During follow-up, there was no graft-specific lethal complication, such as rupture, thromboembolism, or aneurysm formation. In one patient, the tissue-engineered graft was replaced with a polytetrafluoroethylene patch 2 months after the original surgery because of unexpected slower tissue growth on the patch used for lateral tunnel procedure, which had caused massive right-to-left shunting. This patient recovered quickly after this surgical intervention and is currently in New York Heart Association functional class I. A confluent monolayer of luminal cells was present in the TEVG. In the medial layer, there were many collagen fibers and no evidence of calcification. Fever of unknown origin has not been seen in any of the patients. Maximum elevated temperatures were in the range of $37.4°C \pm 0.8°C$ after surgery. Further temperature measurements were performed until discharge without any temperature instability. Transthoracic echocardiography, multislice computed tomography, or magnetic resonance imaging showed calcification to be absent in the tissue-engineered grafts in all patients. Pulmonary angiography showed persistent patency in the peripheral pulmonary artery that was reconstructed with a tissue-engineered patch. Maximal transectional area was calculated and compared with the implanted size in the TCPC group. In patients with azygous connection (in which only hepatic flow goes up through the tissue-engineered graft), the larger grafts implanted tended to decrease in diameter with time. Depending on the flow amount, some grafts decreased in diameter and some increased, which seemed to reflect environmental adaptation of the tissue-engineered grafts.

Although the first few grafts implanted were seeded with mature vascular cells, the cell source in tissue engineering for human clinical applications was changed in 2002 based on work by Noishiki and colleagues who reported that BMCs implanted onto the surface of an artificial graft led to earlier endothelialization in a large animal model.[12] Moreover, it had been reported that some multipotent cells in bone marrow have the potential to differentiate into several cell types *in vivo*. Furthermore, previous studies had demonstrated endothelial progenitor cells derived from bone marrow that contribute to vasculogenesis and angiogenesis, and recent studies have demonstrated that endothelial cell lineage cells have potential in endothelialization. Anticoagulation therapies have been administered to all patients because animal experiments showed that it usually require two weeks to accomplish the complete endothelialization on the inner surface of the grafts. It was assumed that autologous tissue would not necessitate anticoagulation and that patients would be ultimately maintained on no anticoagulants or anti-platelet agents. Shortening the duration of warfarin treatment would improve quality of life, especially for young children in whom the risk of traumatic bleeding would be great and in women desiring pregnancy.

Based on the results of our clinical trial, we concluded that the use of TEVGs was safe and feasible in pediatric cardiovascular surgery and showed excellent hemodynamic performance during intermediate-term follow-up without anticoagulation therapy. It appears that the application of biodegradable scaffold with seeded BMCs will decrease the need for reintervention in pediatric patients. Because the results in both the clinical setting and the experimental model were quite encouraging, the tissue-engineering approach may play an important role as an alternative method to polytetrafluoroethylene grafts or allografts, especially in the field of pediatric cardiovascular surgery. The long-term durability of these tissue-engineered constructs will be determined by additional follow-up.

The underlying mechanism involved in the development of neotissue in tissue-engineered vascular grafts remains poorly understood. Most of the work on TEVGs described thus far has been carried out in large animal models including both ovine and canine models. Even though these are excellent models for the development of TEVGs, there are some significant limitations. One such limitation of this work is cost. Additionally, the large animal model lacks many of the molecular tools and probes trial that are essential for establishing the basic cellular and molecular mechanisms.[13]

1.3. *Post-clinical Studies*

Advances in mouse genetic models have been highly informative in the study of vascular biology, but have been inaccessible to vascular tissue engineers due to technical limitations resulting from size constraints when using mouse recipients. To this end, we developed a method for constructing sub-1mm internal diameter biodegradable scaffolds utilizing a dual cylinder chamber molding system and a hybrid polyester sealant. The development of TEVGs constructed from PCLA/PGA for use as vascular conduits in high-flow,

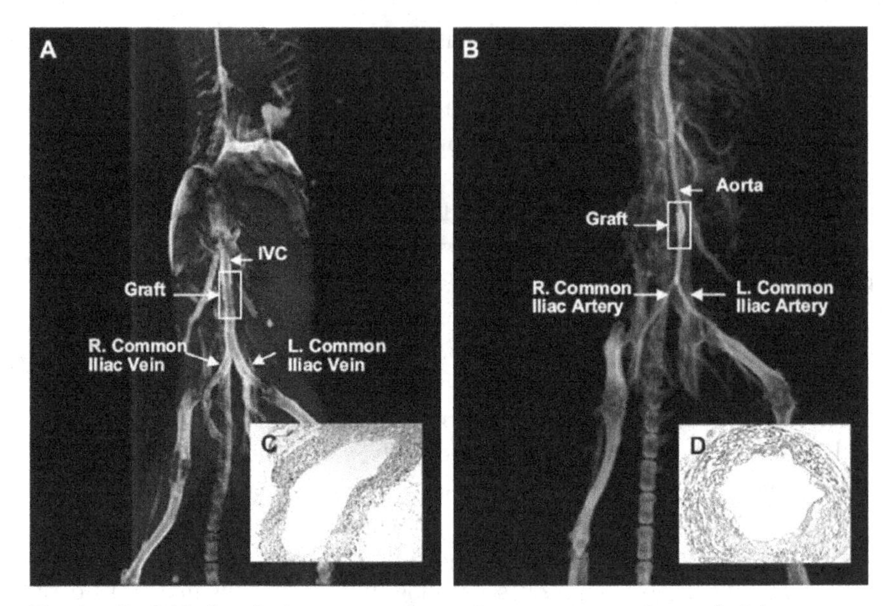

Fig. 3. Scaffolds functioning as vascular grafts at post-operative week 3 in a mouse model. (A) MCT reconstruction of PCLA/PGA scaffold as IVC graft, (B) MCT reconstruction of PCLA/PLA scaffold as aortic graft. By 3 weeks, scaffolds were fully infiltrated with cells. (C) H&E of PCLA/PGA as IVC graft. (D) H&E of PCLA/PLA as aortic graft. Original magnification 100× (C, D).[14]

low-pressure circulatory systems in animal models have demonstrated growth potential and adaptation into the venous system. Unfortunately, the use of this same TEVG as an arterial vascular conduit is associated with aneurysmal dilation and graft failure secondary to rupture. Scaffolds were therefore constructed from either PCLA/PGA or PCLA/PLA. Unseeded PCLA/PGA and PCLA/PLA scaffolds ($n = 7$) were implanted as IVC and aortic interposition grafts, respectively, in female CB-17 severe combined immunodeficient-beige (SCID/bg) mice (Fig. 3).[14]

Despite their gradual biodegradation, PCLA/PGA and PCLA/PLA scaffolds were functional as venous and arterial interposition grafts, respectively, exhibiting no thrombus or aneurysm formation over the course of 6 weeks. The continued biomechanical strength and functionality of the scaffolds over prolonged *in vivo* times are likely secondary to the vascular remodeling of the scaffolds as they slowly degrade. Even without cell seeding prior to implantation, early stages of organized vascular neotissue formation, consisting of partial endothelialization, medial generation and extracellular matrix deposition, were evident by postoperative week 6. At the present time, the mechanism of vascular neotissue formation in these engineered constructs is unknown. The differences in medial generation in the PCLA/PGA arterial grafts and PCLA/PLA venous grafts suggest that different hemodynamic forces between the venous and the arterial circulation may potentially be a contributing factor to the recruitment and proliferation of alpha-smooth muscle actin (αSMA) expressing cells in TEVGs. Additionally, a significant macrophage infiltration was evident within the walls of both scaffolds, implicating a possible role for inflammation in vascular neotissue formation. Studies are underway to determine the specific role of seeded cells, immune responses, and hemodynamic forces in the development of tissue engineered vascular grafts using these small-diameter scaffolds in mouse models. The ability to study tissue engineered vascular grafts in the mouse model will provide a powerful experimental tool for answering the mechanistic and developmental questions in vascular tissue engineering.

We used the SCID mouse model to develop a seeded vascular graft that can withstand high arterial pressures thereby allowing for expansion of this field even further as numerous congenital cardiac defects involve the arterial circuit. We conducted a pilot study in which TEVGs constructed from PCLA/PLA for use as arterial conduits were evaluated.[15] Scaffolds were seeded with human aortic muscle cells and human aortic endothelial cells and were then implanted into the abdominal aorta as interposition grafts in thirteen female SCID/bg mice. After graft fabrication, representative grafts were analyzed by scanning electron microscopy to determine pre-implantation inner diameter and wall thickness. The inner diameters of all grafts measured were less than 1 mm, with wall thicknesses ranging from 200 to 300 μm. Additional analysis of the grafts after cell seeding and culture revealed cell distribution throughout the graft wall and interspersed between polymeric fibers.

All grafts remained patent throughout the study period without evidence of stenosis, thrombus formation, or rupture. There was no clinical evidence of lower extremity ischemia in any of the graft recipients. These findings were confirmed using *in vivo* transabdominal ultrasound and micro-CT. Although slight graft dilatation was noted on imaging, this did not appear to be clinically significant; and all grafts were followed without failure owing to graft rupture. In addition, the explanted grafts grossly resembled that of the surrounding native aorta at the time of explantation.

Explanted grafts stained with hematoxylin and eosin (H&E) revealed neotissue distributed throughout the constructs and a 100% patency rate without evidence of graft rupture. The neotissue that developed was composed of an inner region or neomedia that mimics the media of the native mouse aorta and an outer region containing remaining polymer and tissue. As post-implantation time progressed, the polymeric scaffolds partially degraded; however, polymer was still present one year post-implantation. Neotissue developed within and among the polymeric fibers. The structural integrity of the conduits was maintained by the polymeric scaffold in conjunction with neotissue. As study time progressed, the grafts demonstrated slight dilatation that subsequently retracted as additional remodeling occurred. In addition, a well-defined, concentric, laminated neomedia resembling the media of the native aorta was appreciated in the developing graft one year post-implantation.[16] Grafts explanted at later study time-points reveal increasing amounts of collagen deposition in the neotissue when evaluated by Gomori 1-step trichrome stain. The collagen content one year post-implantation closely resembled that seen in native mouse aorta. Despite an initially unorganized distribution of collagen in the neovessels, collagen and smooth muscle fibers become laminated and are in a well-defined concentric distribution by 1-year post implantation.

In order to better understand the role of cell seeding in neovessel formation, we again turned our attention to the heterogenous bone marrow population as an alternative cell source to smooth muscle cells and endothelial cells in the construction of arterial tissue-engineered grafts. Doing such enabled us to fabricate and implant a graft within a short duration of time, thereby bypassing the need for prolonged culture periods and the associated risks of contamination. Similar to the clinical studies in which autologous bone marrow is extracted from the graft recipient and used to seed a polymeric tubular scaffold, the same approach could be applied in the development of arterial grafts. As such, we again seeded human bone marrow derived mononuclear cells onto scaffolds composed of PCLA/PLA and implanted these as aortic interposition grafts in SCID/bg mice. The mice were maintained without the use of anticoagulant or antiplatelet agents post-operatively. There was no evidence of graft thrombosis or stenosis in any of the graft recipients by one year following implantation. As was seen with the venous grafts constructed and implanted previously, the arterial grafts also demonstrated the formation of a neo-intima containing endothelial cells, a neo-media containing smooth muscle cells and a neo-adventitia containing collagen as is similarly seen in native vessels.

Evaluation of the PCLA/PLA scaffolds in the fabrication of arterial grafts demonstrated a slight increased propensity for the formation of graft dilatation during the remodeling process but without rupture. Although this dilatation retracts as remodeling continues and cellular deposition and proliferation continue, this raises concern for the development of aneurysm formation with the potential for graft failure. Furthermore, weakness of the graft and neovessel wall increases the risk of rupture, a consequence that may be lethal. In order to address such concerns, we developed a TEVG that could be implanted into the arterial system by implementing a technique known as electrospinning. Using this approach, we are able to dissolve a polymer (PLA) into a solvent (in this case, acetone and chloroform). The solution is drawn into a syringe that has a blunt needle tip and is aligned with a collection plate or mandril. As electrostatic forces are induced, the polymeric solution extrudes from the syringe and forms a taylor cone at which time the solvent evaporates, leaving behind polymeric fibers. The fibers are directed onto the rotating collection mandril by means of electrostatic forces and form a tubular, seamless, polymeric construct that can serve as a TEVG scaffold. Fiber size and alignment, porosity, and scaffold dimensions can be altered simply in an electrospinning system by changing the polymer concentration in solution, the speed at which the solution is extruded, or the rotational speed of the mandril.

Similar to the scaffolds previously described for use as TEVGs, the electrospun scaffold can be coated with a PCLA solution and seeded with bone marrow derived mononuclear cells. Our group has constructed such scaffolds that have been implanted in SCID/bg mice as infrarenal aortic interposition grafts. The grafts are able to withstand arterial pressures and do not demonstrate evidence of graft dilatation during the remodeling process. The grafts show evidence, however, of the development of a neovessel containing cellular layers similar to those seen in native arteries; a luminal endothelial monolayer surrounded by a concentric smooth muscle cell layer and an outer collagen-containing adventitia.

2. Conclusion

The development of tissue-engineered vascular conduits and grafts hold great promise in further advancing the fields of pediatric cardiothoracic and vascular surgery. We have demonstrated successful long-term clinical results after the implantation of such grafts in various animal models with the development of neovessels that histologically resemble native vessels. To date, implantation of such grafts in human patients has also been successful and has presented us with an exciting, rapidly advancing field. Findings described thus far support continued research in the development of tissue-engineered grafts.

References

1. Shin'oka, T., Matsumura, G., Hibino, N., Naito, Y., Watanabe, M., Konuma, T., Sakamoto, T., Nagatsu, M., and Kurosawa, H. (2005) Midterm clinical result of tissue-engineered vascular autografts seeded with autologous bone marrow cells. *The Journal of Thoracic and Cardiovascular Surgery* **129**, 1330–1338.
2. Conte, M. S. (1998) The ideal small arterial substitute: a search for the Holy Grail? *FASEB J* **12**, 43–45.
3. Weinberg, C. B., and Bell, E. (1986) A Blood Vessel Model Constructed From Collagen and Cultured Vascular Cells. *Science* **231**, 397–400.
4. Fuchs, J. R., Nasseri, B. A., and Vacanti, J. P. (2001) Tissue engineering: a 21st century solution to surgical reconstruction. *The Annals of Thoracic Surgery* **72**, 577–591.
5. Shinoka, T., Shum-Tim, D., Ma, P. X., Tanel, R. E., Isogai, N., Langer, R., Vacanti, J. P., and Mayer, J. E. (1998) Creation of Viable Pulmonary Artery Autografts Through Tissue Engineering. *J Thorac Cardiovasc Surgery* **115**, 536–546.
6. Watanabe, M., Shin'oka, T., Tohyama, S., Hibino, N., Konuma, T., Matsumura, G., Kosaka, Y., Ishida, T., Imai, Y., Yamakawa, M., Ikada, Y., and Morita, S. (2001) Tissue-Engineered Vascular Autograft: Inferior Vena Cava Replacement in a Dog Model. *Tissue Engineering* **7**, 429–439.
7. Matsumura, G., Miyagawa-Tomita, S., Shinoka, T., Ikada, Y., and Kurosawa, H. (2003) First evidence that bone marrow cells contribute to the construction of tissue engineered vascular autografts *in vivo*. *Circulation* **108**, 1729–1734.
8. Matsumura, G., Ishihara, Y., Miyagawa-Tomita, S., Ikada, Y., Matsuda, S., Kurosawa, H., and Shinoka, T. (2006) Evaluation of tissue-engineered vascular autografts. *Tissue Eng* **12**, 1–9.
9. Hibino, N., Shinoka, T., Matsumura, G., Ikada, Y., and Kurosawa, H. (2005) The tissue engineered vascular graft using bone marrow without culture. *J Thorac Cardiovasc Surg* **129**, 1064–1070
10. Brennan, M. P., Dardik, A., Hibino, N., Roh, J. D., Nelson, G. N., Papademitris, X., Shinoka, T., and Breuer C. K. (2008) Tissue engineered vascular grafts demonstrate evidence of growth and development when implanted in a juvenile animal model. *Ann Surg* **248**, 370–377.

11. Shin'oka, T., Imai, Y., and Ikada Y. (2001) Transplantation of a tissue-engineered pulmonary artery. *N Engl J Med* **344** 532–533.
12. Noishiki, Y., Tomizawa, Y., Yamane, Y., and Matsumoto A. (1996) Autocrine angiogenic vascular prosthesis with bone marrow transplantation. *Nat Med* **2**, 90–93.
13. Lopez-Soler, R. I., Brennan, M. P., Goyal, A., Wang, Y., Fong, P., Tellides, G., Sinusas, A., Dardik, A., and Breuer, C. (2007) Development of a mouse model for evaluation of small diameter vascular grafts. *J Surg Res* **139**, 1–6.
14. Roh, J. D., Nelson, G. N., Brennan, M. P., Mirensky, T. L., Yi, T., Hazlett, T. F., Tellides, G., Sinusas, A. J., Pober, J. S., Saltzman, W. M., Kyriakides, T. R., and Breuer, C. K. (2007) Small-Diameter biodegradable scaffolds for functional vascular tissue engineering in the mouse model. *Biomaterials* **29**, 1454–1463.
15. Isomatsu, Y., Shin'oka, T., Matsumura, G., Hibino, N., Konuma, T., Nagatsu, M., and Kurosawa, H. (2003) Extracardiac total cavopulmonary connection using a tissue-engineered graft. *J Thorac Cardiovasc Surgery* **126**, 1958–1962.
16. Mirensky, T. L., Nelson, G. N., Brennan, M. P., Roh, J. D., Hibino, N., Yi, T., Shinoka, T., and Breuer, C. K. (2009) Tissue-engineered arterial grafts: long-term results after implantation in a small animal model. *J Pediatr Surg* **44**, 1127–1132.

Chapter 11

DESIGN IMPLICATIONS FOR ENDOVASCULAR STENTS AND THE ENDOTHELIUM

JUAN M. JIMÉNEZ* and PETER F. DAVIES*,†,‡
*Institute for Medicine and Engineering

†Department of Pathology and Laboratory Medicine

‡Department of Bioengineering, University of Pennsylvania
Philadelphia, PA 19104, USA

1010 Vagelos Research Laboratories, 3340 Smith Walk,
Philadelphia, PA 19104-6383
pfd@pobox.upenn.edu

The multifocal distribution of atherosclerotic lesions throughout the cardiovascular system correlates with arterial geometries that promote regions of disturbed flow. Disturbed blood flow develops due to the local boundary conditions and is more prevalent near branches and areas of small radii of curvature, arterial sites susceptible to lesion formation. Endothelial cells exposed to disturbed flow exhibit an atheroprone phenotype. Thus disturbed flow is a contributor to the development of arterial disease regardless of the physical length scale of the vessel. This should be considered when designing implantable endovascular devices that can change the local blood flow characteristics. Stenotic regions of arteries are mechanically opened through the deployment of commercial stents that introduce boundary conditions that also promote flow separation and flow reversal, conditions present at arterial sites where atherosclerosis develops and where there is increased risk of thrombosis. This chapter considers how the merger of aerodynamic theory and local vessel hemodynamic conditions can serve as a design paradigm for a new generation of streamlined stent struts that inhibit the development of disturbed flow within the stented segment of a blood vessel.

1. Stent Deployment and the Endothelium

1.1. *Stent Struts Promote Disturbed Flow*

Bare metal stents (BMS) have been approved for clinical use since the 1990's to restore perfusion distal to stenosed vessels by mechanically expanding the vessel luminal area. Stents are deployed after initial expansion of the lumen by angioplasty. The stent, either self-expandable or balloon expandable, is placed over the area of interest, and once expanded, the radial forces of the metal scaffold preserve the effective lumen cross-sectional area. Immediately after deployment, the vessel wall boundary condition is changed from a stenotic lesion to a modified compressed, disrupted or displaced lesion with protruding metal struts on the surface (Fig. 1). In general, the vessel wall boundary condition is modified from the converging-diverging luminal trajectory of a stenotic lesion to that of a relatively constant luminal diameter vessel occasionally interrupted by the protruding stent struts. Although stent deployment increases the mean lumen diameter throughout the lesion, the vessel wall boundary condition is not reconstituted to a smooth topographic pre-lesion boundary condition. Only vessel wall topographic variations much greater than the height of an endothelial cell ($5 - 8\mu$m) become an important determining factor of flow quality in the near vessel wall boundary region.

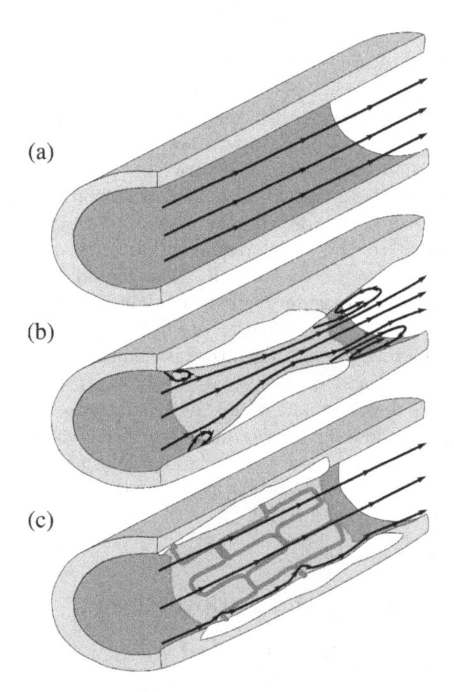

Fig. 1. Streamlines denoting mean bulk flow through a (a) healthy, (b) stenotic, and (c) stented vessel.

The Reynolds number (Re), the nondimensional parameter that quantifies the ratio of inertial forces (ρU) to viscous forces (μ/D), provides an insight into the likelihood that vessel wall irregularities such as protruding stent struts will contribute to the development of disturbed flow. The variables ρ and μ correspond to the density and dynamic viscosity of the blood, respectively. The bulk blood flow velocity is denoted by U and the blood vessel diameter by D. Although atherosclerotic lesions develop at different sites corresponding to a wide range of physiologic Reynolds numbers, the inertial forces have to be much greater than the viscous forces for small physical perturbations to promote the development of disturbed flow. As the Reynolds number increases, the physical length scale of objects that can potentially perturb the flow decrease in size. Likewise, as Re increases, arterial radii of curvature and vessel wall boundary condition variations that can lead to the development of disturbed flow decrease in size. Given the relatively high Reynolds number flow environment present in medium sized vessels like the coronary and carotid arteries, the protruding stent struts create flow disturbances that modify the local flow patterns generating local pockets of disturbed flow.[1–5] For antegrade flow, as the blood along the vessel wall approaches a stent strut, it encounters a local adverse pressure gradient and it separates from the wall creating a flow recirculation zone proximally of the stent strut. Due to the inertial forces, the flow traveling tangentially to the luminal strut surface separates from the distal edge since it cannot follow the abrupt change in geometry. This distal flow separation is much larger than the proximal flow separation. Both flow separation zones are characterized by slower moving flow, longer particle residence time, and lower wall shear stress levels than vessel wall areas away from the struts with attached flow. These flow characteristics correspond to atheroprone and procoagulant flow conditions[6–11] that can disrupt the convective transport of nutrients, waste, and oxygen, and lead to the entrapment of molecules and cells inside the vortex leading to longer residence times.

The vessel wall shear stress corresponds to the tangential frictional force exerted on the vessel wall by the blood flow. The wall shear stress is defined by the following,

$$\begin{aligned}\tau_w &= \mu\left(\frac{\partial u}{\partial r} + \frac{\partial v}{\partial x}\right)\\ &= \mu\dot{\gamma}, \qquad (1.1)\end{aligned}$$

where $\dot{\gamma}$ is the shear strain rate, and u and v are the axial and radial velocity components, respectively. The variables x and r are the streamwise and radial spatial coordinates, respectively. The flow separation and reattachment points correspond to the point along the wall where the velocity gradient in the direction normal to the wall equals zero. Fluid flow streamlines at these points are perpendicular to the surface.

Figure 2a shows a diagram of flow about the cross-section of an individual stent strut. The upstream separation distance (S_{ux}) corresponds to the distance along the vessel wall between the flow separation point and the upstream strut side-wall. The downstream separation distance (S_{dx}) is the length between the downstream strut side-wall and the

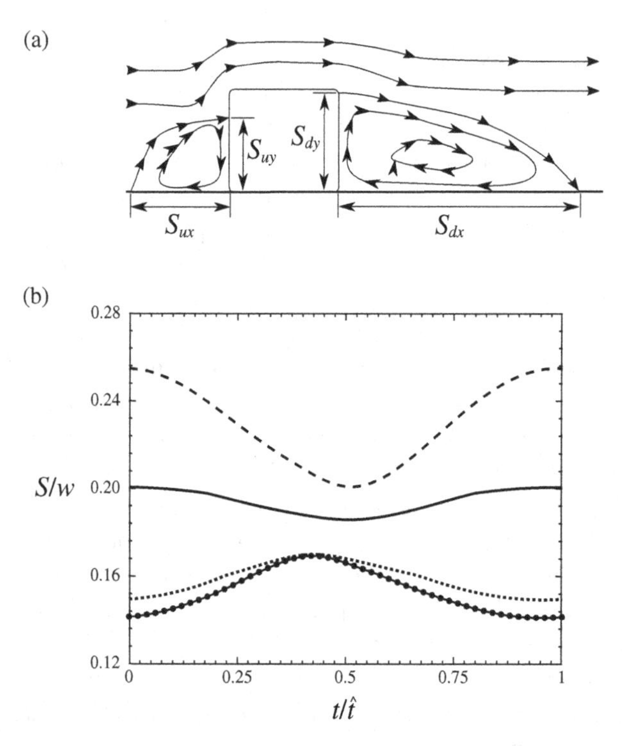

Fig. 2. Flow separation about a stent strut. (a) Diagram of separation and reattachment distances along the upstream vessel wall (S_{ux}), upstream strut side surface (S_{uy}), downstream strut side surface (S_{dy}), and downstream vessel wall (S_{dx}), of a rectangular stent strut. (b) Separation and reattachment distances S_{ux}, —•—; S_{uy}, ···; S_{dy}, ——; S_{dx}, - - -; normalized by the stent strut width (w) for a rectangular stent strut of AR = 4:1 for one pulsatile time period. From Jiménez and Davies.[4]

flow reattachment point. Figure 2a further shows the reattachment and separation points along the upstream and downstream strut side-walls, respectively, and their corresponding distances along the walls are denoted by S_{uy} and S_{dy}. All these distances are dependent on the Reynolds number. For example, as shown in Fig. 2b in the presence of pulsatile flow, upstream (S_{ux}) and downstream (S_{dx}) separation distances along the wall in the vicinity of a rectangular cross-section strut (200 μm wide by 50 μm high) are inversely proportional and proportional, respectively, to the instantaneous Reynolds number.[4] The instantaneous Reynolds number is a function of the instantaneous bulk flow mean velocity. For the data shown in Fig. 2b, the instantaneous Reynolds number was varied from 86 to 400 during the nondimensional pulsatile time period, $t/\hat{t}$, where $\hat{t}$ is the total length of time of the pulsatile period. Furthermore, the upstream reattachment (S_{uy}) and downstream separation (S_{dy}) distances on the side-walls of the strut behave similarly to the corresponding distances along the vessel wall demonstrating inversely proportional and proportional relationships to the instantaneous Reynolds number, while exhibiting smaller distance fluctuations throughout the period. The separation and reattachment distances upstream and downstream can become more similar in magnitude if the stent is implanted at a site where the bulk flow reverses, as occurs in certain sites of the coronary arteries.[12] The extent of the flow separation will depend on the instantaneous flow direction and magnitude. Given that the size of the recirculation zone is proportional to Re, the proximal recirculation zone may temporarily become as large as the distal recirculation zone if the peak retrograde flow magnitude matches the peak forward flow magnitude.

1.2. *Stent Deployment Compromises Endothelium*

Unregulated thrombus growth and smooth muscle cell-extracellular matrix related neointimal hyperplasia (NH) are the primary causes of stent restenosis. The endothelium, a single-cell lining extending throughout the cardiovascular system, maintains vascular wall and blood homeostasis. Each endothelial cell serves as a local nonthrombogenic barrier between the blood and extracellular matrix and modulates local antagonistic elements of vascular homeostasis. However, the deployment of stents can result in partial endothelial denudation[13] exposing the highly thrombogenic extracellular matrix (ECM), enabling platelet activation and adhesion, and exposing membrane-bound tissue factor (TF) and release of TF by subendothelial cells.[14] The resulting platelet shape change and sequential release of secretory granules in combination with tissue factor activates the coagulation cascade. Polymerized fibrin and platelets aggregate to form a thrombus at the site of injury. The growth of the thrombus may not be properly regulated due to the absence of endothelial cells that express and release fibrinolytic and anticoagulant molecules. These molecules include tissue plasminogen activator (tPA), thrombomodulin, tissue factor pathway inhibitor (TFPI), heparin-like molecules, and adenosine diphosphatase (ADPase). Tissue plasminogen activator, a key component of the fibrinolytic pathway, activates plasmin promoting dissolution of the newly formed thrombus. The absence of endothelial cells also voids the presence of the surface receptor thrombomodulin, a co-factor in the thrombin induced activation of protein C, a clotting inhibitor that proteolytically cleaves factors Va and VIIIa. Similarly, TFPI, an endothelial surface protein, inhibits factors VIIa and Xa. Moreover, the absence of the endothelium facilitates the adhesion of platelets to the exposed ECM via von Willebrand factor (vWF).

The expansion of the vessel lumen through stent deployment not only can partially denude the endothelium, but it also disrupts the internal elastic lamina (IEL) and causes damage to the tunica media. If severe enough, the disruption to the vessel wall can extend to the tunica adventitia. The disruption of the endothelium activates the natural healing response promoting smooth muscle cell (SMC) migration from the tunica media to the intima, followed by SMC proliferation, and ECM synthesis and deposition. However, an over-compensatory response to such injury can lead to neointimal hyperplasia (NH). The degree of NH correlates with the severity of the disruption to the vessel wall.[15] If severe enough, NH can lead to restenosis of a stented vessel. Conversely, endothelialization of the affected site can arrest SMC proliferation and migration. Therefore, the degree of restenosis is inversely proportional to the rate of endothelialization. Regions that are rapidly re-covered by endothelial cells display decreased intimal thickening compared to those that do not.[16–19] The rate of endothelialization is proportional to the local flow rate (shear stress) with slower moving flow in a recirculation zone yielding lower shear stress levels and retarding endothelialization.[20,21]

Current nonstreamlined strut designs abet the development of distal and proximal regions of disturbed flow. Endothelial cells that remain after stent deployment and are consequently exposed to disturbed flow synthesize less endothelial nitric oxide (NO) and prostacyclin (PGI_2), molecules linked to the inhibition of SMC proliferation and migration, and the inhibition of platelet aggregation. In contrast, the endothelial secretion of vWF, a required cofactor of platelet binding to the extracellular matrix (ECM), and plasminogen activator inhibitor type 1 (PAI-1), a depressor of fibrinolysis, are inversely proportional to the local shear stress level. On average, disturbed flow yields low shear stress levels, bolstering the secretion of vWF[22] and PAI-1.[7] Furthermore, disturbed flow also promotes the endothelial production of endothelin-1, a SMC mitogen.[23]

Local inflammation in the stented region can also play a role in restenosis. ECs exposed to disturbed flow translocate P-selectin to the cell membrane,[24] a crucial factor in leukocyte recruitment and migration. Disturbed flow also promotes upregulation of vascular adhesion molecule-1 (VCAM-1) and intracellular adhesion molecule-1 (ICAM-1) in endothelial cells,[10] which facilitate the migration of leukocytes across the endothelium. In addition, cytokines secreted and acting on endothelial cells mediate interactions between the endothelium and leukocytes. The flow field generated by stent struts transports leukocytes from the blood mainstream to the vessel wall. The slow moving recirculation zone increases the monocyte-to-endothelial cell interaction[25] promoting transmigration and peri-strut presence of macrophages.[26,27] Macrophages not only influence the formation of atherosclerotic lesions, but also release growth factors and inflammatory mediators that in concert with SMC migration and proliferation contribute to the vascular lesion locally after stent deployment.[28]

1.3. *Stent Design Properties Affecting Restenosis*

In vitro, *in vivo*, and computational studies have addressed different physical properties of stents that influence restenosis including strut thickness, strut surface roughness, number of strut-strut intersections, effective number of struts per cross-section, interstrut spacing, postdeployment stent orientation, strut amplitude, and strut radius of curvature among others.[1,29–37] The ISAR-STEREO and ISAR-STEREO 2 clinical trials reported a proportional relationship between strut thickness and angiographic restenosis.[31,33] The ISAR-STEREO trial considered the influence of stent strut thickness for two identical stents differing in thickness and a minor difference in the number of inter-ring articulations, while preserving a strut width of 100 μm and similar architecture for both stents. The strut thickness was 50 μm for the thin strut stent and 140 μm for the thick strut stent. The angiographic restenosis rates after 6 months were 42% lower for the randomly selected patients that received the thinner strut stent. The ISAR-STERE0 2 trial found similar decreased angiographic restenosis results for the thinner strut stent group, even though the stents differed architecturally. In addition to larger scale properties like strut thickness, small length scale properties are also important. For instance, strut surface roughness about 1/100 of typical endothelial length scales have been linked to lower rates of angiographic restenosis when compared to electrochemically polished stents.[35] This surface roughness length scale promotes faster endothelialization than the much smaller surface roughness length scales present in the electrochemically polished stents. Furthermore, *in vivo* experiments showed that a change in strut-strut intersection, while maintaining the total mass and surface area constant, yielded different levels of vascular injury, thrombosis, and neointimal hyperplasia.[29] Neointimal hyperplasia and mural thrombus levels were decreased when the effective number of struts per cross-sectional area was increased by 50%, recreating more closely a circular lumen than the polygonal shape seen in lower strut number cases.[30] For a review on general aspects of stent design the reader is referred to Sangiorgi *et al.*[38]

With the availability of clinical and *in vitro* data and the resulting association of disturbed flow with a shift of the endothelium towards a procoagulant and atherosusceptible phenotype,[6–10] computational studies have provided high resolution approximations of the flow field in the cardiovascular system that have been instrumental in the improvement of stents. For example, numerical simulation results have shown that inter-ring strut connectors should be kept to a minimum.[36] Although inter-ring strut connectors are generally aligned with the bulk blood flow direction, their presence generates local axially distributed regions of low wall shear stress. These regions of low wall shear stress increase in size as the orientation of the connector varies from a parallel to perpendicular configuration with respect to the bulk flow. An additional design parameter studied, the distance between struts, is a compromise between fluid and mechanical forces. As the interstrut distance increases, the extent of disturbed flow between struts decreases.[36] However, the degree of interstrut vascular tissue prolapse increases, as well as the mechanical force exerted by the struts hence creating large, local nonphysiological stresses on the vessel wall. If the interstrut distance is on the order of one strut thickness or less, the proximal and distal recirculation zones merge yielding a discrete, recirculating stagnant zone.[1,36] In general, recirculation zones disrupt the natural transport of nutrients, waste, and oxygen, while extending the monocyteto-to-endothelial cell interaction and the residence time of coagulation factors. In the absence of an intact endothelium, when local anticoagulation factors are exhausted, recirculation zones can become nidi for thrombus formation. The net volume of entrapped blood and endothelial cells exposed to disturbed flow is greater in a discrete merged recirculating zone than that present in individual proximal and distal recirculation zones for struts placed farther apart.

1.4. *Drug Eluting Stents (DES) and the Endothelium*

The recurring problem of in-stent restenosis due to neointimal hyperplasia (NH) was addressed through the introduction of drug-eluting stents (DES). These stents are coated with an anti-proliferative drug that is eluted over a period of weeks to months. The rate of drug elution is partially dependent on fluid mechanical forces acting on the luminal side of the strut and by diffusion on the abluminal side. The drugs control any over-compensatory injury response that may arise due to the deployment of the stent, the potential NH, and subsequent restenosis. A randomized clinical trial comparing two architecturally identical stents, one DES and the other BMS, showed that 6 months after deployment restenosis occurred in 25.9% of BMS recipients, while none of the DES recipients demonstrated restenosis.[39] Meta-analysis results of 17 clinical trials reported a decrease in reinterventions when patients received a DES instead of BMS.[40] However, the use of DES have not reduced total mortality when compared to BMS.[40,41] A meta-analysis of four randomized trials comparing DES and BMS showed a 1.3% greater survivability rate with BMS than with DES.[42] Two other meta-analyses have suggested that DES recipients suffer from increased rates of death and myocardial infarction.[41] Although decreased rates of restenosis are seen with DES, they are linked to late-stent thrombosis (LST),[43] a different and distinct type of response to injury at the site of stent deployment. Lack of endothelialization, endothelial dysfunction, and hypersensitivity to the stent coating, have been implied as possible factors in LST.[44–52]

DES are coated with drugs that indiscriminately inhibit cell proliferation and migration. Although SMC are the main target for these drugs, an unintended consequence is the prevention of endothelialization of the stent struts and denuded vessel wall regions. The arrest of cell proliferation and migration preserves the post-stent deployment modified vessel wall boundary condition where the struts protrude into the lumen. The protrusion of the stent struts promotes the development of disturbed flow regions that result in local atheroprone and procoagulant flow conditions. Contrary to BMS where intimal thickening eventually buries the stent struts, DES are designed to inhibit restenosis. If the degree of intimal thickening is minimal, but sufficient to bury the stent struts, as occurs with successful BMS stents, the presence of disturbed flow is eliminated due to the change of the vessel wall boundary condition. However, after DES implantation, drug-induced delayed arterial healing results in uncovered stent struts months to years later, promoting chronic procoagulant and atheroprone flow, and increased risk of LST. Consistent with this mechanism, histology and imaging confirm that thrombosis colocalizes with uncovered stent struts.[43,50,53]

1.5. *Elimination and Minimization of Disturbed Flow in the Vicinity of Stent Struts*

Disturbed flow occurs in natural arterial geometries such as the inner arch of the aorta and the sinus of the carotid artery (Fig. 3(a)–3(b)). Although the dimensions and geometry of these vessels are quite different, the boundary conditions promote the development of disturbed flow and the underlying endothelium displays an atheroprone and procoagulant phenotype.[9–11,54] Similarly, as shown in Fig. 3c and although much smaller in length scale, the struts of current commercial nonstreamlined stents promote the development of local atheroprone and procoagulant flow conditions that retard endothelialization, decrease secretory rates of NO, tPA, and PGI_2, and increase secretion of vWF and PAI-1. During the early stages of BMS post-deployment, and possibly indefinitely for DES, struts that protrude into the lumen promote disturbed flow proximally and distally maintaining a procoagulant milieu and a local procoagulant and atheroprone endothelial phenotype. Restenosis, re-narrowing of the vessel lumen, due to neointimal hyperplasia occurs in 30 to 40% of BMS recipients,[29] while DES recipients are susceptible

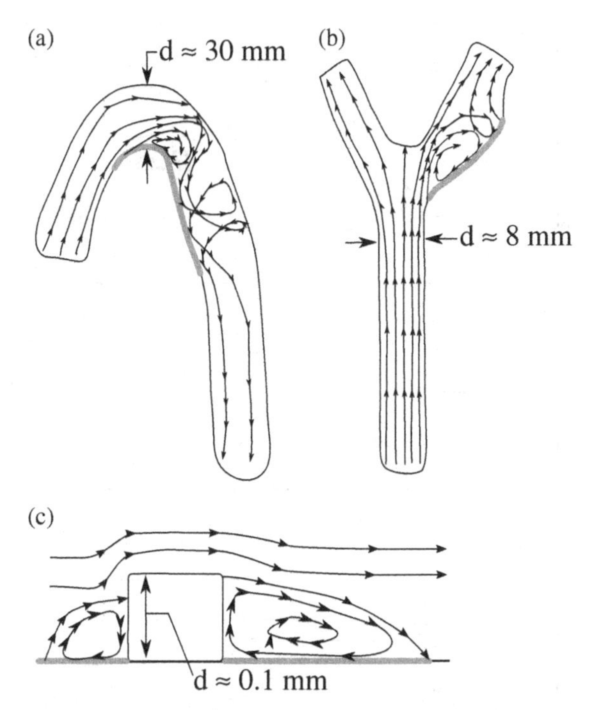

Fig. 3. Examples of disturbed flow in vessels differing in dimensions. Examples include (a) the aortic arch and (b) the sinus of the carotid artery, and flow disturbances promoted by (c) elements of implantable devices such as stents. Regions that experience disturbed flow are highlighted in gray.

to chronic nonendothelialization of stent struts and consequential LST.[43]

The spatial extent of the flow disturbances can be minimized by decreasing the stent strut thickness $(h)^4$, which may be a reason why patients from the ISAR-STERE0 and ISAR-STERE0 2 demonstrated lower angiographic restenosis rates with thinner stent struts.[31,33] Figure 4(a)–4(c) shows that as the thickness of the strut decreases, while keeping the strut width (w) constant, the spatial extent of the disturbed flow region decreases nonlinearly. The recirculation zone can be further decreased by rounding the cross-sectional geometry while keeping the aspect ratio (AR = $w : h$) constant (Fig. 4(a) and 4(d)). This minor modification in geometry can lead to a significant reduction in cross-sectional area for the upstream and downstream recirculation zones.[4] In addition, endothelialization is

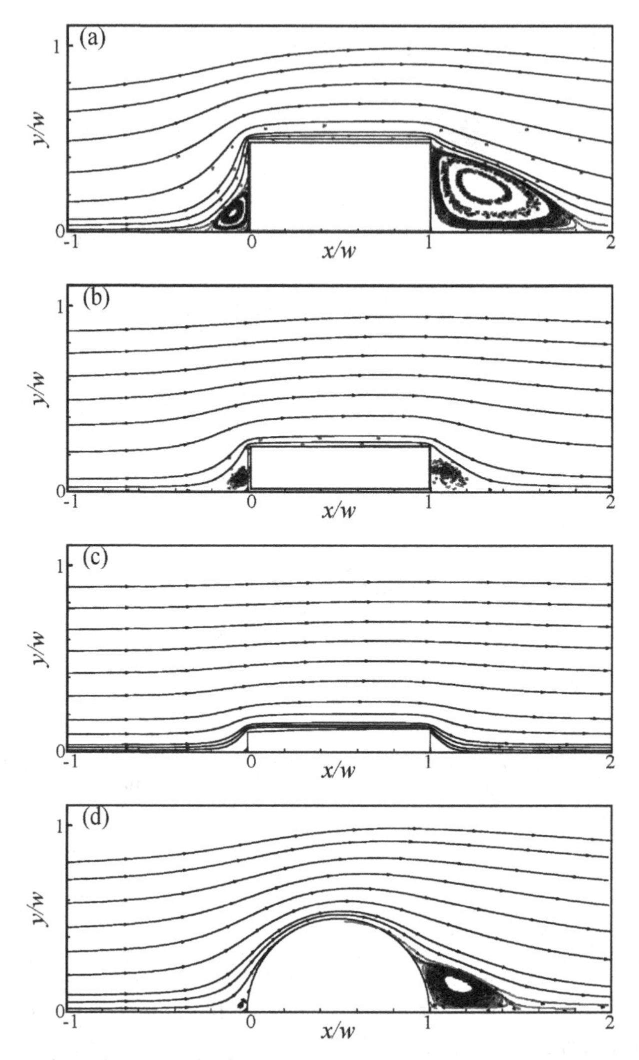

Fig. 4. Streamlines denoting the fluid path about rectangular stent strut cross-sectional geometries with AR = (a) 2:1 (b) 4:1, (c) 8:1, and a (d) circular arc stent strut cross-sectional geometry of AR = 2:1. Aspect ratio (AR) equals $w : h$, where w is the width of the strut and h is the thickness of the strut. Data from Jiménez and Davies.[4]

dependent on the strut thickness and the spatial extent of the flow disturbance. The rate of endothelialization decreases as the strut thickness increases.[55] EC migration rates are higher on the upstream side of stent struts where the recirculation zone is smaller, as opposed to the distal

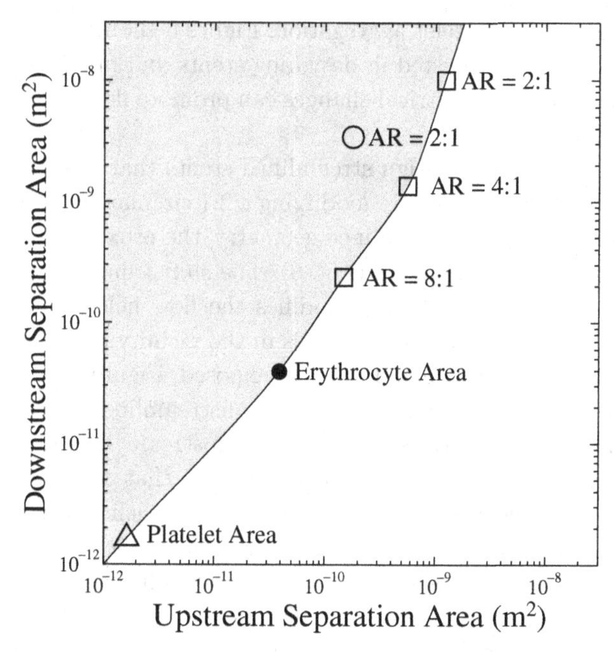

Fig. 5. Stent strut design plane based upon recirculation zone cross-sectional areas of rectangular, □, and circular arc ○, stent struts with corresponding AR $= w : h$ ($w = 200\,\mu$m), and the typical cross-sectional area of an erythrocyte, ●, and a platelet, △. Data from Jiménez and Davies.[4]

side, which is characterized by a much larger recirculation zone and slower endothelial migration rates.[55]

Figure 5 shows a design plane for different stent strut geometrical cross-sections. The design plane shows that as the aspect ratio (AR $= w : h$) changes from 8:1 to 4:1 to 2:1 the cross-sectional area of the upstream and downstream recirculation zones increases nonlinearly for rectangular struts. Holding constant the aspect ratio at 2:1 while changing the cross-sectional geometry to a circular arc, the upstream recirculation zone is decreased below that of the rectangular 4:1. The geometries shown on Fig. 5 are nonstreamlined, since they promote flow separation for physiological Reynolds numbers present in arteries. Even the cross-sectional area of the upstream and downstream recirculation zones in the vicinity of the 8:1 rectangular strut is an order of magnitude greater than the cross-sectional area of an erythrocyte (Fig. 5). The difference is much greater when compared to the cross-sectional area of a platelet, emphasizing the spatial potential for platelet aggregation. Figure 5 should serve as a design paradigm for those interested in designing stents and provides insight into how dimensional or geometrical changes can promote flow disturbances and affect the endothelium.

An alternative is to design streamlined stents that passively eliminate or minimize flow separation. By modifying a 2:1 circular arc nonstreamlined geometry to a 4:1 or 8:1 streamlined geometry, the proximal and distal flow separation zones are eliminated (Fig. 6). The shift from nonstreamlined to streamlined geometries not only modifies the flow field qualitatively, but affects the vessel wall shear stress levels in the vicinity of the strut and the shear rate levels to which blood cells are exposed. Figure 7 shows the shear stress distribution over streamlined and nonstreamlined strut geometries. The vessel wall shear stress immediately upstream and downstream of the nonstreamlined struts is much lower than that for the streamlined geometries. Low shear stress levels decrease endothelialization rates. The shear rates and spatial shear rate gradients along the luminal surface of the nonstreamlined struts reach much greater values than those for the streamlined stents. High shear rate flow fields activate platelets[56] and if high enough, promote ADP release by erythrocytes, which induces platelet aggregation.[57]

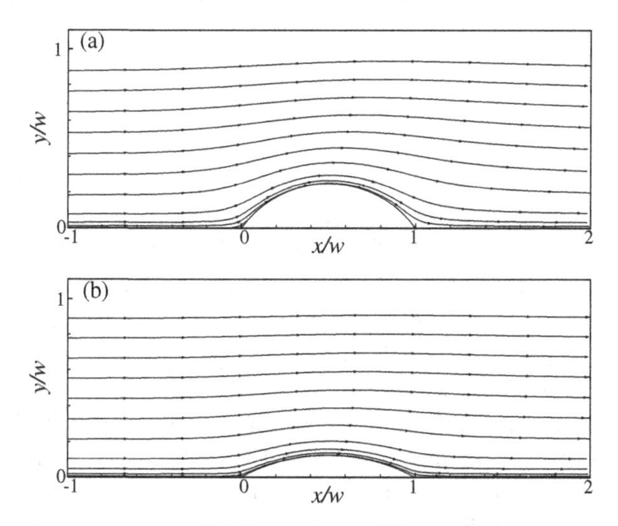

Fig. 6. Streamlines denoting the fluid path about circular arc stent strut cross-sectional geometries with AR = (a) 4:1 and (b) 8:1. No flow separation is observed in the vicinity of these two streamlined geometries. Data from Jiménez and Davies.[4]

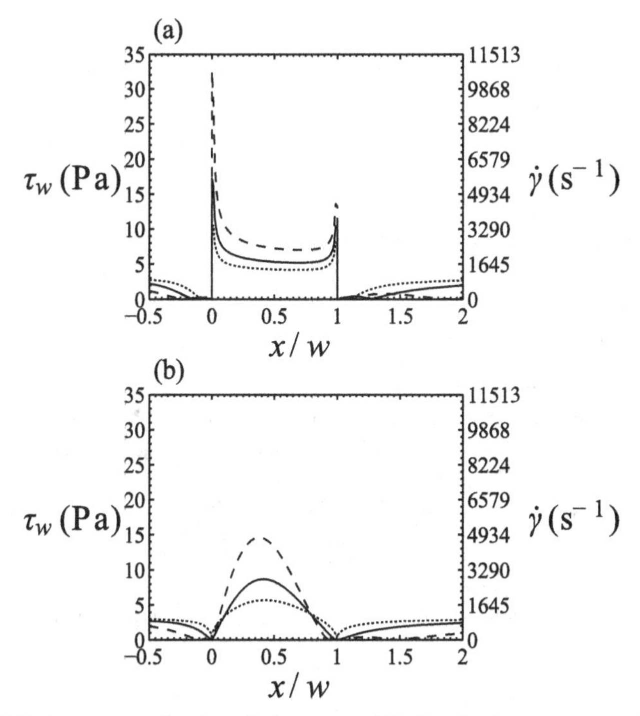

Fig. 7. Wall shear stress (τ_w) and shear rate ($\dot{\gamma}$) distributions corresponding to (a) rectangular and (b) circular arc stent struts for aspect ratios, AR = 2:1, - - -, 4:1, ——, and 8:1, ... From Jiménez and Davies.[4]

The gradual changes in slope along the surface of a 4:1 or 8:1 circular arc enable a smooth transition for blood traveling tangentially from the vessel wall to the stent strut surface (Fig. 8). The absence of recirculation zones promotes a flow environment conducive to endothelialization of the stent strut surface and adjacent vessel wall, and restores anticoagulative properties around the struts. Furthermore, the absence of recirculating flow enables the natural wash out of blood in these regions, shortening residence times of leukocytes, platelets, and coagulation factors that tend to accumulate at recirculation sites promoting coagulation[58] and inflammation. The combination of aerodynamic theory and hemodynamics yields a streamlined geometry that when incorporated into stent design creates conditions that promote faster endothelialization and reduce the probability of thrombogenesis, two important indicators of clinical success.

(a)

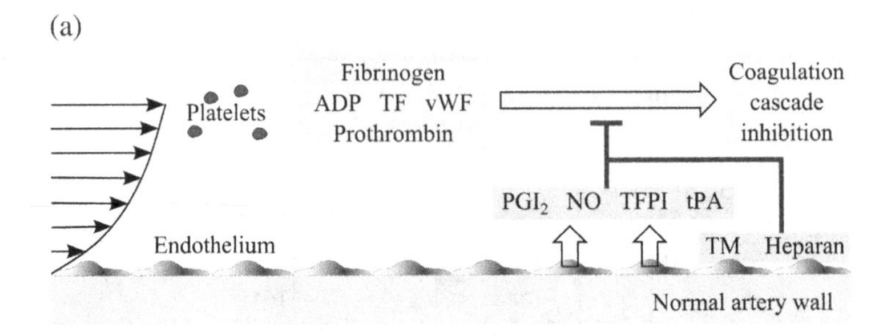

(b)

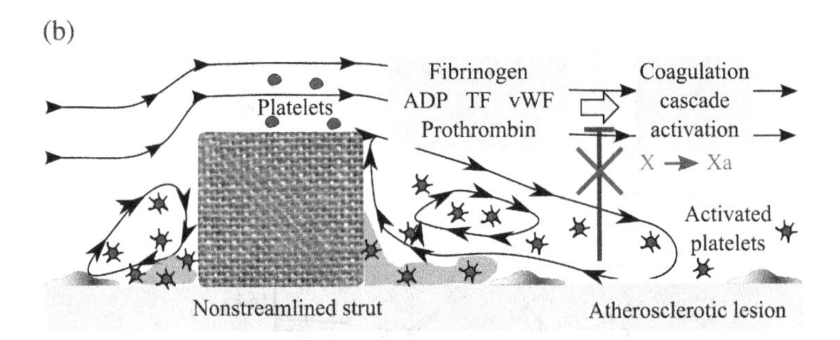

(c)

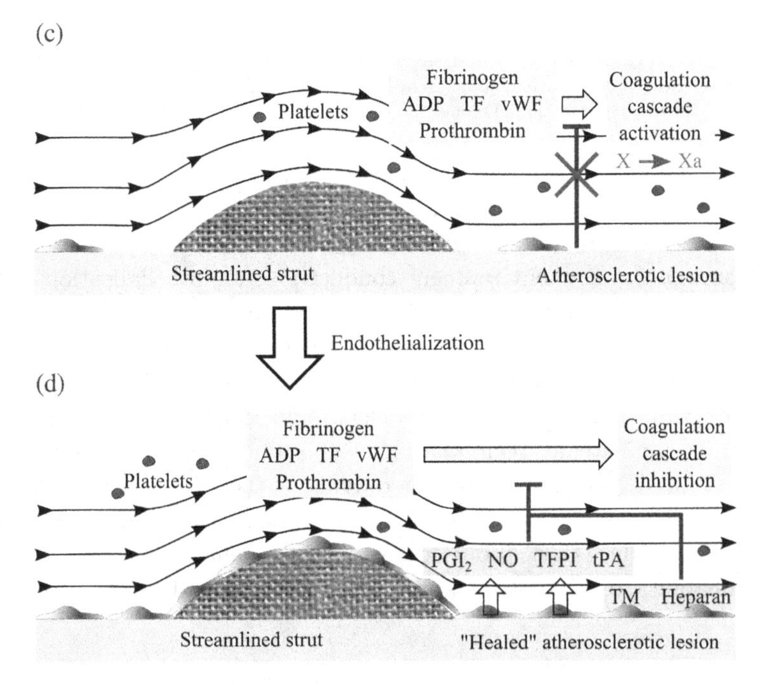

Fig. 8. (See figure caption on facing page.)

References

1. Berry, J. L., Santamarina, A., Moore, J. E., Jr., Roychowdhury, S., and Routh, W. D. (April, 2000) Experimental and computational flow evaluation of coronary stents. *Ann Biomed Eng* **28**(4), 386–398.
2. LaDisa, J. Jr., Guler, I., Olson, L., Hettrick, D., Kersten, J., Warltier, D., and Pagel, P. (Sep, 2003) Three-dimensional computational fluid dynamics modeling of alterations in coronary wall shear stress produced by stent implantation. *Ann Biomed Eng* **31**(8), 972–980.
3. Seo, T., Schachter, L., and Barakat, A. (Apr, 2005) Computational study of fluid mechanical disturbance induced by endovascular stents. *Ann Biomed Eng* **33**(4), 444–456.
4. Jiménez, J. M., and Davies, P. F. (August, 2009) Hemodynamically driven stent strut design. *Ann Biomed Eng* **37**(8), 1483–1494.
5. Mejia, J., Ruzzeh, B., Mongrain, R., Leask, R., and Bertrand, O. (2009) Evaluation of the effect of stent strut profile on shear stress distribution using statistical moments. *BioMedical Engineering OnLine* **8**(1), 8.
6. Frangos, J., Eskin, S., McIntire, L., and Ives, C. (1985) Flow effects on prostacyclin production by cultured human endothelial cells. *Science* **227**(4693), 1477–1479.

Fig. 8. Blood contains multiple procoagulant proteins as well as natural anticoagulants that together with the endothelium normally maintain a non-coagulation state. (a) In the normal artery wall the secreted and surface-presented anticoagulant molecules of the endothelium help maintain hemostatic balance. ADP, adenosine diphosphate; TF, tissue factor; vWF, von Willebrand factor; PGI_2, prostacyclin; NO, nitric oxide; TFPI, tissue factor pathway inhibitor; tPA, tissue plasminogen activator; TM, thrombomodulin. (b) The deployment of current commercial (nonstreamlined) stents promotes flow separation in the proximal and distal regions of the strut. Procoagulant conditions are greatly increased around the stent strut by the following: (i) accelerated flow over the strut edges yields shear rate magnitudes that can activate platelets some of which will enter the distal flow separation zone, (ii) recirculation zones retain activated platelets and procoagulant factors that can reach critical concentrations for activation of the coagulation cascade, (iii) the removal of endothelium during angioplasty and stenting eliminates anticoagulant mechanisms and exposes the highly thrombogenic extracellular matrix surface. Furthermore, (iv) low flow velocity (shear stress) inhibits endothelialization of the vessel and strut surface. (c) A streamlined stent strut inhibits fluid flow separation and high shear rate peaks that can activate platelets. Furthermore, a streamlined geometry will be less likely to generate recirculation zones therefore decreasing the residence time of procoagulant molecules and the probability of thrombogenesis despite the absence of endothelium. Undisturbed flow proximal and distal to the streamlined strut favors endothelialization of the vessel and strut surface. (d) An endothelialized vessel and strut surface provide an anticoagulant environment that helps maintain hemostatic balance and protect against stent-related thrombosis. From Jiménez and Davies.[4]

7. Diamond, S., Eskin, S., and McIntire, L. (1989) Fluid flow stimulates tissue plasminogen activator secretion by cultured human endothelial cells. *Science* **243**(4897), 1483–1485.
8. Dai, G., Kaazempur-Mofrad, M. R., Natarajan, S., Zhang, Y., Vaughn, S. Blackman, B. R., Kamm, R. D., García-Cardeña, G., and Gimbrone, M. A. (2004) Distinct endothelial phenotypes evoked by arterial waveforms derived from atherosclerosis-susceptible and -resistant regions of human vasculature. *P Natl Acad Sci USA* **101**(41), 14871–14876.
9. Passerini, A. G., Polacek, D. C., Shi, C., Francesco, N. M., Manduchi, E., Grant, G. R., Pritchard, W. F., Powell, S., Chang, G. Y., Stoeckert, C. J., and Davies, P. F. (2004) Coexisting proinflammatory and antioxidative endothelial transcription pro- files in a disturbed flow region of the adult porcine aorta. *P Natl Acad Sci USA* **101**(8), 2482–2487.
10. Suo, J., Ferrara, D. E., Sorescu, D., Guldberg, R. E., Taylor, W. R., and Giddens, D. P. (2007) Hemodynamic shear stresses in mouse aortas: Implications for atherogenesis. *Arterioscler Thromb Vasc Biol* **27**(2), 346–351.
11. Won, D., Zhu, S.-N., Chen, M., Teichert, A.-M., Fish, J. E., Matouk, C. C., Bonert, M., Ojha, M., Marsden, P. A., and Cybulsky, M. I. (2007) Relative reduction of endothelial nitric-oxide synthase expression and transcription in atherosclerosis-prone regions of the mouse aorta and in an *in vitro* model of disturbed flow. *Am J Pathol* **171**(5), 1691–1704.
12. Voci, P., Pizzuto, F., and Romeo, F. (2004) Coronary flow: a new asset for the echo lab?, *Eur Heart J* **25**, 1867–1879.
13. Rogers, C., Tseng, D. Y., Squire, J. C., and Edelman, E. R. (1999) Balloon-artery interactions during stent placement: a finite element analysis approach to pressure, compliance, and stent design as contributors to vascular injury. *Circ Res* **84**(4), 378–383.
14. Stampfuss, J.-J., Censarek, P., Fischer, J. W., Schror, K., and Weber, A.-A. (2006) Rapid release of active tissue factor from human arterial smooth muscle cells under flow conditions. *Arterioscler Thromb Vasc Biol* **26**(5), e34–e37.
15. Schwartz, R., Huber, K., Murphy, J., Edwards, W., Camrud, A., Vlietstra, R., and Holmes, D. (1992) Restenosis and the proportional neointimal response to coronary artery injury: results in a porcine model. *J Am Coll Cardiol* **19**(2), 267–274.
16. Schwartz, S., Stemerman, M., and Benditt, E. (1975) The aortic intima. II. Repair of the aortic lining after mechanical denudation. *Am J Pathol* **81**(1), 1542.
17. Tada, T., and Reidy, M. (1987) Endothelial regeneration. IX. Arterial injury followed by rapid endothelial repair induces smooth-muscle-cell proliferation but not intimal thickening. *Am J Pathol* **129**(3), 429–433.
18. Rogers, C., Parikh, S., Seifert, P., and Edelman, E. R. (1996) Endogenous cell seeding: remnant endothelium after stenting enhances vascular repair. *Circulation* **94**(11), 2909–2914.

19. Doornekamp, F. N. G., Borst, C., and Post, M. J. (1997) The influence of lesion length on intimal hyperplasia after fogarty balloon injury in the rabbit carotid artery: Role of endothelium. *J Vasc Res* **34**(4), 260–266.
20. Sprague, E., Luo, J., and Palmaz, J. (1997) Human aortic endothelial cell migration onto stent surfaces under static and flow conditions. *J Vasc Interv Radiol* **8**(1), 83–92.
21. Wentzel, J. J., Krams, R., Schuurbiers, J. C. H., Oomen, J. A., Kloet, J., van der Giessen, W. J., Serruys, P. W., and Slager, C. J. (2001) Relationship between neointimal thickness and shear stress after wallstent implantation in human coronary arteries. *Circulation* **103**(13), 1740–1745.
22. Galbusera, M., Zoja, C., Donadelli, R., Paris, S., Morigi, M., Benigni, A., Figliuzzi, M., Remuzzi, G., and Remuzzi, A. (1997) Fluid shear stress modulates von Willebrand Factor release from human vascular endothelium. *Blood* **90**(4), 1558–1564.
23. Yoshizumi, M., Kurihara, H., Sugiyama, T., Takaku, F., Yanagisawa, M., Masaki, T., and Yazaki, Y. (Jun, 1989) Hemodynamic shear stress stimulates endothelin production by cultured endothelial cells. *Biochem Biophys Res Commun* **161**(2), 859–864.
24. Moore, K., Patel, K., Bruehl, R., Li, F., Johnson, D., Lichenstein, H., Cummings, R., Bainton, D., and McEver, R. (1995) P-selectin glycoprotein ligand-1 mediates rolling of human neutrophils on p-selectin. *J Cell Biol* **128**(4), 661–671.
25. Chiu, J., Chen, C., Lee, P., Yang, C., Chuang, H., Chien, S., and Usami, S. (December, 2003) Analysis of the effect of disturbed flow on monocytic adhesion to endothelial cells. *J Biomech* **36**(12), 1883–1895.
26. Bayes-Genis, A., Campbell, J. H., Carlson, P., Holmes, D. R. Jr., and Schwartz, R. S. (July, 2002) Macrophages, myofibroblasts and neointimal hyperplasia after coronary artery injury and repair. *Atherosclerosis* **163**(1), 89–98.
27. Nakatani, M., Takeyama, Y., Shibata, M., Yorozuya, M., Suzuki, H., Koba, S., and Katagiri, T. (2003) Mechanisms of restenosis after coronary intervention: Difference between plain old balloon angioplasty and stenting. *Cardiovasc Pathol* **12**(1), 40–48.
28. Miller, D., Karim, M., Edwards, W., and Schwartz, R. (Aug, 1996) Relationship of vascular thrombosis and inflammatory leukocyte infiltration to neointimal growth following porcine coronary artery stent placement. *Atherosclerosis* **124**(2), 145–155.
29. Rogers, C., and Edelman, E. R. (1995) Endovascular stent design dictates experimental restenosis and thrombosis. *Circulation* **91**(12), 2995–3001.
30. Garasic, J. M., Edelman, E. R., Squire, J. C., Seifert, P., Williams, M. S., and Rogers, C. (2000) Stent and artery geometry determine intimal thickening independent of arterial injury. *Circulation* **101**(7), 812–818.
31. Kastrati, A., Mehilli, J., Dirschinger, J., Dotzer, F., Schuhlen, H., Neumann, F.-J., Fleckenstein, M., Pfafferott, C., Seyfarth, M., and Schomig, A. (2001) Intracoronary stenting and angiographic results : Strut thickness

effect on restenosis outcome (ISAR-STEREO) trial. *Circulation* **103**(23), 2816–2821.

32. Auriti, A., Cianfrocca, C., Pristipino, C., Greco, S., Galeazzi, M., Guido, V., and Santini, M. (Septmeber, 2003) Improving feasibility of posterior descending coronary artery flow recording by transthoracic doppler echocardiography. *Eur J Echocardiogr* **3**(3), 214–220.
33. Pache, J., Kastrati, A., Mehilli, J., Schühlen, H., Dotzer, F., Hausleiter, J., Fleckenstein, M., Neumann, F.-J., Sattelberger, U. Schmitt, C., Muller, M., Dirschinger, J., and Schömig, A. (2003) Intracoronary stenting and angiographic results: Strut thickness effect on restenosis outcome (ISAR-STEREO-2) trial. *J Am Coll Cardiol* **41** (8), 1283–1288.
34. Chen, M., Lu, P., Chen, J., and Hwang, N. (Jul-Aug, 2005) Computational hemodynamics of an implanted coronary stent based on three-dimensional cine angiography reconstruction. *ASAIO J* **51**(4), 313–320.
35. Dibra, A., Kastrati, A., Mehilli, J., Pache, J., von Oepen, R., Dirschinger, J., and Schömig, A. (2005) Influence of stent surface topography on the outcomes of patients undergoing coronary stenting: A randomized double-blind controlled trial. *Catheter Cardiovasc Inte* **65**(3), 374–380.
36. He, Y., Duraiswamy, N., Frank, A. O., and Moore, J. E. Jr. (2005) Blood flow in stented arteries: A parametric comparison of strut design patterns in three dimensions. *J Biomech Eng-T ASME* **127**(4), 637–647.
37. LaDisa, J. Jr., Olson, L., Hettrick, D., Warltier, D., Kersten, J., and Pagel, P. (Oct, 2005) Axial stent strut angle influences wall shear stress after stent implantation: Analysis using 3d computational fluid dynamics models of stent foreshortening. *Biomed Eng Online* **4**(59).
38. Sangiorgi, G., Melzi, G., Agostoni, P., Cola, C., Clementi, F., Romitelli, P., Vir-mani, R., and Colombo, A. (2007) Engineering aspects of stents design and their translation into clinical practice. *Ann Ist Super Sanita* **43**(1), 89–100.
39. Serruys, P., Ong, A., Piek, J., Neumann, F., van der Giessen, W., Wiemer, M., Zeiher, A., Grube, E., Haase, J., Thuesen, L., Hamm, C., and Otto-Terlouw, P. (May, 2005) A randomized comparison of a durable polymer Everolimus-eluting stent with a bare metal coronary stent: The SPIRIT first trial. *Euro Interv* **1**(1), 58–65.
40. Kastrati, A., Mehilli, J., Pache, J., Kaiser, C., Valgimigli, M., Kelbaek, H., Menichelli, M., Sabate, M., Suttorp, M. J., Baumgart, D., Seyfarth, M., Pfisterer, M. E., and Schomig, A. (2007) Analysis of 14 trials comparing sirolimus-eluting stents with bare-metal stents. *N Engl J Med* **356**(10), 1030–1039.
41. Nordmann, A., Briel, M., and Bucher, H. (December, 2006) Mortality in randomized controlled trials comparing drug-eluting vs. bare metal stents in coronary artery disease: A meta-analysis. *Eur Heart J* **27**(23), 2784–2814.
42. Spaulding, C., Daemen, J., Boersma, E., Cutlip, D. E., and Serruys, P. W. (2007) A pooled analysis of data comparing sirolimus-eluting stents with bare-metal stents. *N Engl J Med* **356**(10), 989–997.

43. Finn, A. V., Nakazawa, G., Joner, M., Kolodgie, F. D., Mont, E. K., Gold, H. K., and Virmani, R. (2007) Vascular responses to drug eluting stents: Importance of delayed healing. *Arterioscler Thromb Vasc Biol* **27**(7), 1500–1510.
44. Babinska, A., Markell, M., Salifu, M., Akoad, M., Ehrlich, Y., and Kornecki, E. (1998) Enhancement of human platelet aggregation and secretion induced by rapamycin. *Nephrol Dial Transplant* **13**(12), 3153–3159.
45. McFadden, E., Stabile, E., Regar, E., Cheneau, E., Ong, A. T., Kinnaird, T., Suddath, W. O., Weissman, N. J., Torguson, R., Kent, K. M., Pichard, A. D., Satler, L. F., Waksman, R., and Serruys, P. W. (2004) Late thrombosis in drug-eluting coronary stents after discontinuation of antiplatelet therapy. *Lancet* **364**(9444), 1519–1521.
46. Sianos, G., Hofma, S., Ligthart, J., Saia, F., Hoye, A., Lemos, P., and Serruys, P. (January, 2004) Stent fracture and restenosis in the drug-eluting stent era. *Catheter Cardiovasc Interv* **61**(1), 111–116.
47. Virmani, R., Guagliumi, G., Farb, A., Musumeci, G., Grieco, N., Motta, T., Mihalcsik, L., Tespili, M., Valsecchi, O., and Kolodgie, F. D. (2004) Localized hypersensitivity and late coronary thrombosis secondary to a sirolimus-eluting stent: Should we be cautious?, *Circulation* **109**(6), 701–705.
48. Scheller, B., Grandt, A., Wnendt, S., Lorenz, G. Böhm, M., and Nickenig, G. (July, 2005) Comparative study of tacrolimus and paclitaxel stent coating in the porcine coronary model. *Z Kardiol* **94**(7), 445–452.
49. Hofma, S. H., van der Giessen, W. J., van Dalen, B. M., Lemos, P. A., McFadden, E. P., Sianos, G., Ligthart, J. M., van Essen, D., de Feyter, P. J., and Serruys, P. W. (2006) Indication of long-term endothelial dysfunction after sirolimus-eluting stent implantation. *Eur Heart J* **27**(2), 166–170.
50. Joner, M., Finn, A. V., Farb, A., Mont, E. K., Kolodgie, F. D., Ladich, E., Kutys, R., Skorija, K., Gold, H. K., and Virmani, R. (2006) Pathology of drug-eluting stents in humans: Delayed healing and late thrombotic risk. *J Am Coll Cardiol* **48**(1), 193–202.
51. Nebeker, J. R., Virmani, R., Bennett, C. L., Hoffman, J. M., Samore, M. H., Alvarez, J., Davidson, C. J., McKoy, J. M., Raisch, D. W., Whisenant, B. K., Yarnold, P. R., Belknap, S. M., West, D. P., Gage, J. E., Morse, R. E., Gligoric, G., Davidson, L., and Feldman, M. D. (2006) Hypersensitivity cases associated with drug-eluting coronary stents: A review of available cases from the research on adverse drug events and reports (radar) project. *J Am Coll Cardiol* **47**(1), 175–181.
52. Daemen, J., Wenaweser, P., Tsuchida, K., Abrecht, L., Vaina, S., Morger, C., Kukreja, N., Jüni, P. Sianos, G., Hellige, G., van Domburg, R., Hess, O., Boersma, E., Meier, B., Windecker, S., and Serruys, P. (February, 2007) Early and late coronary stent thrombosis of sirolimus-eluting and paclitaxel-eluting stents in routine clinical practice: data from a large two-institutional cohort study. *Lancet* **369**(9652), 667–678.
53. Jiménez-Valero, S., Moreno, R., and Sánchez-Recalde, A. (September, 2009) Very late drugeluting stent thrombosis related to incomplete stent

endothelialization: *In-vivo* demonstration by optical coherence tomography. *J Invasive Cardiol* **21**(9), 488–490.
54. Civelek, M., Manduchi, E., Riley, R., Stoeckert, C. Jr., and Davies, P. (Aug, 2009) Chronic endoplasmic reticulum stress activates unfolded protein response in arterial endothelium in regions of susceptibility to atherosclerosis. *Circ Res* **105**(5), 453–461.
55. Simon, C., Palmaz, J., and Sprague, E. (2000) Influence of topography on endothelialization of stents: Clues for new designs. *J. Long-Term Eff Med* **10**(1–2), 143–151.
56. Shankaran, H., Alexandridis, P., and Neelamegham, S. (2003) Aspects of hydrodynamic shear regulating shear-induced platelet activation and self-association of von willebrand factor in suspension. *Blood* **101**(7), 2637–2645.
57. Alkhamis, T., Beissinger, R., and Chediak, J. (Jul-Sep, 1988) Red blood cell effect on platelet adhesion and aggregation in low-stress shear flow. Myth or fact?, *ASAIO Trans* **33**(3), 868–873.
58. Hathcock, J. J. (2006) Flow effects on coagulation and thrombosis. *Arterioscler Thromb Vasc Biol* **26**(8), 1729–1737.

Chapter 12

VASCULAR MIMETIC MICROFLUIDIC SYSTEMS FOR THE STUDY OF ENDOTHELIAL ACTIVATION AND LEUKOCYTE RECRUITMENT IN MODELS OF ATHEROGENESIS

R. MICHAEL GOWER and SCOTT SIMON*

Department of Biomedical Engineering, University of California, Davis
451 Health Sciences Dr. Room 3216, GBSF Building
University of California Davis, Ca 95616
** sisimon@ucdavis.edu*

Monocyte recruitment to inflamed endothelium is an early event in atherogenesis and occurs at focal regions where the average shear stress is on the order of one dyne/cm^2. Applying soft lithography to fabricate microfluidic channels that assemble above a living endothelial monolayer grown in culture, we have produced a vascular mimetic system that enables detailed studies of the influence of inflammation, hydrodynamics, and dietary lipid on the expression and function of vascular adhesion molecules.

1. Shear Stress Modulates Endothelial Adhesion Molecule Expression

The focal nature of inflammation can be observed by histological examination of atherosclerotic lesions in aorta and arteries.[1] Plaques and atheromata develop preferentially within characteristic geometries, such as curvatures and bifurcations that exhibit disturbed flow characteristics.[2,3] A hallmark of atherogenesis is the upregulation of endothelial cellular adhesion molecules (CAMs) and concomitant recruitment of monocytes, which rapidly emigrate across inflamed EC and over time differentiate into foam cells within the vessel intima.

Shear stress imparted by the viscous flow of blood plays a significant role in the homeostasis of vascular structure and function in part through the action of the mechanically-responsive endothelium. The presence of low fluid shear (i.e $\sim$1 dyne/cm^2), high gradients of stress, and flow disturbances all correlate with atherogenesis, whereas steady laminar shear is required to maintain vessel homeostasis.[4] Thus, the magnitude of fluid shear stress and the level of cytokine stimulation tightly regulate where and when in arteries monocyte recruitment occurs. Elevatedlevels of shear stress as observed in arteries of healthy human subjects (i.e. $\sim$15 dyne/cm^2) are atheroprotective. This is in part attributed to the mechanical influence of shear force acting on endothelium that results in attenuation of VCAM-1 expression, despite the fact that ICAM-1 expression is upregulated at high shear stress. Conversely, preconditioning EC at low shear stress (i.e. $\sim$2 dyne/cm^2) as associated with regions of flow disturbance at bifurcations and the inner curvature of the aorta, results in pro-atherogenic conditions. For instance, arterial regions of low shear stress and large spatial gradients exhibit amplified upregulation of VCAM-1 and E-selectin, which in turn increase the efficiency of monocyte capture even at very low concentrations of cytokine stimulation (i.e. TNF-α 0.1 ng/ml).[5–8] Thus, differential regulation of CAM transcription could result in changes that are both pro- and anti-inflammatory in the context of leukocyte recruitment.[9–12] Since atherosclerosis is a focal disease that typically develops at vascular sites of bifurcations and curved arteries that harbor steep shear stress gradients, a detailed study of how CAM expression and monocyte recruitment maps on inflamed endothelium exposed to shear is of keen interest for thorough understanding of disease.

2. Monocyte Recruitment During Atherosclerosis

Monocyte capture, rolling, activation, and arrest to nascent atherosclerotic plaques is a coordinated effort by selectins, integrins, and their respective ligands. Capture from the free stream of blood is supported by P-selectin glycoprotein-1 (PSGL-1) and other glycosylated ligands on the monocyte which bind P-selectin, and E-selectin on inflamed endothelium.[13,14] Monocyte capture is an important first step of atherosclerosis. Hypercholesterolemic mice lacking these molecules are atheroprotected.[15,16] Selectins enable leukocytes to be recruited and roll along the endothelium due to their exceptionally high on and off rates, which govern how quickly bonds are formed and broken.[17] P- and E-selectin require a threshold level of shear stress on the order of 1 dyne/cm^2 to initiate tethering through receptor tension; interruption of the shear field causes rolling leukocytes to detach.[18] This is due to their catch bond nature,[19] the force imparted by the fluid flow strengthens the bond. This phenomenon in conjunction with presentation of additional ligand to selectins as the monocyte rolls allows new bonds to form before old ones are broken.[20]

Integrins are responsible for decelerating the rolling leukocyte and mediating firm adhesion through binding Ig superfamily members expressed on the endothelial membrane. The $\beta 1$ integrin, very late antigen-4 (VLA-4 or $\alpha_4\beta_1$), is activated on the monocyte through inside-out signaling following ligation of chemokines such as MCP-1 and subsequently binds vascular cell adhesion molecule-1 (VCAM-1). VCAM-1 expression is detected at early plaques on hypercholesterolemic rabbits and its expression precedes macrophage accumulation.[21] In addition, hypercholesterolemic mice lacking a VLA-4 binding domain in VCAM-1 have decreased atherosclerosis.[22] It is controversial whether VCAM-1 expressed at athero-susceptible sites is an initiating event in monocyte recruitment and plaque formation.

The $\beta 2$ (CD18) integrins also play a role in monocyte trafficking to atherosclerotic lesions as CD18$^{-/-}$ mice have decreased atherosclerosis (Nageh *et al.*, 1997). The β_2 integrin, lymphocyte functional agntigen-1 (LFA-1 or $\alpha_1\beta_2$) binds ICAM-1 on the endothelium and their interactions are important for atherogenesis (Kitagawa *et al.*, 2002). Recently, CD11c/CD18 has been reported to bind VCAM-1 during monocyte firm arrest on inflamed endothelium.[23] Furthermore, CD11c$^{-/-}$ hypercholesterolemic mice have decreased atherosclerosis and their monocytes exhibit a defect in recruiting to recombinant VCAM-1 and E-selectin in shear flow.[24] A cooperative process appears to underlie recruitment of monocytes in response to activation and VCAM-1 ligation of VLA-4 and CD11c. In both humans and mouse models, a high fat diet can induce upregulation of CD11c and enhanced efficiency of monocyte recruitment to VCAM-1 in shear flow (Gower *et al.*, Unpublished data).

During inflammation the endothelium drastically alters its adhesive phenotype increasing the expression of E-selectin, ICAM-1, and VCAM-1 allowing monocytes that come in contact with the vessel wall to capture, roll, firm arrest, and emigrate into the tissue. These dynamic endothelial-leukocyte interactions are crucial for immune surveillance, however, when this process becomes dysregulated, chronic inflammatory disease ensues. To examine how hydrodynamic shear superposes with inflammatory insult to promote monocyte recruitment, we have developed microfluidic networks that allow us to study these interactions in real-time using small sample volumes that enable of the study of limited and expensive biological specimens and reagents.

3. Design and Fabrication of Vascular Mimetic Microfluidic Chambers

In vitro models that mimic physiological parameters of blood vessels such as shear stress and geometry are powerful tools to study the molecular and cellular events associated with inflammation occurring at the membrane of the endothelium. Conventional parallel-plate flow chambers (PPFC) have been implemented to assay the endothelial or leukocyte response to defined magnitudes of shear stress.[25] The shear stress at the endothelial membrane in a PPFC may be approximately by:

$$\tau_w = \frac{6\mu Q}{wh^2}. \tag{3.1}$$

Where μ is the fluid viscosity, Q is the volumetric flow rate, w is the channel width, and h is the channel height. Owing to their macro-scale dimensions, PPFC require large volumes to infuse cell media or buffer solution at constant flow rates. Assuming the viscosity of water (1 cP), a typical PPFC[9,26] with a height of 300 μm and a width of 2 cm requires flow rates on the order of 40 ml/min to maintain a shear stress of 20 dyn/cm^2; the stress present at the endothelial membrane at regions of the coronary artery that are athero-protected.[2] Thus, these devices have limited utility in assays requiring limited reagents such as small molecule inhibitors, antibodies, or sparse leukocyte populations such as monocytes.

To address the need for smaller working volumes in assays studying leukocyte or endothelial mechanobiology in shear flow, we designed novel microfluidic devices capable of delivering fluid with precisely controlled chemical composition and flow rate. The general design of the flow device consists of two major components: (I) microfluidic flow channels and (II) a vacuum channel network. As shown in Fig. 1, the vacuum channel network is a spider web-like pattern that serves to seal the device to a glass coverslip in the absence of adhesives or chemistries that are incompatible with cells or proteins. These microchannels have heights between 50 and 100 μm and a variety of widths ranging from 200 μm to 2 mm. We have coined these devices vascular mimetic microfluidic chambers (VMMC) in contrast to their generic macro-scale counter parts, PPFC.

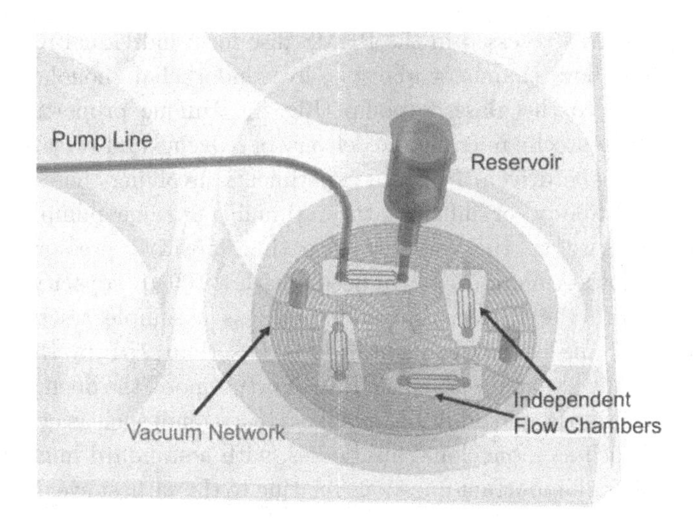

Fig. 1. Schematic of the vascular mimetic microfluidic device. Four independent chambers containing microchannels are recessed into a PDMS disc and assemble above an endothelial monolayer (here grown in a 6-well tissue culture plate). The network of vacuum channels resembles a spider-web. When connected to house vacuum through access ports punched into the PDMS, the device is sealed to the biological substrate. A blunt 20-gauge needle hub serves as a reservoir for monocyte suspensions, chemokines, or antibodies. A syringe pump applying negative pressure at the outlet drives flow. From Schaff UY *et al.* (2007) Lab Chip (4): 448–456. Reproduced by permission of the Royal Society of Chemistry.

Standard methods of soft lithography[27] are applied to create the VMMC. The network of microchannels are designed in CAD (Autodesk, San Rafael, CA) and printed at 5000 dpi on a transparency. Negative photoresist (SU8, Micro Chem, Newton, MA) is spun onto a silicon wafer at a user-defined thickness between 50 to 100 μm. The transparency is than overlayed on the coated wafer and exposed to UV light. During development photoresist that is not polymerized by the incident UV light is removed and a positive replica (master mold) of the design remains on the wafer. Polydimethylsiloxane (PDMS) (Sylgard 184) prepolymer is poured over the master mold and cured. A disc containing the design is excised and access ports are punched with a hollow blunt needle into the PDMS (Fig. 1). The VMMC's small profile allows for incorporation of multiple microfluidic designs into a single master mold. This yields a practical advantage of batch production and because PDMS is inexpensive, the flow chamber can be discarded if soiled by chemicals or deteriorated.

Microchannels recessed in the PDMS disc form individual micro-scale parallel plate flow chambers above a live endothelial monolayer when vacuum-sealed to the glass coverslip (Fig. 1). Unique properties of our VMMC include precise microfluidic delivery of reagents and versatility with which flow can be driven. In acute experiments involving the addition of leukocytes, antibody, or inflammatory stimuli a syringe pump applying negative pressure to the outlet rather than positive pressure to the inlet drives flow. A blunt 20-gauge needle with a $100\,\mu$L capacity is press-fit directly into the PDMS disc and serves as a sample reservoir. The inlet dead volume of this configuration is less than $2\,\mu$L, a value three orders of magnitude smaller than a PPFC. Furthermore, the open "on-chip" reservoir facilitates rapid addition of leukocytes, stimuli such as cytokine, or antagonists such as monoclonal antibodies, with a standard micropipette. Thus a number of important questions relating to the earliest events of acute inflammation may be addressed by controlling the cellular and chemical composition entering the VMMC in real time.[28]

Depending on the design, two to eight independent and vacuum-isolated VMMC are integrated into each PDMS device and are addressed by sequential connection to a syringe pump and perfused with separate suspensions of leukocytes or soluble inflammatory agonists. This makes it possible to apply multiple experimental conditions to a single endothelial monolayer, allowing for higher experimental throughput and less variability. In contrast, a conventional PPFC requires an individual glass slide coated with cells for every experimental condition due its much larger footprint.

In experiments that require long term culture (i.e. to orient EC in the direction of flow ~24 hours) of the endothelial monolayer in shear flow, a syringe pump infusing fluid into the inlet of the VMMC drives flow. Cell media can be collected at the outlet and assayed for chemokines or other soluble agents released by the endothelium. The feasibility of this configuration is owed to the dimensions of our VMMC. A microchannel that is $75\,\mu$m in height and 2 mm wide requires less that 60 mL of fluid to apply $20\,\text{dyn/cm}^2$ at the endothelial membrane for 4 hours. Use of a peristaltic pump that circulates a constant volume of buffer over the monolayer can be used in place of the syringe pump. In order to simulate conditions associated with inflammation, TNF-α or other inflammatory stimuli is premixed with cell media. Following shear conditioning the outlet tubing is removed and a reservoir is inserted in its place. Running the syringe pump in withdraw mode an assay measuring leukocyte adhesion efficiency on the monolayer is carried out.

PDMS is transparent so that cellular interactions within the VMMC can be imaged from below with an inverted DIC-fluorescence microscope coupled to a CCD camera and image analysis system. This system represents a virtual lab on a chip since it affords up to 8 separate experiments in which HAEC are preconditioned by defined shear regimes, activated by cytokines, and treated with inhibitors under static or shear flow conditions. Inflammatory responses are detected *in situ* by immunofluorescent imaging of CAM up-regulation or transcription factor activation or by adhesive interactions with leukocytes.[28–31]

4. Adhesion Molecule Expression on Cultured Aortic Endothelium Studied in a Linear Gradient of Shear Stress

Hemodynamics exerts a significant influence in the inflammatory response of vascular endothelium to cytokine.[32,33] The relationship between the magnitude of shear stress and upregulation of endothelial CAMs has been widely studied using PPFC to produce a constant shear rate and defined average shear stress.[34–37] In order to examine the focal nature by which atherosclerotic plaques form within defined regimes of shear stress in the vasculature, we produced a modified version of our VMMC that delivers a linear decrease in shear stress from the inlet to the outlet. This flow channel was used to study endothelial response along a channel consisting of a continuous human aortic endothelial cell (HAEC) monolayer. The design of the flow chamber was adapted from Hele-Shaw flow theory.[38] A linear decrease in shear stress magnitude along the centerline of the channel, parallel to the longitudinal axis, was achieved by designing the sidewalls of the flow chamber to coincide with the streamlines of a two dimensional stagnation flow and making the end of the channel shaped to match the iso-potential lines. Using this design it was possible to expose the HAEC to a physiological range of shear stress with high spatial resolution while maintaining a constant shear gradient.[31] The generated wall shear stress (τ_w) along the channel centerline at the endothelial membrane is given by:

$$\tau_w = \frac{6\mu Q}{h^2 w_1}\left(1 - \frac{x}{L}\right), \tag{4.1}$$

where μ is the flow medium viscosity, Q is the volumetric flow rate, h is the channel height, w_1 is the entrance channel width, L is the total channel length, and x is the length measured from the entrance at any point down the channel. The dimension of the flow chamber used in this study consisted of the following parameters: $h = 100\,\mu$m, $w_1 = 2$ mm, $L = 20$ mm. The linearity of shear stress with distance down the flow chamber, as defined by Equation 2, was previously validated experimentally based on streamline analysis.[38]

The Hele-Shaw chamber was applied to determine the relative importance of the magnitude versus the gradient of shear stress as endothelial cells respond to stimulation by TNF-α. To gauge the response to shear stress we measured the change in expression of endothelial ICAM-1, VCAM-1 and E-selectin under static and flow conditions. Endothelial CAM expression was measured as a function of distance down the flow channel, in which shear stress decreased linearly from 16 dyne/cm^2 at the inlet to essentially zero at the exit. This shear stress range was chosen to model the transition from atheroprotective (i.e. $\geq$12 dyne/cm^2) to athero-prone (i.e. $\leq$4 dyne/cm^2) arterial regions as defined in previous studies.[7] CAM expression after 4 hours of TNF-α in the presence of laminar shear stress was detected by immunofluorescence of antibody conjugated quantum dots and quantified by image analysis over distinct 0.1 mm^2 regions, corresponding to an area on the monolayer containing 50 HAEC.

The relative change in E-selectin and VCAM-1 expression as a function of the magnitude of shear stress over discrete areas is plotted in Fig. 2A and B as the percent of unstimulated endothelial MFI under static conditions. ICAM-1 was also presented in this study and found to increase to maximum level at ~12 dyne/cm^2. Addition of TNF-α (0.3 ng/mL) under static conditions stimulated upregulation of VCAM-1 by 350%, and ICAM-1, and E-selectin by 150% and 250%, respectively. Shear alone elicited a 100% increase in ICAM-1 expression at high SS, whereas VCAM-1 and E-selectin expression was not significantly upregulated at any position along the gradient.

In the presence of shear stress and TNF-α, ICAM-1 expression increased linearly with shear stress rising to 450% of the unstimulated static condition, before reaching a plateau. The greatest change in CAM expression on inflamed HAEC occurred within the low range in shear stress from 2–4 dyne/cm^2, correlating with shear stress values found within vascular regions prone to atherogenesis.[7] In contrast, TNF-α stimulated

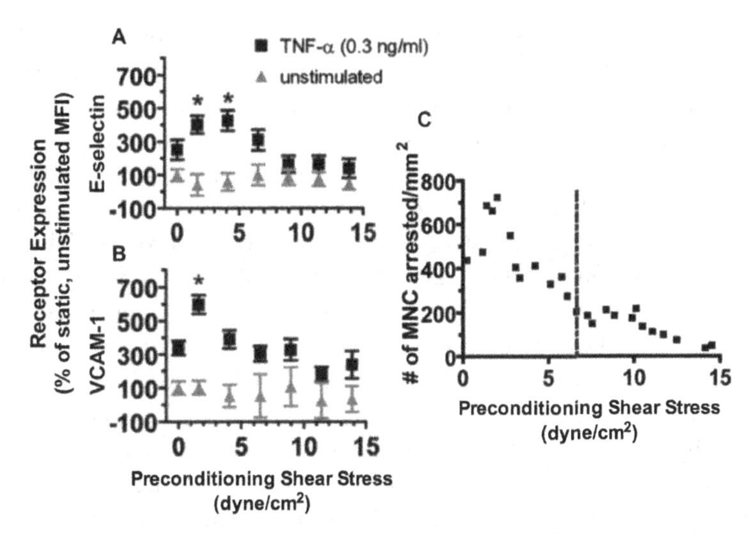

Fig. 2. Cellular adhesion molecule expression and monocyte recruitment as a function of shear stress down the Hele-Shaw chamber. Monocyte adhesion assay was conducted at 2dyn/cm^2. Adapted from Tsou JK *et al.* Microcirculation (2008) 15(4): 311–323. Reprinted by permission of the publisher (Taylor & Francis Ltd, http://www.tandf.co.uk/journals).

CAM expression was invariant at shear stress greater than 10 dyne/cm^2, which reflects the quiescence of inflammatory response within straight unperturbed arterial regions (i.e. 12–17 dyne/cm^2). The rate of change of CAM expression was steepest between 2–8 dyne/cm^2, which suggests a mechanotransduction signaling pathway that modulates inflammation within this range of SS. Although the precise mechanisms by which shear stress superposes with cytokine to regulate inflammatory gene expression have yet to be determined, it is clear that they act through distinct, often converging pathways to modulate the activity of transcription factors associated with inflammation including NFκB, AP-1, GATA, specificity protein-1 (SP-1), and IFN regulatory factor-1 (IRF-1).[32,39–43]

5. Monocyte Recruitment on Vascular Mimetics

Monocyte activation and recruitment to lesions is a harbinger of atherosclerosis. For instance, monocytes from individuals with hypercholesterolemia exhibit upregulated expression of integrins[44] and increased adhesion.[45–47] In response to insult, endothelium and monocytes produce cytokines and chemokines that in turn upregulate the expression of CAMs on adjacent endothelial cells. Adhesion is mediated by coordinate ligation of membrane receptors on monocytes and their cognate ligands on the inflamed endothelium. Direct observation of monocyte recruitment in microfluidic channels on TNF-α stimulated endothelium shear conditioned in the Hele-shaw chamber was performed to examine the importance of a linear gradient of shear stress on this multi-step process. The level cytokine stimulation and the magnitude of fluid shear stress tightly regulate monocyte recruitment. As depicted in Fig. 2 we examined monocyte arrest on a monolayer that was aligned parallel to the direction of shear stress preconditioning, in which HAEC were exposed to 0–16 dyne/cm^2. Monocytes were infused at a constant shear stress of 2 dyne/cm^2, and adhesive interactions were video recorded. These data reveal the effect of the shear stress gradient on CAM expression and in turn its significant impact on monocyte recruitment. Monocyte recruitment efficiency was found to vary as a function of position down the flow channel. This essentially provides a map of recruitment efficiency as a function of the differential expression of CAMs that are modulated by the superposition of cytokine activation and shear stress. A shear stress of 7 dyne/cm^2 emerged as a critical value for altering CAM expression and favoring monocyte arrest, as recruitment efficiency increased significantly below this threshold. This observation is consistent with the fact that both E-selectin and VCAM-1 expression begin to rise from the baseline at this shear stress. Significantly, E-selectin reached the greatest rate of change in expression between 6–9 dyne/cm^2. Thus, HAEC ligands that support monocyte capture and arrest are critical for optimum transition to stable adhesion and transmigration.

6. Lipid Primes Endothelium for an Enhanced Response to Inflammation and Increases Monocyte Recruitment

In a separate set of studies, we used the VMMC to examine the role of dietary lipids (triglyceride rich lipoprotein, TGRL consisting of vLDL and chylomicron remnants) and TNF-α stimulation on monocyte recruitment to HAEC.[30] HAECs were treated with TGRL (2.5 mg/dL) for 2 hours a day for 1, 2 or 3 days, followed by a 4 hour TNF-α exposure (0.3 ng/mL) after the last TGRL treatment. This was meant to simulate the repetitive injury sustained by endothelium during consumption of a high fat diet. E-selectin

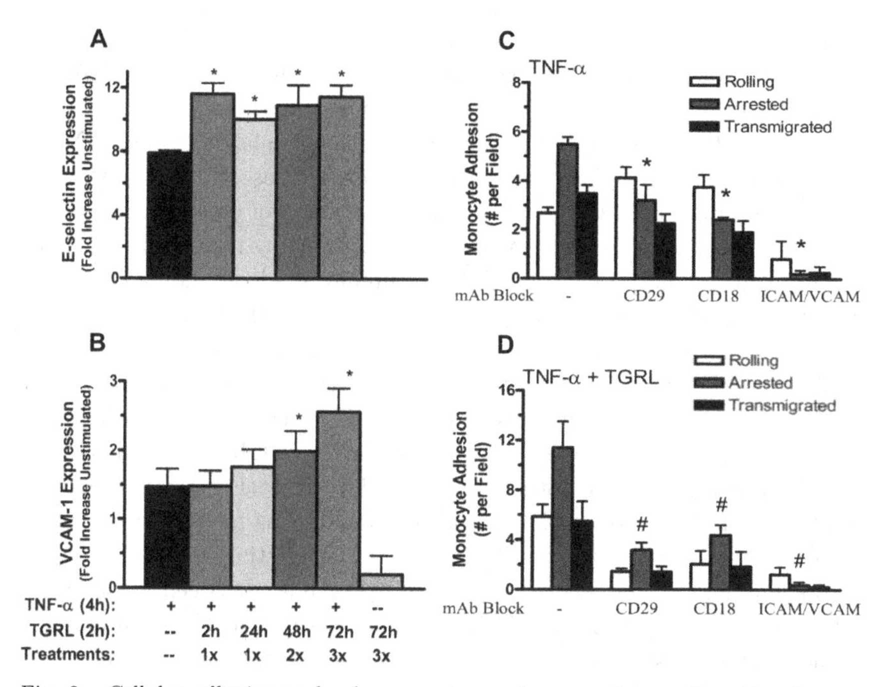

Fig. 3. Cellular adhesion molecule expression and monocyte recruitment on human aortic endothelium exposed to triglyceride rich lipoprotein (TGRL) for 3 days, followed by TNF-α treatment. TNF-α concentration for all panels is 0.3 ng/mL. TGRL concentration is 2.5 mg/dL. Adapted from Ting HJ *et al.* (2007) Circulation Research 100(3): 381–390.

expression was significantly higher after a single TGRL treatment followed by TNF-α compared to TNF-α alone (Fig. 3A). ICAM-1 expression did not change with lipid treatment (data not shown). VCAM-1 expression was significantly increased over TNF-α alone after 2 days of TGRL pretreatment, but 3 days of TGRL treatment in the absence of TNF-α did not affect VCAM-1 expression (Fig. 3B). Thus we find superposition of lipid and cytokine or low shear stress and cytokine (Fig. 2A, B) can potentiate expression of two endothelial CAMs obligatory for monocyte arrest.

Recruitment of monocytes to HAECs at 2 dyn/cm^2 was imaged by phase contrast microscopy in order to gauge the effect of the amplification of VCAM-1 over cytokine stimulation by TGRL. Monocytes were categorized as rolling, arrested, or transmigrated across the endothelial monolayer. The number of adherent monocytes increased over a range of TNF-α

stimulation and 0.3 ng/mL was a concentration at which 50% of maximum monocyte interaction was observed (data not shown). Pretreating HAECs with TGRL for 3 days and subsequently stimulating them for 4 hours with TNF-α effectively doubled monocyte recruitment efficiency over TNF-α alone, whereas neutrophil recruitment did not increase.[30] Consistent with CAM upregulation, TGRL treatment alone did not support monocyte recruitment. We next examined the CAMs supporting increased monocyte recruitment. In the presence of TNF-α stimulation alone, monocyte arrest and transmigration was supported by β1 and β2 integrins, as blocking each with antibody added up to the control level of 6 monocytes per field (Fig. 3C). ICAM-1 and VCAM-1 supported firm adhesion; however, capture and rolling required expression of E-selectin, as determined by antibody inhibition. Monocyte recruitment on TGRL treated HAEC remained dependent on both β1 and β2 integrins (Fig. 3D). However, inhibition of β2 integrins blocked proportionally less monocyte arrest on TGRL-primed HAECs versus TNF-α alone, suggesting that β1 integrin is predominant. Interestingly, greater cooperativity between β1 and β2 integrins was apparent for the TGRL primed HAECs, as the total number of monocytes arrested was 30% greater than the sum of monocytes recruited when blocking integrins individually. These data reveal that priming with vLDL lipids increases monocyte recruitment to inflamed HAECs in a β1- and β2-integrin dependent manner.

Summary

Design and implementation of a custom microfluidic flow channel that reversibly bonds to a glass coverslip or plastic tissue culture plate containing a living endothelial monolayer we denote vascular mimetic microvascular chambers (VMMC) was presented. This device allows the study of both acute exposure to inflammatory molecules that upregulate CAMs over hours, as well as more chronic studies using shear flow to mechanically modulate the endothelial response. The combination of a living substrate along with fine tune control of the shear rate and stress distribution throughout the channel allows a variety of biological studies to be performed. We examined how endothelial cells sense a linear gradient of fluid shear stress and transduce signals that regulate membrane expression of cell adhesion molecules and monocyte recruitment. We also demonstrated that repetitive exposure to native dietary lipids prime HAECs for an amplified inflammatory response to TNF-αu Employing our VMMC we showed monocytes were preferentially recruited over neutrophils on HAECs inflamed by both cytokine and dietary vLDL in shear flow. These vascular mimetic models provide an opportunity to perform *ex vivo* studies of the contributions of hyperlipidemia, hemodynamics, and vascular inflammation in the etiology of atherosclerosis.

Acknowledgement

This work was supported by NIH grants HL082689 (S.I.S) and HL086350 (R.M.G.) and a Howard Hughes Medical Institution Med into Grad Fellowship, University of California Davis (R.M.G.).

References

1. Stary, H. C., Chandler, A. B., Dinsmore, R. E., Fuster, V., Glagov, S., Insull, W., Jr., Rosenfeld, M. E., Schwartz, C. J., Wagner, W. D., and Wissler, R. W. (1995) A definition of advanced types of atherosclerotic lesions and a histological classification of atherosclerosis. A report from the Committee on Vascular Lesions of the Council on Arteriosclerosis, American Heart Association. *Circulation* **92**, 1355–1374.
2. Giddens, D. P., Zarins, Z. K., and Glagov, S. (1993) The role of fluid mechanics in the localization and detection of atherosclerosis. *J Biomech Eng* **115**, 588–594.
3. Garin, G., and Berk, B. C. (2006) Flow-mediated signaling modulates endothelial cell phenotype. *Endothelium* **13**, 375–384.
4. Tedgui, A., and Mallat, Z. (2001) Anti-inflammatory mechanisms in the vascular wall. *Circ Res* **88**, 877–887.
5. Dardik, A., Chen, L. L., Frattini, J., Asada, H., Aziz, F., Kudo, F. A., and Sumpio, B. E. (2005) Differential effects of orbital and laminar shear stress on endothelial cells. *J Vasc Surg* **41**, 869–880.
6. Gonzales, R. S., and Wick, T. M. (1996) Hemodynamic modulation of monocytic cell adherence to vascular endothelium. *Annals of Biomedical Engineering* **24**, 382–393.
7. Malek, A. M., Alper, S. L., and Izumo, S. Hemodynamic shear stress and its role in atherosclerosis. *JAMA* **282**, 2035–2042.
8. Mohan, S., Mohan, N., Valente, A. J., and Sprague, E. A. (1999) Regulation of low shear flow-induced HAEC VCAM-1 expression and monocyte adhesion. *Am J Physiol* **276**, C1100–C1107.
9. Chiu, J.-J., Lee, P.-L., Chen, C.-N., Lee, C.-I., Chang, S.-F., Chen, L.-J., Lien, S.-C., Ko, Y.-C., Usami, S., and Chien, S. (2004) Shear Stress Increases ICAM-1 and Decreases VCAM-1 and E-selectin Expressions Induced by

Tumor Necrosis Factor-{alpha} in Endothelial Cells. *Arterioscler Thromb Vasc Biol* **24**, 73–79.
10. Chiu, J. J., Chen, L. J., Lee, P. L., Lee, C. I., Lo, L. W., Usami, S., and Chien, S. (2003) Shear stress inhibits adhesion molecule expression in vascular endothelial cells induced by coculture with smooth muscle cells. *Blood* **101**, 2667–2674.
11. Tsao, P. S., Buitrago, R., Chan, J. R., and Cooke, J. P. (1996) Fluid flow inhibits endothelial adhesiveness. *Circulation* **94**, 1682–1689.
12. Tsuboi, H., Ando, J., Korenaga, R., Takada, Y., and Kamiya, A. (1995) Flow stimulates ICAM-1 expression time and shear stress dependently in cultured human endothelial cells. *Biochemical and Biophysical research communications* **206**, 988–996.
13. Xia, L., Sperandio, M., Yago, T., McDaniel, J. M., Cummings, R. D., Pearson-White, S., Ley, K., and McEver, R. P. (2002) P-selectin glycoprotein ligand-1-deficient mice have impaired leukocyte tethering to E-selectin under flow. *J Clin Invest* **109**, 939–950.
14. Yang, J., Hirata, T., Croce, K., Merrill-Skoloff, G., Tchernychev, B., Williams, E., Flaumenhaft, R., Furie, B. C., and Furie, B. (1999) Targeted gene disruption demonstrates that P-selectin glycoprotein ligand 1 (PSGL-1) is required for P-selectin-mediated but not E-selectin-mediated neutrophil rolling and migration. *J Exp Med* **190**, 1769–1782.
15. Dong, Z. M., Chapman, S. M., Brown, A. A., Frenette, P. S., Hynes, R. O., and Wagner, D. D. (1998) The combined role of P- and E-selectins in atherosclerosis. *J Clin Invest* **102**, 145–152.
16. Johnson, R. C., Chapman, S. M., Dong, Z. M., Ordovas, J. M., Mayadas, T. N., Herz, J., Hynes, R. O., Schaefer, E. J., and Wagner, D. D. (1997) Absence of P-selectin delays fatty streak formation in mice. *J Clin Invest* **99**, 1037–1043.
17. Alon, R., Hammer, D. A., and Springer, T. A. (1995) Lifetime of the P-selectin-carbohydrate bond and its response to tensile force in hydrodynamic flow. *Nature* **374**, 539–542.
18. Lawrence, M. B., Kansas, G. S., Kunkel, E. J., and Ley, K. (1997) Threshold levels of fluid shear promote leukocyte adhesion through selectins (CD62L,P,E). *J Cell Biol* **136**, 717–727.
19. Marshall, B. T., Long, M., Piper, J. W., Yago, T., McEver, R. P., and Zhu, C. (2003) Direct observation of catch bonds involving cell-adhesion molecules. *Nature* **423**, 190–193.
20. Yago, T., Zarnitsyna, V. I., Klopocki, A. G., McEver, R. P., and Zhu, C. (2007) Transport governs flow-enhanced cell tethering through L-selectin at threshold shear. *Biophys J* **92**, 330–342.
21. Cybulsky, M. I., Gimbrone, M. A., Jr. (1991) Endothelial expression of a mononuclear leukocyte adhesion molecule during atherogenesis. *Science* **251**, 788–791.
22. Cybulsky, M. I., Iiyama, K., Li, H., Zhu, S., Chen, M., Iiyama, M., Davis, V., Gutierrez-ramos, J. C., Connelly, P. W., and Milstone, D. S. (2001) A major

role for VCAM-1, but not ICAM-1, in early atherosclerosis. *J Clin Invest* **107**, 1255–1262.

23. Sadhu, C., Ting, H. J., Lipsky, B., Hensley, K., Garcia-Martinez, L. F., Simon, S. I., and Staunton, D. E. (2007) CD11c/CD18: novel ligands and a role in delayed-type hypersensitivity. *J Leukoc Biol* **81**, 1395–1403.
24. Wu, H., Gower, R. M., Wang, H., Perrard, X.-Y. D., Ma, R., Bullard, D. C., Burns, A. R., Paul, A., Smith, C. W., Simon, S. I., and Ballantyne, C. M. (2009) Functional role of CD11c+ monocytes in atherogenesis associated with hypercholesterolemia. *Circulation* **119**, 2708–2717.
25. Gopalan, P. K., Burns, A. R., Simon, S. I., Sparks, S., McIntire, L. V., and Smith, C. W. (2000) Preferential sites for stationary adhesion of neutrophils to cytokine-stimulated HUVEC under flow conditions. *J Leukoc Biol* **68**, 47–57.
26. Ohtsuka, A., Ando, J., Korenaga, R., Kamiya, A., Toyama-Sorimachi, N., Miyasaka, M. (1993) The effect of flow on the expression of vascular adhesion molecule-1 by cultured mouse endothelial cells. *Biochem Biophys Res Commun* **193**, 303–310.
27. Whitesides, G. M., Ostuni, E., Takayama, S., Jiang, X., and Ingber, D. E. (2001) Soft lithography in biology and biochemistry. *Annu Rev Biomed Eng* **3**, 335–373.
28. Schaff, U. Y., Xing, M. M., Lin, K. K., Pan, N., Jeon, N. L., and Simon, S. I. (2007) Vascular mimetics based on microfluidics for imaging the leukocyte–endothelial inflammatory response. *Lab Chip* **7**, 448–456.
29. Green, C. E., Schaff, U. Y., Sarantos, M. R., Lum, A. F., Staunton, D. E., and Simon, S. I. (2006) Dynamic shifts in LFA-1 affinity regulate neutrophil rolling, arrest, and transmigration on inflamed endothelium. *Blood* **107**, 2101–2111.
30. Ting, H. J., Stice, J. P., Schaff, U. Y., Hui, D. Y., Rutledge, J. C., Knowlton, A. A., Passerini, A. G., and Simon, S. I. (2007) Triglyceride-rich lipoproteins prime aortic endothelium for an enhanced inflammatory response to tumor necrosis factor-alpha. *Circ Res* **100**, 381–390.
31. Tsou, J. K., Gower, R. M., Ting, H. J., Schaff, U. Y., Insana, M. F., Passerini, A.G., and Simon, S. I. (2008) Spatial regulation of inflammation by human aortic endothelial cells in a linear gradient of shear stress. *Microcirculation* **15**, 311–323.
32. Dagia, N. M., Harii, N., Meli, A. E., Sun, X., Lewis, C. J., Kohn, L. D., and Goetz, D. J., (2004) Phenyl methimazole inhibits TNF-alpha-induced VCAM-1 expression in an IFN regulatory factor-1-dependent manner and reduces monocytic cell adhesion to endothelial cells. *J Immunol* **173**, 2041–2049.
33. Lan, Q, Mercurius, K. O., and Davies, P. F. (1994) Stimulation of transcription factors NF kappa B and AP1 in endothelial cells subjected to shear stress. *Biochem Biophys Res Commun* **201**, 950–956.
34. Sampath, R., Kukielka, G. L., Smith, C. W., Eskin, S. G., McIntire, L. V. (1995) Shear stress-mediated changes in the expression of leukocyte adhesion

receptors on human umbilical vein endothelial cells *in vitro*. *Ann Biomed Eng* **23**, 247–256.

35. Tsuboi, H., Ando, J., Korenaga, R., Takada, Y., Kamiya, A. (1995) Flow stimulates ICAM-1 expression time and shear stress dependently in cultured human endothelial cells. *Biochem Biophys Res Commun* **206**, 988–996.
36. Korenaga. R., Ando, J., Kosaki, K., Isshiki, M., Takada, Y., Kamiya, A. (1997) Negative transcriptional regulation of the VCAM-1 gene by fluid shear stress in murine endothelial cells. *Am J Physiol* **273**, C1506–1515.
37. Ando, J., Tsuboi, H., Korenaga, R., Takada, Y., Toyama-Sorimachi, N., Miyasaka, M., and Kamiya, A. (1994) Shear stress inhibits adhesion of cultured mouse endothelial cells to lymphocytes by downregulating VCAM-1 expression. *Am J Physiol* **267**, C679–687.
38. Usami, S., Chen, H. H., Zhao, Y., Chien, S., and Skalak, R. (1993) Design and construction of a linear shear stress flow chamber. *Ann Biomed Eng* **21**, 77–83.
39. Ledebur, H. C., and Parks, T. P. (1995) Transcriptional regulation of the intercellular adhesion molecule-1 gene by inflammatory cytokines in human endothelial cells. Essential roles of a variant NF-kappa B site and p65 homodimers. *J Biol Chem* **270**, 933–943.
40. Neish, A. S., Read, M. A., Thanos, D., Pine, R., Maniatis, T., and Collins, T. (1995) Endothelial interferon regulatory factor 1 cooperates with NF-kappa B as a transcriptional activator of vascular cell adhesion molecule 1. *Mol Cell Biol* **15**, 2558–2569.
41. Neish, A. S., Williams, A. J., Palmer, H. J., Whitley, M. Z., and Collins, T. (1992) Functional analysis of the human vascular cell adhesion molecule 1 promoter. *J Exp Med* **176**, 1583–1593.
42. Umetani, M., Mataki, C., Minegishi, N., Yamamoto, M., Hamakubo, T., and Kodama, T. (2001) Function of GATA transcription factors in induction of endothelial vascular cell adhesion molecule-1 by tumor necrosis factor-alpha. *Arterioscler Thromb Vasc Biol* **21**, 917–922.
43. Voraberger, G., Schafer, R., and Stratowa, C. (1991) Cloning of the human gene for intercellular adhesion molecule 1 and analysis of its 5'-regulatory region. Induction by cytokines and phorbol ester. *J Immunol* **147**, 2777–2786.
44. van Oostrom, A. J., Plokker, H. W., van Asbeck, B. S., Rabelink, T. J., van Kessel, K. P., Jansen, E. H., Stehouwer, C. D., and Cabezas, M. C. (2006) Effects of rosuvastatin on postprandial leukocytes in mildly hyperlipidemic patients with premature coronary sclerosis. *Atherosclerosis* **185**, 331–339.
45. de Gruijter, M., Hoogerbrugge, N., van Rijn, M. A., Koster, J. F., Sluiter, W., and Jongkind, J. F. (1991) Patients with combined hypercholesterolemia-hypertriglyceridemia show an increased monocyte-endothelial cell adhesion *in vitro*: Triglyceride level as a major determinant. *Metabolism* **40**, 1119–1121.
46. Jongkind, J. F., Verkerk, A., and Hoogerbrugge, N. (1995) Monocytes from patients with combined hypercholesterolemia-hypertriglyceridemia and isolated hypercholesterolemia show an increased adhesion to endothelial cells

in vitro: II. Influence of intrinsic and extrinsic factors on monocyte binding. *Metabolism* **44**, 374–378.

47. Weber, C., Erl, W., Weber, K. S., and Weber, P. C. (1997) HMG-CoA reductase inhibitors decrease CD11b expression and CD11b-dependent adhesion of monocytes to endothelium and reduce increased adhesiveness of monocytes isolated from patients with hypercholesterolemia. *J Am Coll Cardiol* **30**, 1212–1217.

Chapter 13

MICRO SHEAR STRESS SENSORS: FROM *IN VITRO* TO *IN VIVO* ASSESSMENT OF INFLAMMATORY RESPONSES

LISONG AI*, FEI YU†, ZHOUYUAN ZHANG‡ and TZUNG HSIAI§
University of Southern California, Department of Biomedical Engineering
1042 Downey Way, Denney Research Center (DRB) 172
Los Angeles, CA 90089-1111, USA
* *lisongai@usc.edu*
† *feiyu@usc.edu*
‡ *zhouyuaz@usc.edu*
§ *hsiai@usc.edu*

To date, developing a translatable strategy to detect secondary flow in the athero-prone regions *in vivo* remains a challenge. To address this need, we have developed the MEMS thermal sensors to assess intravascular voltage (IVV) changes in the New Zealand White (NZW) rabbits on high fat/cholesterol diet. The MEMS thermal sensors were capable of sensing secondary flow as recorded by the significantly elevated time-averaged voltage values (V_{ave}) and the time-varying component ($\delta V/\delta t$) in the lesion-prone regions. These voltage profiles were distinct between the control and treated groups, corresponding to the histopathological findings for atheromas and foam cell infiltration. In this chapter, the heat transfer strategy will be introduced as a potential entry point to assess inflammatory responses, to demonstrate spatial and temporal variations in shear stress under a low Reynolds number flow in an arterial bifurcation model, and to detect sense secondary flow developed in the athero-prone regions of fat-fed NZW rabbits.

1. Overview and Clinical Relevance

In the athero-prone regions, flow separation and secondary flow develop. In response to cardiac contraction, the migrating stagnation points generate low and oscillating flow.[1] Mounting evidence supports that hemodynamics, specifically, fluid shear stress, is intimately involved in vascular oxidative stress,[2] inflammatory responses, and atherosclerosis.[3–6] In the arterial regions where flow separation develops, secondary flow, low and oscillatory wall shear stress predict the progression of atherosclerosis,[7] vessel wall remodeling,[8] and development of abdominal aortic aneurysm.[9,10]

Intravascular strategy has emerged to detect unstable plaque. The combination of three dimensional intravascular ultrasound (IVUS) images and finite element analysis have been reported to assess plaque size, shape, expansive remodeling, calcification, and lipid core.[11] By using IVUS, biplane coronary angiography, and coronary blood flow measurements, Stone *et al.* demonstrated the effects of endothelial shear stress on the progression of coronary artery disease, vascular remodeling, and in-stent re-stenosis in humans.[12] Recently, Jaffer *et al.* demonstrated the use of real-time near-infrared fluorescence catheter to sense arterial inflammation in proteolytically active atherosclerosis.[13]

The advent of microelectromechanical systems (MEMS) thermal sensors has provide an entry point to assess the non-obstructive atherosclerotic lesions with high spatial (1/10th of a string of hair) and temporal resolution (kilo Hz).[14] The operational principle is based on convective cooling of a heated sensing element as fluid flows over the sensing element surface. The heat transfer from the heated surface to the fluid depends on the flow characteristics in the viscous region of the boundary layer.[15] Based on heat transfer principle, the heat dissipation from the sensors to the blood flow alters the resistance of the sensing elements in response to instantaneous fluctuation in temperature, from which voltage changes are acquired and calibrated to shear stress.[16] The MEMS sensors can be packaged to the coaxial wire for intravascular interrogation (Fig. 1).

In this chapter, the readers will embark on a journey starting from the application of MEMS sensors to assess monocyte-endothelial cell interaction *in vitro*, low Reynolds number flow in the arterial bifurcation model, followed by intravascular shear stress assessment in the New Zealand White (NZW) rabbits.

1.1. *MEMS Shear Stress Sensors to Assess Monocyte Recruitment*

The important interplay between blood circulation and vascular cell behavior warrants the development of highly sensitive but small sensing systems. The emerging Micro Electro Mechanical Systems (MEMS) technology, thus, provides the high spatiotemporal resolution to link biomechanical forces on the micro-scale with large-scale physiology. We fabricated MEMS sensors, comparable to the endothelial cells (EC) in size,

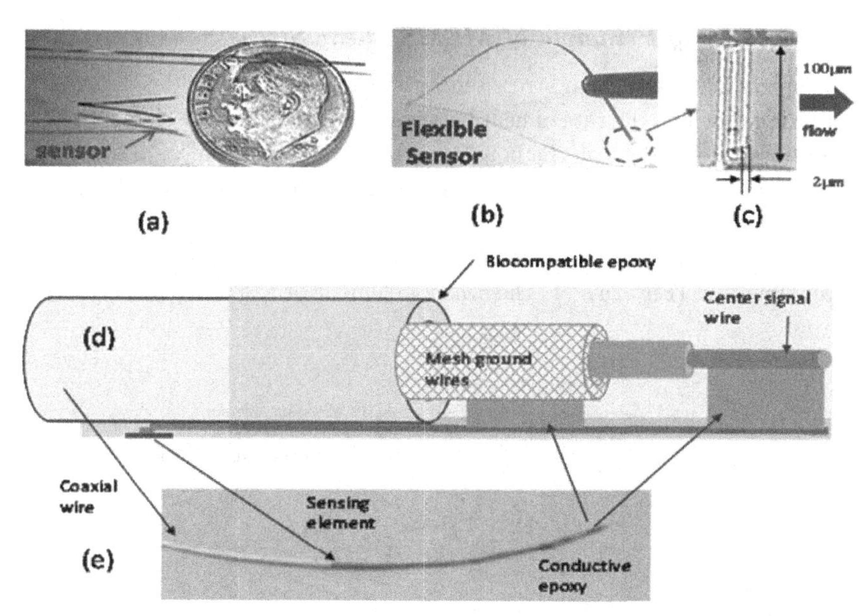

Fig. 1. Flexible MEMS sensors. (a) The sensor can be folded in a zigzag fashion without structural or functional damage. (b) The flexible polymer coated sensor is 320 μm in width and 21 μm in thickness as indicated by the dotted circle. (c) The sensing element at terminal end of the sensor was made of a 2 μm wide Ti/Pt strip with a span wise dimension of 100 μm. (d) A schematic diagram depicts the packaging of the polymer sensor to the coaxial wire. The sensor was connected to the electrical coaxial wire with conductive epoxy and covered with biocompatible epoxy to prevent electrical current leakage. The distance between the sensing element and the tip of the catheter is 4 cm. (e) The photograph shows a packaged sensor to the coaxial wire.

to link real-time shear stress with monocyte/endothelial cell interactions in an oscillatory flow environment, simulating the moving and unsteady separation point at arterial bifurcations. In response to oscillatory shear stress (τ) at $\pm 2.6\,\text{dynes/cm}^2$, time-averaged shear stress (τ_{ave}) $=$ 0 at 0.5 Hz, individual monocytes displayed unique to-and-fro trajectories, undergoing rolling, binding and dissociation with other monocyte, followed by solid adhesion on EC. Incorporating with cell tracking velocimetry, we visualized that these real-time events occurred over a dynamic range of oscillating shear stress between $\pm 2.6\,\text{dynes/cm}^2$ and Reynolds numbers between 0 and 22.2 in the presence of activated adhesion molecule and chemokine mRNA expression.

1.2. *Operating Principle of MEMS Shear Stress Sensors*

The operation of the shear stress sensor is based on the fully developed flow condition in which the rate of heat loss from a heated resistive element to the fluid-flow is dependent on the boundary–layer velocity profile.[15] The change in temperature of the local flow milieu leads to the change in resistivity of the sensors.

The dynamic performance of the sensors is characterized by a three-layer structure (Fig. 2a): (1) the sensing element or the film layer is the top

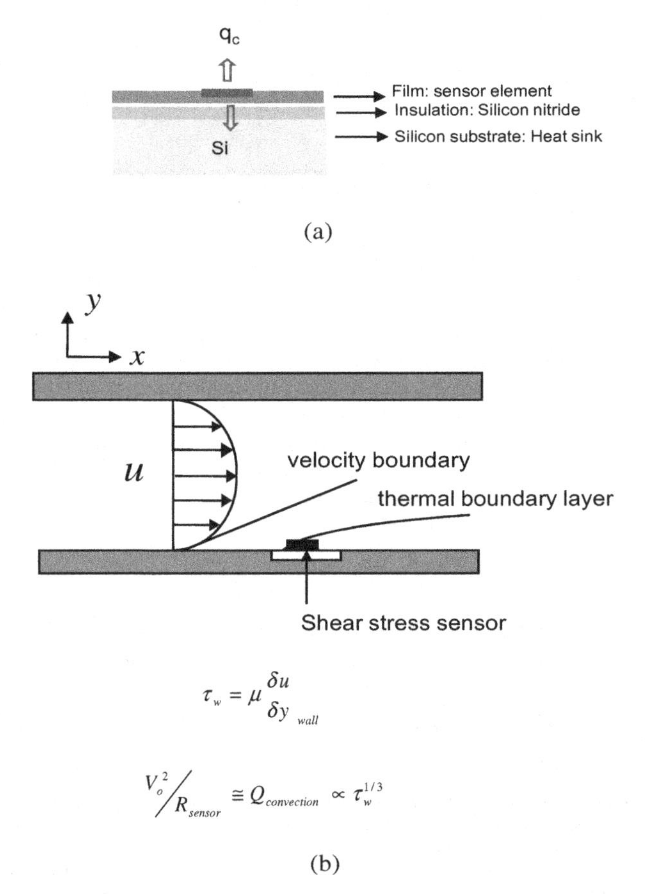

Fig. 2. Principle of thermal shear stress sensors. (a) Three-layer model for heat transfer with "q_c" referring to convective heat transfer. (b) The thermal element resides within a velocity boundary layer. Thus, the rate of heat loss from a heated resistive element to the fluid flow is dependent on the velocity profile in the boundary layer. A linear relation is obtained as $V^2/R \propto \tau^{1/3}$ based on heat transfer principles.

layer; (2) the silicon nitride diaphragm in the middle serves as an insulation layer, and (3) the silicon substrate at the bottom provides heat sink. From Fig. 1a, the energy balance equation is expressed as:[17]

$$P = I^2R = c_f m_f \frac{dT_f}{dt} + c_i m_i \frac{dT_i}{dt} + h(u_\tau)\mathrm{A}(T - T_0), \tag{1.1}$$

where h denotes the heat transfer coefficient. The subscripts f, i, and c represent the convective heat transfer from the film and insulation layer to the fluid, respectively. The terms "c" is defined as specific heat and "m" as mass. T is the temperature of the sensor element and T_0 the heat sink. "**A**" denotes the cross-sectional area of the sensor as $A = WL$, where W and L represent the width and length. The convective heat transfer coefficient is represented by $h(u_\tau)$, which is a function of shear velocity, denoted as u_τ. The relation between the shear velocity and the wall shear stress is $\tau_w = u_\tau^2 \rho$, where ρ is the measured fluid density. The product of the square of current, I^2, and the resistor sensor, R, gives rise to the heating power, P, as i^2R. At a low frequency of cardiac cycles, the two unsteady terms in Eq. (1.1) are negligible. Thus, Eq. (1.1) can be simplified to set power dissipation equal to the convective heat transfer term (from the heated sensor to the ambient fluid). The heating power for the sensor is related to the wall shear stress as:[15]

$$P = h(u_\tau)\mathrm{A}(T - T_o) = (A + B\tau^{\frac{1}{3}})(T - T_o), \tag{1.2}$$

where A and B are calibration constants. The resistance, R, of the semiconductor sensing element is a function of change in temperature:

$$R = R_o[1 + \alpha(T - T_o)] \tag{1.3}$$

where R_o is the resistance at room temperature T_o and alpha, α, is the temperature coefficient of resistance (TCR). An important feature governing the thermal shear-stress sensor operation is the temperature over heat ratio, α_T, defined as the relative change of sensor temperature compared with the ambient temperature:

$$\alpha_T = (T - T_o)/T_o \tag{1.4}$$

It is also commonly defined as resistance over-heat ratio as, α_R, which reflects the relative change of sensor resistance compared with the resistance at the ambient temperature,

$$\alpha_R = (R - R_o)/R_o \tag{1.5}$$

The resistance over heat ratio was set at 0.12 in order to minimize natural convection by the heating of the resistive element. It has been demonstrated by Huang *et al.* that the higher the over-heat ratio, the higher the sensitivity.[18,19]

The MEMS sensors are operated by either constant temperature (CT) or constant current (CC) driving circuit. For constant CT mode, the sensor resistance, R, is kept constant by a Wheatstone bridge feedback circuit. The power can be expressed as $P = V^2/R$, where V is the voltage across the sensor and R, the sensor resistance, Eq. (1.2) becomes

$$V^2/R = (A_T + B_T\tau^{\frac{1}{3}}). \tag{1.6}$$

The temperature coefficient of resistance (TCR or α in Eq. (1.3) can be adjusted by changing the doping concentration of boron into the polysilicon strip. In a fully developed channel flow, the shear stress determines the rate of heat transfer from a heated resistive element to the surrounding fluid field. The heating power is proportional to convective heat transfer. The thickness of thermal boundary layer is likely to be smaller than that of velocity boundary layer. Thus, a linear relation between V^2 and $\tau_w^{1/3}$ is established (Fig. 2b).

1.3. *Unique Aspects of MEMS Shear Stress Sensor Fabrication*

The schematic diagram of the sensor (Fig. 3) features the polysilicon as the heating and sensing element across the center of a cavity diaphragm. The polysilicon, measuring $2\,\mu$m wide, $0.5\,\mu$m high, and $80\,\mu$m long, was uniformly doped with boron at $10^{16}/\text{cm}^2$ at 60 keV of energy to give rise a positive TCR of 0.1%/°C and a typical sheet-resistance of $50\,\Omega/\square$,[19] or a resistance between 1.25 $\sim$ 5 kΩ at room temperature. This resistance was higher than that of the traditional metal sensor (5 to 50 Ω). After doping, the wafer was annealed at 1000°C to activate the dopant and to reduce the intrinsic stress on the polysilicon. The resistance of the sensing element could be adjusted by changing the doping levels.

An array of resistors was fabricated on a single chip. The individual sensing elements were lying across the diaphragm (Fig. 3b).[20] The diaphragm was separated from the bottom of the cavity by an approximately $2\,\mu$m gap. The pressure inside the cavity was equal to 300 mTorr (0.04 Pa), at which the oxide layer ($1.2\,\mu$m) and silicon-nitirde

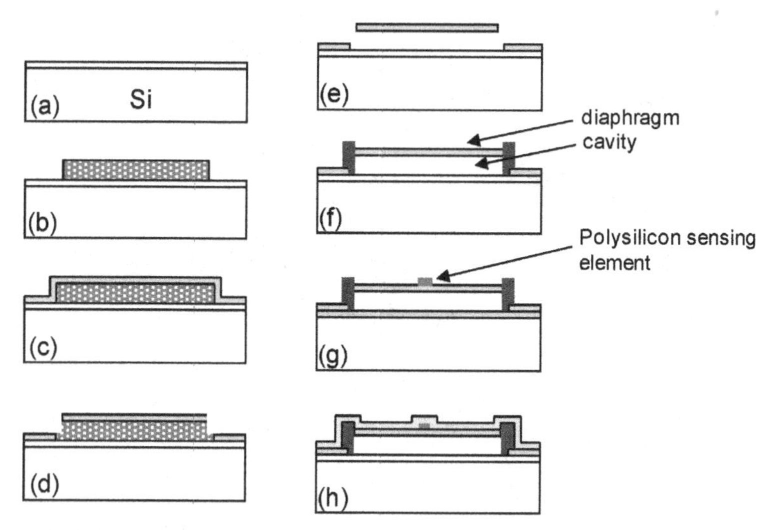

Fig. 3. Fabrication steps of the micro thermal shear stress sensor: (a) thermal oxidation and Si_3N_4 deposition; (b) poly-silicon deposition and patterning; (c) thermal oxidation and Si_3N_4 deposition; (d) opening etching holes; (e) removing the sacrificial poly-Si layer; (f) blocking the etching holes; (g) poly-Si deposition, ion-implantation with boron and patterning; (h) Aluminum deposition and pattering for electrodes, and SiO_2 deposition for water proof. A vacuum was created to optimize convective heat transfer from the heated sensor to the ambient fluid. Refer to Fig. 4(b) for the photos of sensors.

layer (300 nm) were deposited in Fig. 3(f). Thermal evaporation of the aluminum metalization (300 nm in height and 10 μm in width) formed the leads connecting the polysilicon resistor or the sensing element to the external electronics. The vacuum cavity allowed for effective thermal isolation between the heated element and the substrate, thereby minimizing the heat conduction from the diaphragm to the substrate through the gap.[15]

1.4. *Interfacing MEMS Sensors with a Pulsatile Flow Channel*

A pulsatile flow system was used to deliver well-defined flow profiles simulating the flow conditions in the arterial circulation (Fig. 4).[16] This unique configuration ensured velocity uniformity and absence of flow separation across the width of the channel during flow reversal. Due to the symmetry of the rectangular flow channel, we were able to flush-mount the sensor opposite to the EC monolayers (Fig. 4a), which were seeded

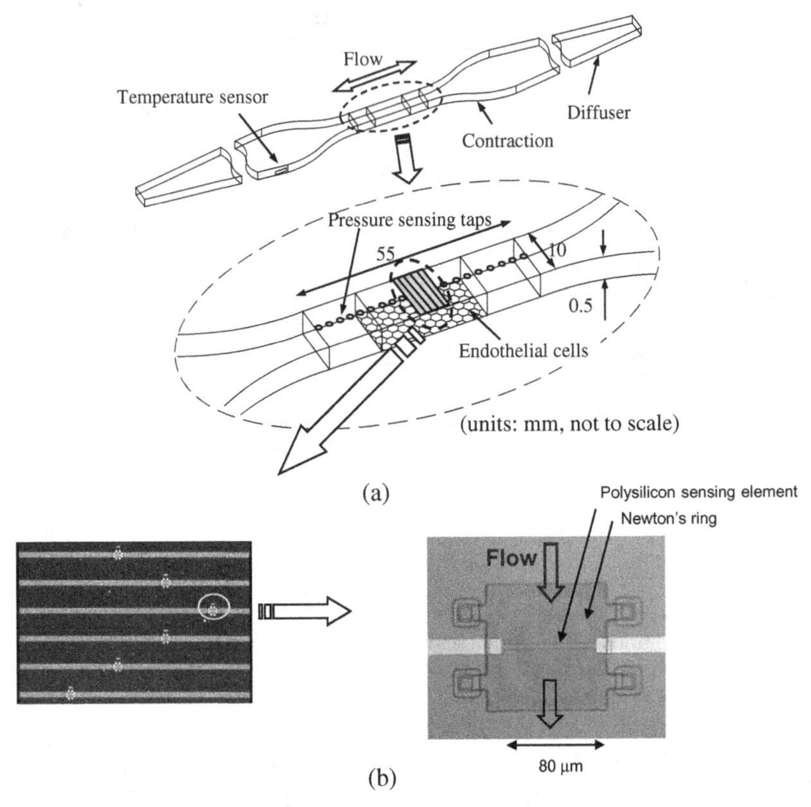

Fig. 4. (a) The MEMS sensor array was flush-mounted on the upper wall of the pulsatile flow channel. Confluent BAEC monolayes were seeded on the bottom. (b) A photograph of individual shear stress sensors illustrate the polysilicon as a sensing element. The diaphragm (refer to 2(f)) was bent down by the external atmospheric pressure giving rise to an optical interference patterns referred as Newton rings.

on the bottom parallel plate. This approach circumvented the local flow disturbance introduced by conventional probes.

Two flow profiles representative of different sites at vascular branching points were generated: oscillatory and pulsatile flow. Real-time pulsatile vs. oscillatory shear stresses that were delivered to endothelial cells at $37.0 \pm 0.15°C$ (Figs. 5a and 5b). The oscillatory shear stress at an arbitrary periodicity of 0.5 Hz simulated the flow pattern seen at the reattachment points. The time-averaged shear stress (τ_{ave}) was 50 dynes/cm^2 for pulsatile flow. The flow reversal was recorded as upward deflection as rectified signals (Fig. 5b).

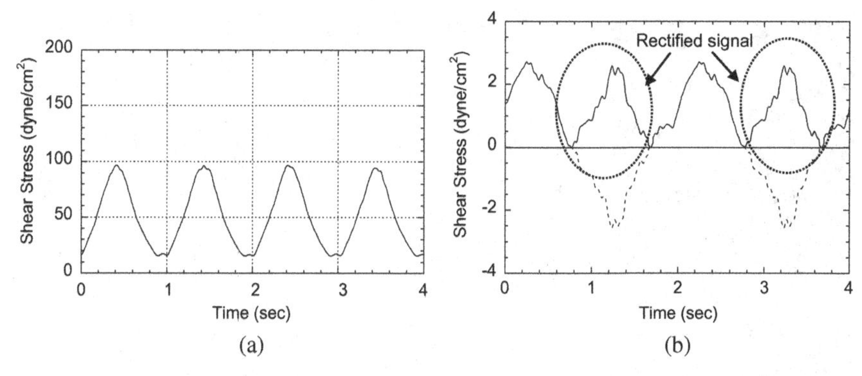

Fig. 5. Shear stress measurement by the micro thermal shear stress sensors: (a) pulsatile flow; (b) oscillatory flow to simulate the outer wall of arterial bifurcations at the reattachment point. The rectified signal reflected flow reversal.

Overall, the micro-shear stress sensor offers three particularly novel design characteristics: (1) the heat-insulation features a free standing diaphragm on a vacuum cavity, which minimizes heat loss to the substrate; (2) the semi-conductor material serves as a high performance heating/sensing element providing a much higher resistivity than metal which is used in conventional thermal sensors; and (3) the high sensitivity of sensing element allows for real-time shear stress measurements (frequency >10 kHz) and a fine spatial resolution comparable to the length of an elongated endothelial cell (<100 μm). The transient voltage response was measured at 85 μs, or 11.7 kHz. This high frequency response enabled us to measure oscillating shear stress otherwise difficult with the conventional Bernoulli's Principle using an orifice.[16]

1.5. *Nonlinear Displacement of Monocyte Locomotion in Response to Oscillatory Flow*

The paths followed by monocyte locomotion were traced by cell tracking velocimetry, revealing diverse modes of cell-cell interactions in response to oscillating flow. A sequence of images reveals two monocytes undergoing attachment; separation, short-lived reattachment, and re-separation with one another were captured (Fig. 6a–e). Both monocytes briefly established adhesion on EC (Fig. 6b). Monocyte 2 then separated from monocyte 1, which eventually established solid adhesion on EC as illustrated at 0 reference point on the y axis (Fig. 6d). The corresponding trajectories

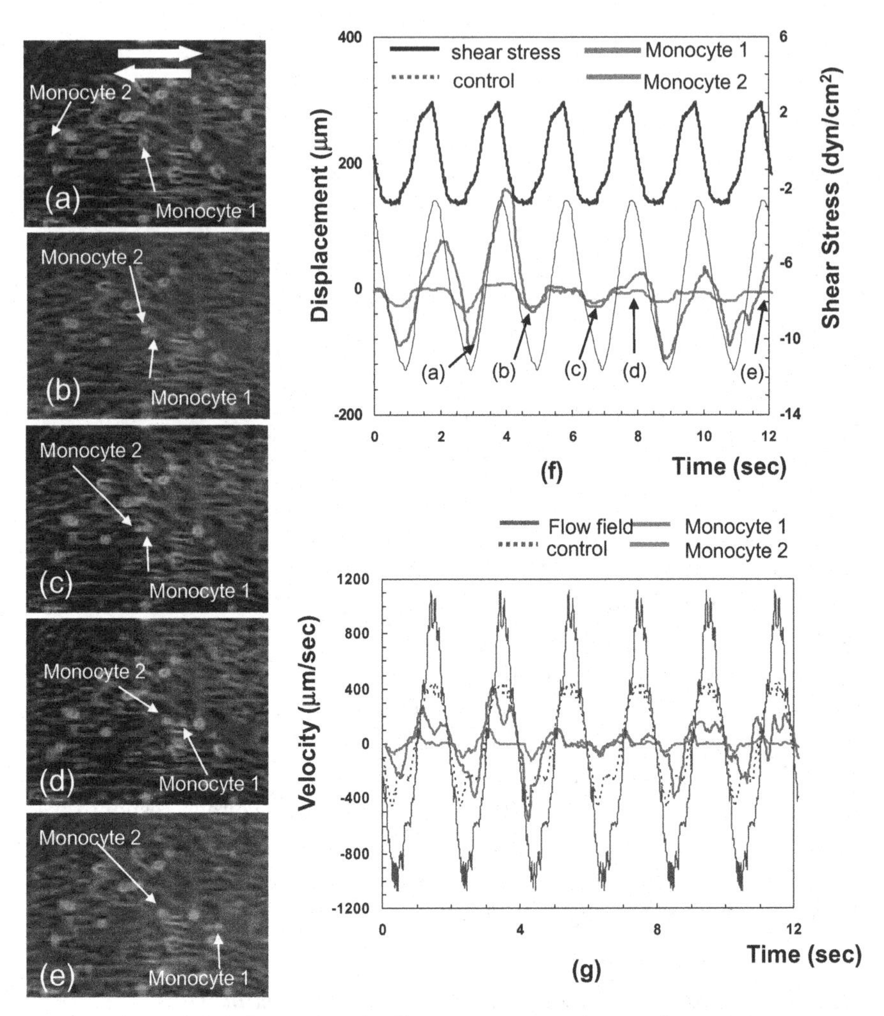

Fig. 6. Captured images of cell-cell interactions under oscillatory shear stress: (a) monocyte 1 was undergoing tethering while monocyte 2 in to-and-for locomotion; (b) monocytes 1 and 2 established binding; (c) monocytes 1 and 2 started to separate; (d) monocytes 1 and 2 were apart; (e) monocyte 2 resumed to-and-for locomotion while monocyte 1 remained attached to EC. (f) The dark blue profile reflects the real-time oscillatory shear stress. The trajectories of monocytes 1 and 2 from the captured images (a–e) are superimposed with the dotted blue trajectory of the non-viable monocyte (control); (g) Velocity profiles of monocytes 1 and 2 are compared with that of the non-viable monocyte (control) in relation to the velocity of oscillating flow field.

of these two individual monocytes were captured using cell tracking velocimetry (Fig. 6f). Monocyte 1 was observed to undergo tethering, characterized as abrupt halt in locomotion alternating with resumption of to-and-for motion. Despite the identical magnitude of oscillatory shear stress, the absolute displacement, velocities and direction of monocytes were nonlinear, and non-random, suggesting the dynamics of molecular interactions underlying the cell-cell binding kinetics. The rolling velocities of individual monocytes were distinct from the average hydrodynamic velocity of the flow field (Fig. 6g). Once in contact with the EC monolayers, the locomotion of individual monocytes was retarded. The trajectory of the non-viable monocytes which were buoyant above the EC monolayer, contrasted those of monocytes 1 and 2 (Fig. 6f). The trajectory of non-viable monocyte followed the direction of shear stress; whereas, the motion of monocytes was influenced by the EC monolayers.

Therefore, the patterns of displacement facilitate the identification of cell-cell binding, monocyte rolling, transient adhesion and solid adhesion to endothelial cells. The velocity profiles of individual monocytes provide clues to monocytes undergoing dynamic changes in displacement.

1.6. *Monocyte Binding to Bovine Aortic Endothelial Cells (BAEC) in Response to Pulsatile vs. Oscillatory Flow*

After 4 hour of pulsatile vs. oscillatory flow conditions, monocyte adhesion assays were performed. The number of monocyte binding to the BAEC after unidirectional pulsatile flow exposure was significantly attenuated (4 ± 1 monocytes/high power field (HPF), $P < 0.05$). In contrast, the distribution and probability of monocytes binding to EC exposed to oscillatory flow was enhanced (static control = 5 ± 2 monocytes/HPF, oscillatory flow = 36 ± 5, $P < 0.05$) (Fig. 7). Hence, the up-regulation of adhesion molecule and chemokine expression in response to oscillatory shear stress implicated their roles in recruiting monocytes as the initiating events in inflammatory responses.

Section 1 introduces MEMS shear stress sensors and cell tracking velocity as novel tools for real-time quantification and visualization of monocyte adhesion events. We demonstrated the distinct behaviors of monocyte/EC binding kinetics in response to oscillatory shear stress with high temporal and spatial resolution. The induction of adhesion molecules and chemokines from BAEC in the presence of an oscillatory shear environment modulated the duration of monocyte tethering, and

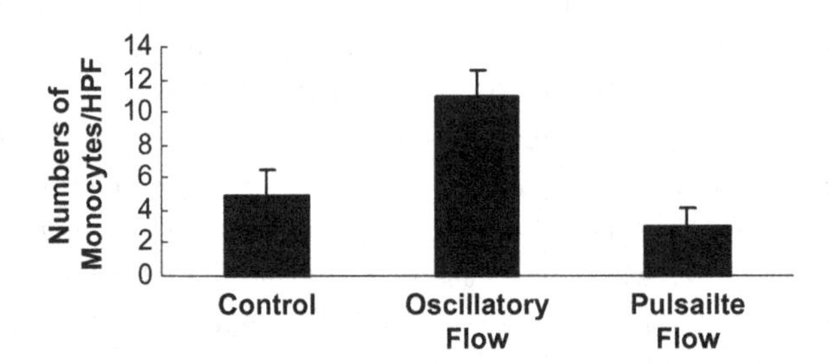

Fig. 7. Effects of pulsatile vs. oscillatory flow on monocyte binding to BAEC by monocyte adhesion assay at 4 hours. Oscillatory flow induced a statistically significant increase in the number of adherent monocytes by 1.2 fold per high power field (HPF) (oscillatory: 11 ± 1.2, control: 5 ± 1.5, $P < 0.05$, $n = 5$). Pulsatile flow attenuated the number of monocyte bound by 1.6-fold (pulsatile flow: 3 ± 1.5). Data (mean $\pm$ SD) are based on five separate experiments.

subsequent attachment. The increase in residence time was conducive to monocyte receptors binding to sufficient ligands such as P-selectin and ICAM-1.

2. Assess Low Reynolds Number Flow in the Arterial Bifurcations

2.1. *A Novel Backside Wire Bonding for Biomedical Applications*

To gain entry into arterial geometry, we developed backside wire bonding to insulate the micro-circuitry from the flow field. Such a technique is critical to advance the MEMS sensors for biomedical applications (Fig. 8). The sensing element was made of polysilicon, measured at $2\,\mu$m (width) $\times$ $0.5\,\mu$m (height) $\times$ $80\,\mu$m (length), and was uniformly doped with phosphorous at $10^{16}/\text{cm}^2$ at 60 keV. This doping resulted in a negative temperature coefficient of resistance (TCR) of $-2.081\%/°$C between 20 and 40°C (Fig. 8a) and a sheet-resistance of $50\,\Omega/\square$,[19] or resistance of $2.5\,\text{k}\Omega$ at room temperature.

When an electric current passed through the heated element, the heat convection from a resistively-heated element to the flowing fluid was measured as the change in voltage across the element, from which a value for shear stress was inferred.[21] The resistance vs. temperature plot

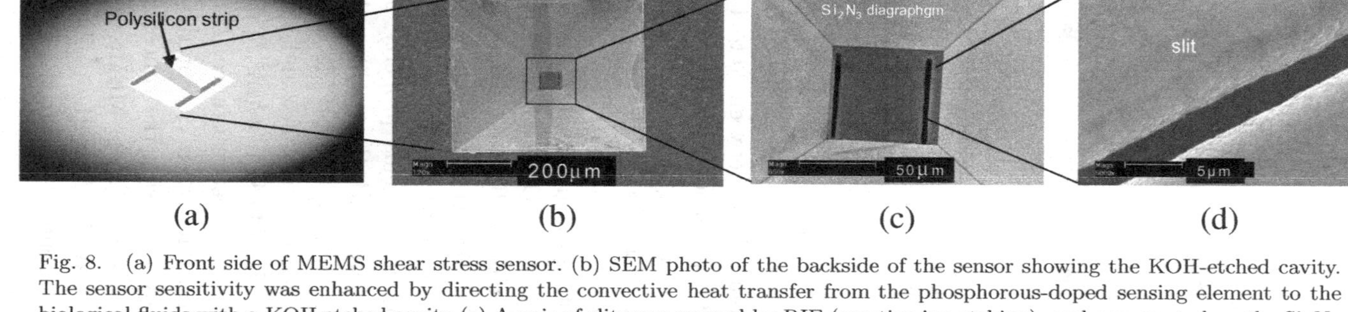

Fig. 8. (a) Front side of MEMS shear stress sensor. (b) SEM photo of the backside of the sensor showing the KOH-etched cavity. The sensor sensitivity was enhanced by directing the convective heat transfer from the phosphorous-doped sensing element to the biological fluids with a KOH-etched cavity (c) A pair of slits was opened by RIE (reactive ion etching), and was created on the Si_2N_3 diaphragm at 0.4 μm in thickness. (d) Electric contact side was established via a pair of slits between the aluminum metallization on the back side and the sensing element on the front.

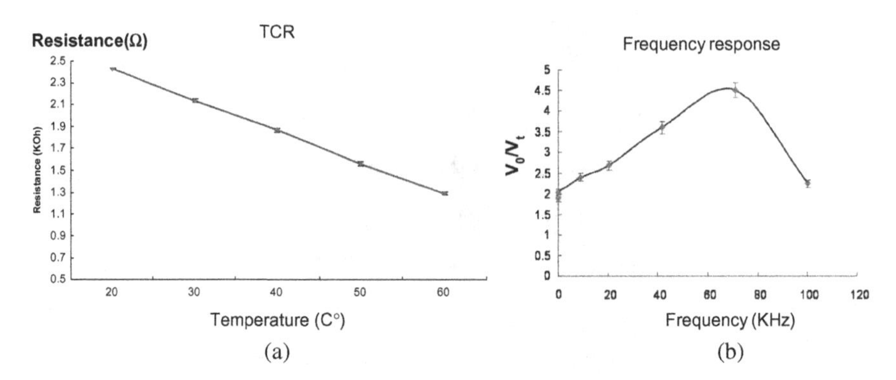

Fig. 9. (a) Resistance vs. temperature measurement for the phosphorous-doped polysilicon sensing element. The negative slope or TCR denotes phonon scattering ($n = 3$). (b) Frequency response diagram illustrates the gain amplitude at around 71 KHz. The error bars reflected the square of standard deviation values ($n = 3$).

demonstrates a negative TCR from 20 to 60°C, suggesting the phonon scattering effect.[22] A linear relation was established between the resistance and temperature. The absolute TCR between 20 to 40°C was estimated to be 0.9937, an ideal value for physiologic testing (Fig. 9a). The frequency response was obtained by measuring the magnitude of the voltage gain over a range of frequency (Fig. 9b). We introduced sine waves through E_t terminal of the constant temperature (CT) mode circuit (Fig. 10), and measured the gain by adjusting the amplitude of the sine wave input signal, Vt, using a feedback amplifier (AI-OP21). The frequency response of the sensors was based on a slope of −2 dB at 71 kHz.

The sensitivity of the MEMS sensor was dependent on the resistivity of the sensing element, which, in turn, was determined by the concentration of phosphorous-doped polysilicon. This property provided an elevated resistance up to 10 kΩ compared with the traditional metal sensors (from 5 to 50 Ω), and also accounted for the MEMS sensor's high frequency response.[23] The relation between resistance and sheet-resistance can be expressed as follows: $\boldsymbol{R} = \boldsymbol{R}_s\ (\boldsymbol{L}/\boldsymbol{W})$, where R denotes the resistance of the sensing element, R_s the sheet-resistance, L the length of sensing element, and W the width. The sensitivity of the shear stress sensors can be further enhanced by increasing the concentration of doping and altering the L/W ratio. The sensitivity for MEMS sensors was determined by $(\Delta v/v)/(\text{dynes/cm}^2)$ or $\Delta v/\Delta\tau$ from the calibration curves, where v denotes voltage and τ represents shear stress. The reported sensitivity

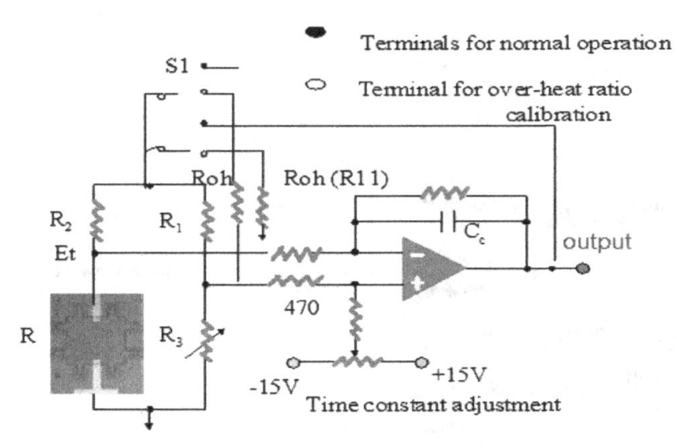

Fig. 10. The constant temperature mode is utilized to drive the MEMS sensor. The resistor (R) in the Wheatstone bridge is coupled to an operational amplifier to form a feedback circuit.

from Sheplak was in the range of 11 mV/Pa or 1.1/(dynes/cm^2).[24] Huang reported a sensitivity of 7 mV/(dynes/cm^2).[23,25] Based on our calibration curve,[21,26] the sensitivity was 17.1 mV/(dynes/cm^2).

2.2. *Integrating MEMS Sensors to Resolve Spatial Variations in Shear Stress in a 3-D Bifurcation Model*

To demonstrate spatial variations in shear stress ($\partial\tau/\partial x$), we constructed a 3-D bifurcation model (Fig. 11a). The MEMS sensors were embedded upstream and downstream in the interior wall of the model. The devices were embedded in the inner wall so that the individual sensing elements, which were 0.5 μm in height, were exposed to the flow field in the lumen while the backside bonding allowed for connection to the external electric circuit. The surface of the MEMS device was at the even level with the surface of the lumen, facilitating precise wall shear stress measurement.

To validate the experimental data, we used a Navier–Stokes solver from FLUENT® and the GAMBIT software to construct a digital representation of the 3-D bifurcation model.[26] The preliminary data demonstrated the feasibility of MEMS sensors to resolve circumferential shear stress at the microcirculation level under low Reynolds number flow. The direct measurements closely agreed with the Computational Fluid Dynamics (CFD) code at steady state ($\partial\tau/\partial t = 0$) (Fig. 11e–g).

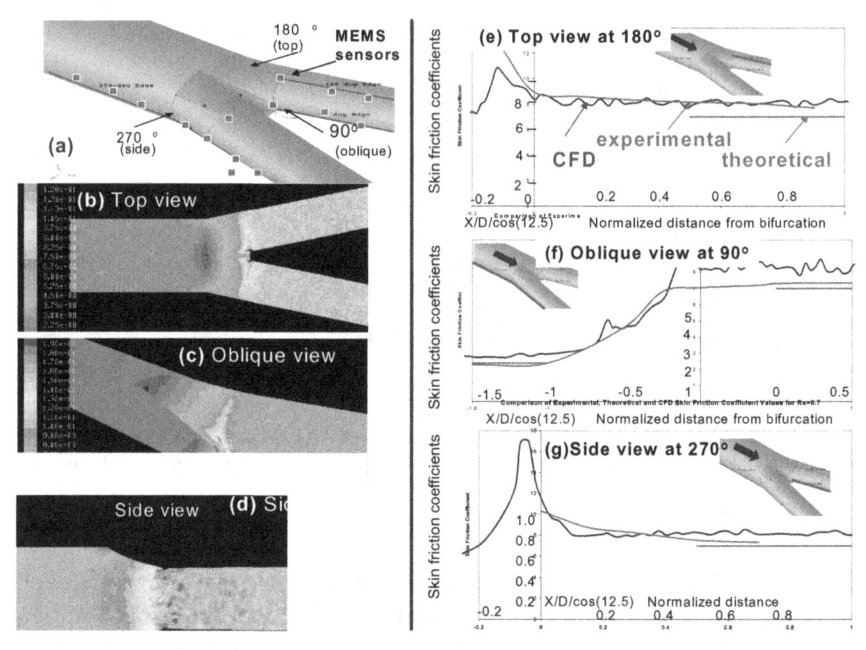

Fig. 11. (a) The bifurcation model was constructed using measurements from angiogram according to Ku *et al.* and Zarin.[27] Red squares are representative of sensor placement. (b) **CFD** solutions for skin friction coefficient (C_f) at Reynolds number Re $= 6.7$. C_f values are shown along the interior surface of bifurcation. (b) Top view. (c) Oblique view or **medial wall**. (d) Side view along the 90° line or **lateral wall**. (e) Comparison of the CFD (in blue), experimental (in green), and theoretical (in red) skin friction for the 270° edge. At a Reynolds number of 6.7, experimental C_f found in the bifurcation region along the 270° edge was distinct from the values along the 180° and 90° lines. $X/D/\cos$ (12.5) is the x distance normalized to the diameter of the inlet pipe and parallel to the centerline of the outlet pipes. Hence, the measured skin friction coefficients at various positions correlated well with values derived from the exact Navier–Stokes solution of the flow within the bifurcation.

The wall-shear stress values were normalized to skin friction coefficient (C_f), defined as:[1]

$$C_f = \frac{\tau}{\frac{1}{2}\rho U^2} \tag{2.1}$$

where C_f, for the experimental values was calculated by dividing the measured shear stress (τ) by the dynamic pressure in the constant area tube ahead of the bifurcation:

$$q = \frac{\rho U^2}{2} \tag{2.2}$$

In addition to comparison between experimental shear stress values and numerical values, the asymptotic values for a straight tube of diameter D in laminar flow were calculated as:

$$C_{\text{fasym}} = \frac{\tau}{\frac{1}{2}\rho U^2} = \frac{16}{\rho UD/\mu} = 16/\text{Re}, \qquad (2.3)$$

where ρ is the scaling density and U_{ave} is the scaling velocity. Both these values can be specified in the *reference values* menu in Fluent. Re denotes Reynolds number.

Skin friction coefficient values (C_f) varied by a factor of two or more depending upon the circumferential position within the bifurcation. At a low Reynolds number of 6.7, skin friction coefficient on the lateral wall along the 270° plane of the bifurcation was $C_f = 7.1$ (corresponding to a shear stress value of 6.1×10^{-3} dynes/m^2); along the 180° plane, C_f was 13 (7.9×10^{-3} dynes/cm^2); at the medial wall along the 90° plane, C_f was 10.3 (9.12×10^{-3} dynes/cm^2). The margin of error between the CFD solutions and the experimental values for skin friction was within 6–10%. However, it is possible to improve the agreement by refining the grid used in the CFD model. Overall, the MEMS sensors provided precise measurement of spatial variations in shear stress ($\partial\tau/\partial x$) at the medial and lateral walls of bifurcation.

We demonstrate that MEMS sensors were capable of resolving small incremental variation in shear stress simulating bifurcation flow at low Reynolds numbers. To our best knowledge, direct measurements of the spatial variation in shear stress in a 3-D bifurcation model simulating microcirculation have not been previously reported. In addition to the high spatial resolution of the sensors for microcirculation at steady state, the micro-dimension also provided high temporal resolution on the order of 71 kHz in response to unsteady flow or pulsatile flow at high Reynolds numbers ranging from 100 to 1,500 as previously reported.

3. Intravascular Shear Stress Sensors in the New Zealand White Rabbits

Detection of non-obstructive, albeit inflammatory atherosclerotic lesions remains an unmet clinical need. In the athero-prone regions, flow separation and secondary flow develop. In response to cardiac contraction, the migrating stagnation points generate low and oscillating flow.[1] Mounting evidence supports that hemodynamics, specifically, fluid shear stress, is intimately involved in vascular oxidative stress,[2] inflammatory responses, and atherosclerosis.[3–6] In the arterial regions where flow separation develops, secondary flow, low and oscillatory wall shear stress predict the progression of atherosclerosis,[7] vessel wall remodeling,[8] and development of abdominal aortic aneurysm.[9,10]

Intravascular strategy has emerged to detect unstable plaque. The combination of three dimensional intravascular ultrasound (IVUS) images and finite element analysis have been reported to assess plaque size, shape, expansive remodeling, calcification, and lipid core.[11] By using IVUS, biplane coronary angiography, and coronary blood flow measurements, Stone *et al.* demonstrated the effects of endothelial shear stress on the progression of coronary artery disease, vascular remodeling, and in-stent re-stenosis in humans.[12] Recently, Jaffer *et al.* demonstrated the use of real-time near-infrared fluorescence catheter to sense arterial inflammation in proteolytically active atherosclerosis.[13] Our laboratories have developed the microelectromechanical systems (MEMS) thermal sensors to assess secondary flow in the athero-prone regions.[14,28,29]

In the last section of this chapter, a heat transfer strategy will be discussed as a means of sensing secondary flow in the athero-prone regions. The development of MEMS sensors provides an entry point to assess the non-obstructive atherosclerotic lesions with high spatial (1/10th of a string of hair) and temporal resolution (kilo Hz).[14] The heat transfer from the heated surface to the fluid depends on the flow characteristics in the viscous region of the boundary layer.[15] As the heat dissipation from the sensors to the blood flow, the resistance of the sensing elements is altered in response to instantaneous fluctuation in temperature, from which the voltage changes can be acquired and calibrated to shear stress.[16] The MEMS sensors can be packaged to the coaxial wire for intravascular interrogation (Fig. 1). By deploying the MEMS thermal sensors into the aorta of NZW rabbits, we will able to acquire distinct intravascular voltage signals and temporal gradients accompanied with pulse amplitudes. In short, the readers will develop an appreciation for the application of heat transfer strategy to assess secondary flow developed in the athero-prone regions.

3.1. *Deployment of MEMS Sensors into Rabbit Aortas*

Angiograms revealed the corresponding *en face* rabbit aortas from the control and diet-treated animals (Fig. 12). The aortas from fat-fed rabbits had significantly greater atherosclerotic lesion size and frequency

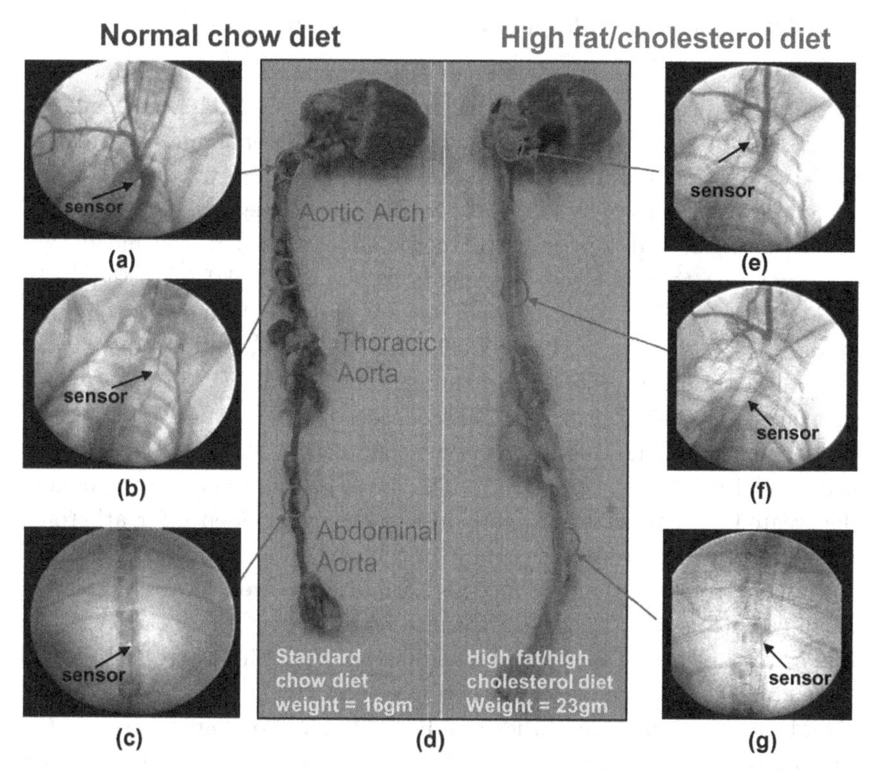

Fig. 12. Angiograms and cardiovascular issues *en face* isolated from adult rabbits after 8 wks on a control or high fat/high cholesterol diet. (a) Contrast dye delineated the contour of aortic arch, innominate and carotid arteries. Arrow indicates the position of MEMS sensor immediately downstream from the aortic arch. (b) Fluoroscope revealed the coaxial wire being deployed to the thoracic aorta. Arrow indicates the position of the sensor in relation to the ribs and cardiac silhouette. (c) Coaxial wire was in the abdominal aorta. (d) Fat-fed rabbits developed myocardial hypertrophy, vessel wall remodeling, and atherosclerotic plaques as evidenced by greater size (radius, R) and weights in abdominal aortas, left ventricles, and aortic arches. (e) Fluoroscope coupled with contrast dye illustrated the position of the sensor in the aortic arch. (f) The sensor was positioned in the thoracic aorta. (g) Fluoroscope revealed the position of the sensor in the abdominal aorta. Present in the background were renal arteries.

compared to the control. The MEMS sensors were deployed to interrogate intravascular voltages (IVV) in the abdominal, thoracic, descending, and ascending aortic arch. Tissues were isolated (n=3/group) after 8 weeks on a control or high fat/high cholesterol diet. This figure provides the basis to correlate the specific arterial histopathology with the IVV measurements (Fig. 16).

3.2. *Intravascular Voltages in the Descending Aorta*

Representative intravascular voltage (IVV) between the control and fat/-fed rabbits were comapred. The mean heart rate was 194 ± 14 beats per minutes (bpm) for the control, and was 157 ± 18 bpm for the treated. Signal processing and filtering removed the ambient and white noises. The red curves represented IVV specific to the arterial segments as indicated by arrows a, b, and c in Fig. 13. In the treated animal, the mean IVV corresponding to the specific segments were 1.053 ± 0.035 V (Fig. 13d), 0.724 ± 0.057 V (Fig. 13e), 0.144 ± 0.003 V (Fig. 13f), and the temporal gradient ($\delta V/\delta t$) was 0.149 ± 0.009, 0.067 ± 0.009, and 0.119 ± 0.010 V/s, respectively. In the control animal, the mean IVV to the specific segments were 0.122 ± 0.006 V (Fig. 13a), 0.131 ± 0.24 V (Fig. 13d), 0.143 ± 0.004 V (Fig. 13c), and $\delta V/\delta t$ was 0.108 ± 0.029, 0.137 ± 0.018, and 0.114 ± 0.018 V/s, respectively. The mean IVV in the thoracic aorta of the treated animal correlated with histopathologic evidence for atheroma and form cell infiltration (Fig. 16b). In the control animal, the mean IVV and $\delta V/\delta t$ from the thoracic and abdominal aorta were nearly similar in magnitude (Fig. 13a, b, and c). Despite high fat diet, the mean IVV was similar to the control in the abdominal aorta (Fig. 13f) where histological section revealed no evidence of atheromas (Fig. 16).

Mean IVV, pulse amplitudes and $\delta V/\delta t$ were compared between the control and treated rabbit (Fig. 14). The mean IVV values (V_{ave}) were significantly elevated in the regions of descending aorta that harbored atherosclerotic lesions in the treated animal (Fig. 14a). In the treated animal, the normalized IVV pulse amplitudes (minimum to peak voltage normalized to mean IVV) and $\delta V/\delta t$ ($\delta V/\delta t$ normalized to mean IVV) were significantly lower compared to the control (Fig. 14b and 14c). Hence, an elevated mean IVV were accompanied with the low normalized pulse amplitude and $\delta V/\delta t$ in distal aortic arch and thoracic aorta where atherosclerotic lesions developed (Fig. 16).

3.3. *Intravascular Voltage Signals in the Aortic Arch*

Representative IVV signals were recorded from both the control and treated animals (Fig. 15). Gross histology revealed the visible plaque formations in the aortic arch of the treated animal (Fig. 15d, e, and f in red). In the control animal, the IVV signals immediately after the greater curvature (Fig. 15a, b, and c in blue) were similar in magnitude to those in the descending

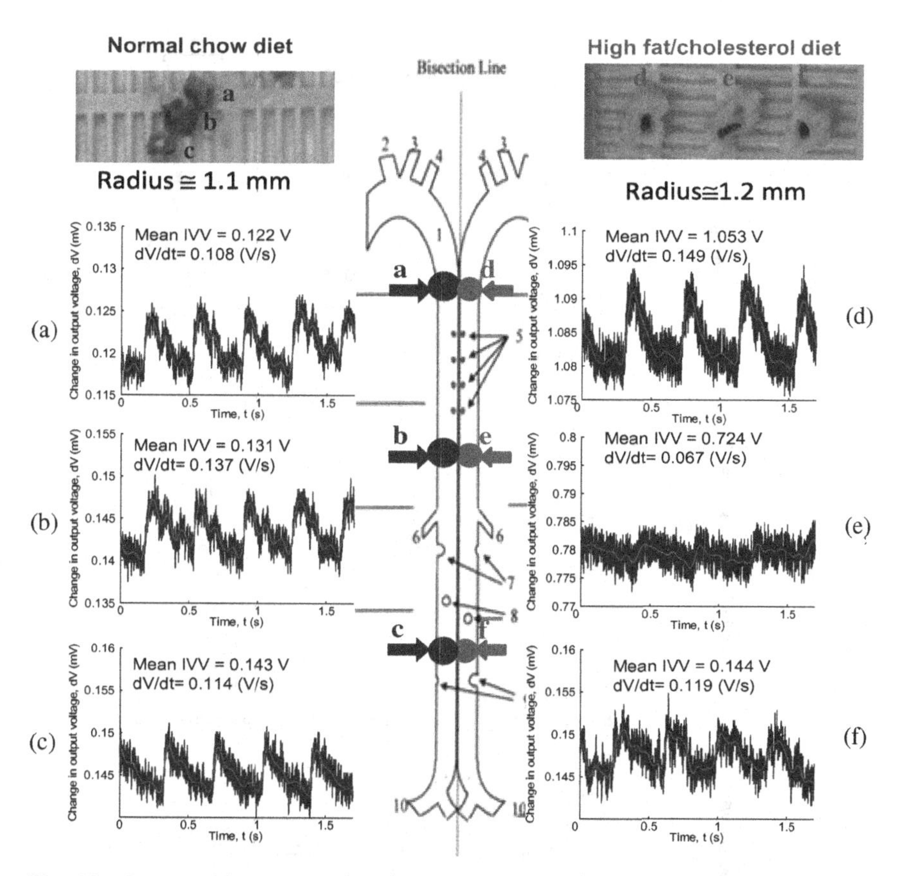

Fig. 13. Intravascular voltage (IVV) signals in the descending aorta. Diagram (not drawn to scale) showing bisection of the aorta, division of aortic segments, and position of aortic tissue sampling. 1 indicates the aorta; 2, brachiocephalic trunk; 3, common carotid artery; 4, left subclavian artery; 5, dorsal intercostal arteries; 6, celiac artery; 7, cranial mesenteric artery; 8, right and left renal arteries; 9, caudal mesenteric artery; and 10, iliac arteries. (a) A representative voltage profiles at the origin of thoracic aorta in the rabbits on normal chow diet. (b) Intravascular voltage (IVV) signals at the distal thoracic aorta. (c) IVV signals in the mid-abdominal aorta. (d)–(f) Representative IVV signals from fat-fed rabbit. Gross pathology for both control and treated animals corresponded to the histopathological sections at which MEMS sensors were positioned as indicated by numbers 1, 2, and 3, respectively.

aorta (Fig. 13a, b, and c). In the treated animal, voltage signal-to-noise ratios increased by 100-fold compared to the descending aorta (Fig. 15a, b, c, versus 15d, e, f). Hence, the heat transfer strategy demonstrated the feasibility to sense secondary flow in the athero-prone regions.

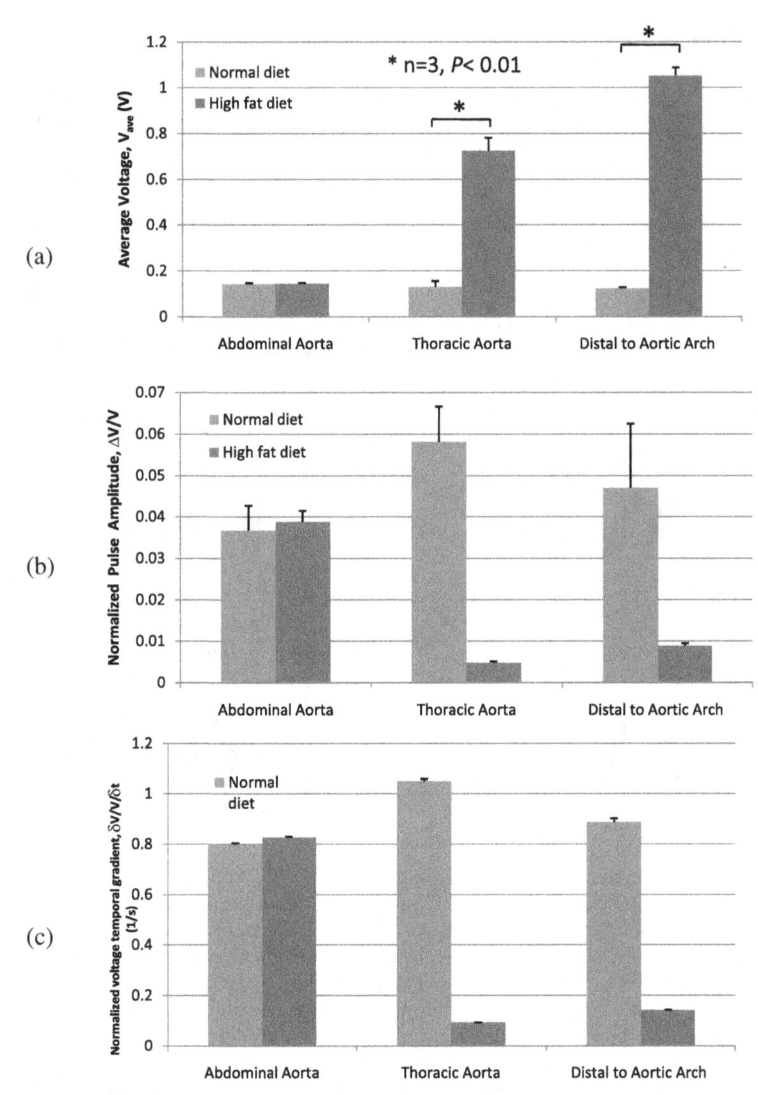

Fig. 14. Comparisons of the mean shear stress, temporal gradients and pulse amplitudes between the signals obtained in the representitive normal rabbit and the treated rabbit. (a) Intravascular voltages between the control and treated animals were compared. Intravascular voltage was elevated in the thoracic and distal aorta where atherosclerotic lesions were present. (b) Normalized pulse amplitudes (minimum to peak voltage) were compared between the control and treated animals. (c) Normalized temporal gradients (dV/dt) were compared between the control and treated animals.

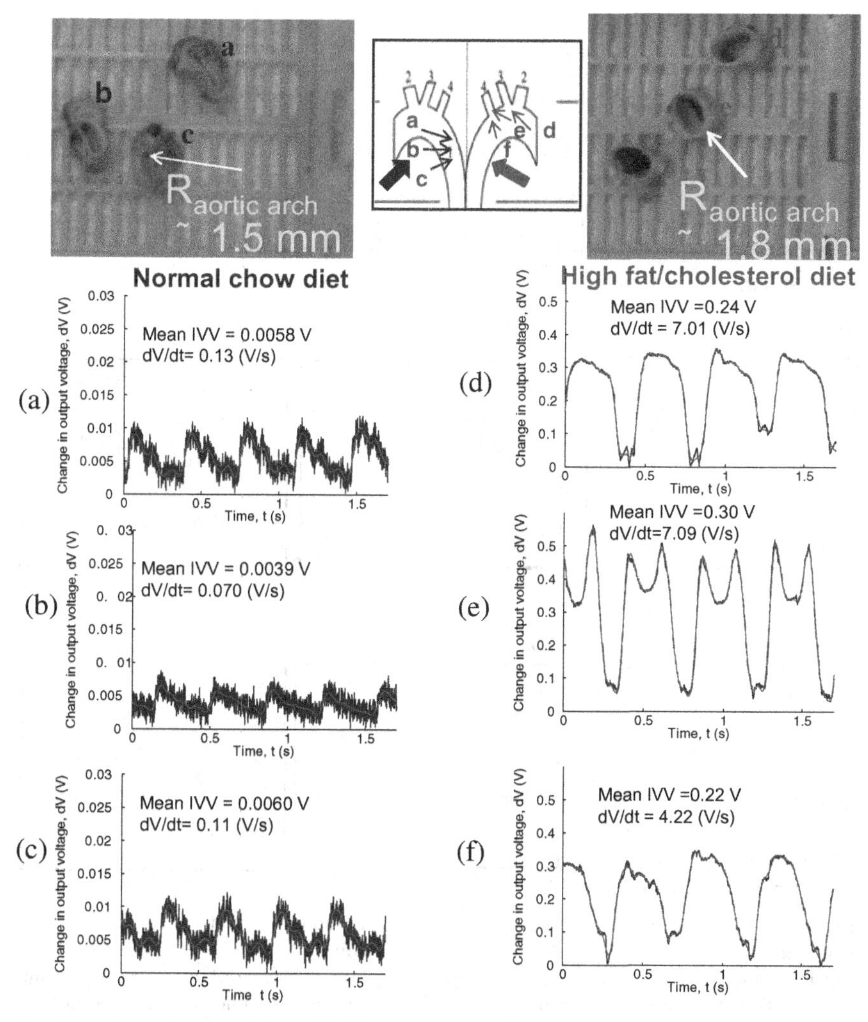

Fig. 15. Intravascular voltage (IVV) signals in the aortic and distal aortic arch. (a)–(c) In the control animals, the voltage signals immediately after the greater curvature were in the similar order of magnitude as those recorded in the descending. The gross pathology revealed patent distal arterial lumens. (d)–(f) In the treated animal, the voltage signal-to-noise ratios were significantly higher than those immediately downstream from the aortic arch in the untreated animal. The gross pathology revealed presence of eccentric lesions.

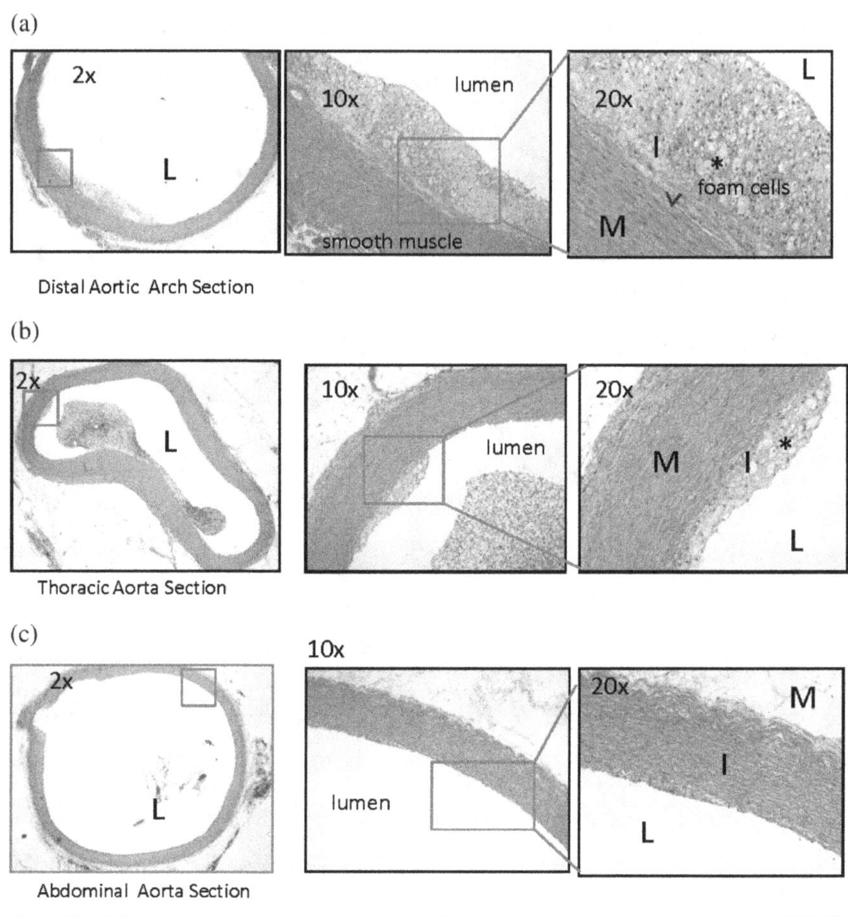

Fig. 16. The aortic tissues were processed for standard hematoxylin-eosin (H&E) staining. (a) Distal Aortic arch section. H&E staining of prominent atheromas from the high fat and high cholesterol-fed rabbit. Note the presence of foam cells (*), and degenerative smooth muscle (arrow) in the thickened intima. L indicates lumen; I, intima; and M, media. Magnification ×20. (b) Thoracic aorta section. Form cell infiltration was present in the atheroma. (c) Abdominal Aorta. Foam cells infiltration was not observed at 20×.

3.4. *Histopathology of Aortas*

Oxidative products, such as oxidized low density lipoprotein (oxLDL), and foam cells play a key role in the initiation of atherosclerosis; however, direct *in vivo* evidence elucidating their link with atherogenic hemodynamics is recently emerging.[30–32] Hematoxylin and eosin (H&E) staining revealed lesions in the arterial cross-sections of distal aortic arch, thoracic and abdominal aorta (Fig. 13). Aortic sections showed the characteristic intimal thickening with foam cell infiltration in the representative distal aortic arch (Fig. 16a and b). Destruction of the internal elastic membrane in the media was also evident (Fig. 16a). Elevated mean IVV signals accompanied with low normalized pulse amplitudes and temporal gradients were also evident in the thoracic arterial regions harboring foam cell infiltrates (Fig. 13d and e). Foam cell infiltration was not observed at 20× magnification in the abdominal aorta section (Fig. 16c), where the IVV signals was similar in magnitude to that of the control. Thus, the histopathology findings support the use of heat transfer strategy to detect secondary flow.

3.5. *Intravascular Shear Stress*

IVV signals were converted to intravascular shear stress (ISS) as previously reported.[14] In the control animal, the time-averaged ISS (τ_{ave}) was $26.9 \pm 1.2\,\text{dynes/cm}^2$ distal to the aortic arch, 28.7 ± 5.0 in the thoracic aorta, and 31.2 ± 0.8 in the abdominal aorta; the corresponding temporal gradient ($\delta\tau/\delta t$) was $21.9 \pm 7.5\,\text{dynes/(cm}^2\cdot\text{s)}$, 29.7 ± 4.2, and 24.6 ± 4.4, respectively. These values were consistent with the previously reported.[28] In the treated animal, τ_{ave} was elevated to $216.3 \pm 6.9\,\text{dynes/cm}^2$ distal to the aortic arch, 150.0 ± 11.0 in the thoracic aorta, and 31.4 ± 0.7 in the abdominal aorta; the corresponding $\delta\tau/\delta t$ was $33.1 \pm 2.5\,\text{dynes/(cm}^2\cdot\text{s)}$, 13.9 ± 1.9, and 23.6 ± 9.6, respectively. In the infra renal segment of the treated animal, atheromas were not observed. Both τ_{ave} ($31.4 \pm 0.7\,\text{dynes/cm}^2$) and $\delta\tau/\delta t$ ($23.7 \pm 5.3\,\text{dynes/(cm}^2\cdot\text{s)}$) were closed to those of the control. τ_{ave} were significantly elevated in the regions of descending aorta that harbored atherosclerotic lesions, consistent with the high IVV signals due to the secondary flow.

In the distal aortic arch of the control animals, τ_{ave} was $26.9 \pm 1.2\,\text{dynes/cm}^2$ and $\delta\tau/\delta t$ was $21.9 \pm 7.5\,\text{dynes/(cm}^2\cdot\text{s)}$. In the aortic arch of the treated animal, τ_{ave} was $29.9 \pm 9.4\,\text{dynes/cm}^2$ and $\delta\tau/\delta t$ was $1{,}250 \pm 358\,\text{dynes/(cm}^2\cdot\text{s)}$. These experimental values overlapped with the computed (Fig. 17) and published results.[33,34] These measurements suggest that heat transfer strategy could also provide a basis to estimate intravascular shear stress.

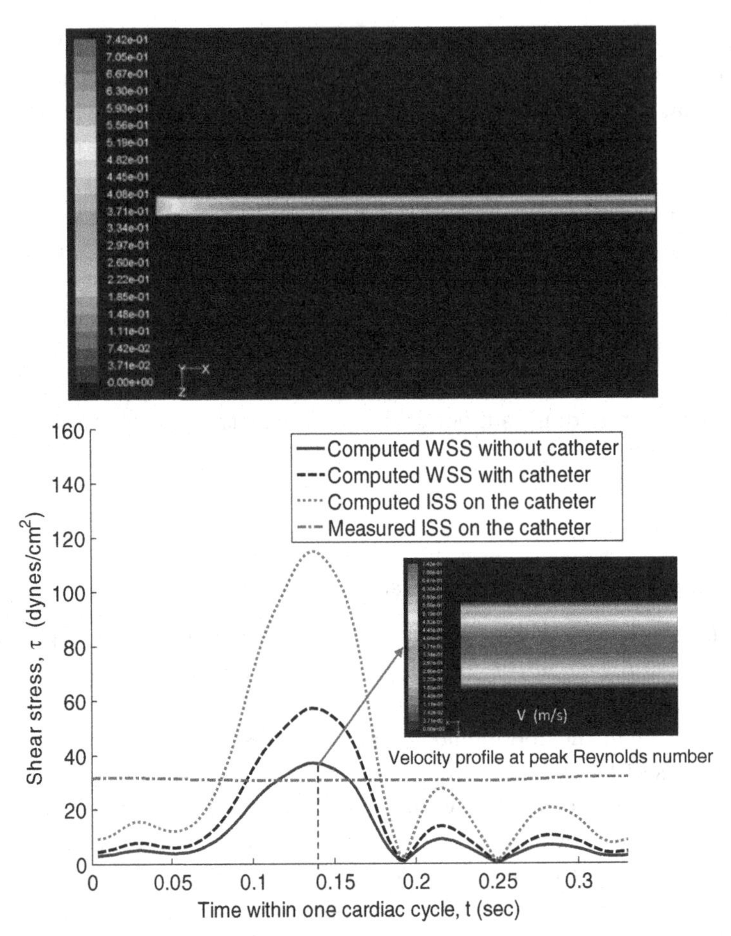

Fig. 17. Comparing wall shear stress (WSS) and intravascular shear stress (ISS). Prior to introducing a catheter-based sensor, the computed mean wall shear stress solved by CFD is 13.4 dynes/cm^2 (blue). After the introducing the catheter, the computed mean wall shear stress is 20.7 dynes/cm^2 (black). The computed mean intravascular shear stress on the catheter located at the center of the artery is 41.5 dynes/cm^2 (green). Our experimentally acquired intravascular shear stress fell within the limit of computed WSS in the presence of catheter (red).

Assessing hemodynamics in the presence of atherosclerotic lesions remains a challenge. We hereby presented a heat transfer strategy to sense secondary flow in the athero-prone regions. By deploying the MEMS thermal sensors into the aorta of NZW rabbits, we were able to acquire distinct intravascular voltage signals and temporal gradients accompanied with pulse amplitudes. These measurements were significantly elevated in the aortic arch where secondary flow developed. These measurements were also distinct between the control and diet-treated groups, corresponding to the histopathologic analyses between the normal and foam cell-infiltrated regions. In the absence of atheromas, the measurements in the abdominal aorta were nearly identical between the control and treated-animals. The voltage profiles could be converted to intravascular shear stress and validated by the computational fluid dynamics results. Taken together, the heat transfer strategy enabled us to assess secondary flow developed in the athero-prone regions.

Overall, detection and characterization of atherosclerotic lesions are of utmost importance in the management of patients with suspected unstable plaques. The heat transfer strategy established a basis to sense secondary flow. Our findings suggest that the MEMS thermal sensors could hold promises to diagnose non-obstructive atherosclerotic lesions.

References

1. Fung, Y. C., *Biomechanics: Circulation*, Second edition ed: Springer, 1997.
2. Madamanchi, N. R., Vendrov, A., and Runge, M. S. (2005) Oxidative stress and vascular disease. *Arterioscler Thromb Vasc Biol* **25**, 29–38.
3. Davies, P. F., Remuzzi, A., Gordon, E. J., Dewey, C. F., and Gimbrone, A. M. J. (1986) Turbulent fluid shear stress induces vascular endothelial cell turnover *in vitro*. *Proc Naatl Acad Sci USA* **83**, 2114–2117.
4. Topper, J. N., Cai, J., Falb, D., and G. M. Jr. (1996) Identification of vascular endothelial genes differentially responsive to fluid mechanical stimuli: Cyclooxygenase-2, manganese superoxide dismutase, and endothelial cell nitric oxide synthase are selectively up-regulated by steady laminar shear stress. *Proc Natl Acad Sci* **93**, 10417–10422.
5. Nerem, R. M., Alexander, R. W., Chappell, D. C., Medford, R. M., Varner, S. E., and Taylor, W. R. (1998) The study of the influence of flow on vascular endothelial biology. *Am J Med Sci* **316**, 169–175.
6. Berk, B. C., Atheroprotective signaling mechanisms activated by steady laminar flow in endothelial cells. *Circulation* **117**, 1082–1089.
7. Stone, P. H., Coskun, A. U., Kinlay, S., Clark, M. E., Sonka, M., Wahle, A., Ilegbusi, O. J., Yeghiazarians, Y., Popma, J. J., Orav, J., Kuntz, R. E., and Feldman, C. L. (2003) Effect of endothelial shear stress on the progression of coronary artery disease, vascular remodeling, and in-stent restenosis in humans — *In vivo* 6-month follow-up study. *Circulation* **108**, 438–444.
8. Chatzizisis, Y. S., Jonas, M., Coskun, A. U., Beigel, R., Stone, B. V., Maynard, C., Gerrity, R. G., Daley, W., Rogers, C., Edelman, E. R., Feldman,

C. L., and Stone, P. H. (2008) Prediction of the localization of high-risk coronary atherosclerotic plaques on the basis of low endothelial shear stress — An intravascular ultrasound and histopathology natural history study. *Circulation* **117**, 993–1002.

9. Taylor, T. W. and Yamaguchi, T. (1994) 3-Dimensional simulation of blood-flow in an abdominal aortic-aneurysm — steady and unsteady-flow cases. *Journal of Biomechanical Engineering — Transactions of the Asme* **116**, 89–97.
10. Raghavan, M. L., Vorp, D. A., Federle, M. P., Makaroun, M. S., and Webster, M. W. (2000) Wall stress distribution on three-dimensionally reconstructed models of human abdominal aortic aneurysm. *Journal of Vascular Surgery* **31**, 760–769.
11. Imoto, K., Hiro, T., Fujii, T., Murashige, A., Fukumoto, Y., Hashimoto, G., Okamura, T., Yamada, J., Mori, K., and Matsuzaki, M. (2005) Longitudinal structural determinants of atherosclerotic plaque vulnerability: a computational analysis of stress distribution using vessel models and three-dimensional intravascular ultrasound imaging. *J Am Coll Cardiol* **46**, 1507–1515.
12. Stone, P. H., Coskun, A. U., Kinlay, S., Clark, M. E., Sonka, M., Wahle, A., Ilegbusi, O. J., Yeghiazarians, Y., Popma, J. J., Orav, J., Kuntz, R. E., and Feldman, C. L. (2003) Effect of endothelial shear stress on the progression of coronary artery disease, vascular remodeling, and in-stent restenosis in humans: *in vivo* 6-month follow-up study. *Circulation* **108**, 438–444.
13. Jaffer, F. A., Vinegoni, C., John, M. C., Aikawa, E., Gold, H. K., Finn, A. V., Ntziachristos, V., Libby, P., and Weissleder, R. (2008) Real-time catheter molecular sensing of inflammation in proteolytically active atherosclerosis. *Circulation* **118**, 1802–1809.
14. Ai, L., Yu, H., Dai, W., Hale, S. L., Kloner, R. A., and Hsiai, T. K. (2009) Real-time intravascular shear stress in the rabbit abdominal aorta. *IEEE Trans Biomed Eng* **56**, 1755–1764.
15. Haritonnidis, J. H. (1989) The Measurement of Shear Stress in Fluid Mechanics Measurements. E. M. G.-e.-H. Springer-Verlag, Ed., pp. 229–236.
16. Hsiai, T. K., Cho, S. K., Honda, H. M., Hama, S., Navab, M., Demer, L. L., and Ho, C. M. (2002) Endothelial cell dynamics under pulsating flows: Significance of high versus low shear stress slew rates (d(tau)/dt). *Ann Biomed Eng* **30** 646–656.
17. Huang, J. B., Tung, S., Ho, C. M., Liu, C., and Tai, Y. C. (1995) Improved Micro Thermal Shear Stress Sensors. in *Proceedings, IEEE Instrumentation and Measurement Conference.* Waltham, MA, pp. 570–574.
18. Huang, J., Ho, C., Tung, S., Liu, C., and Tai, Y. (1995) Microthermal Shear Stress Sensor With and Without Cavity Underneath. presented at IEEE Instrumentation and Measurement Conference, Waltham, MA.
19. Huang, J. B., Tung, S., Ho, C. M., Liu, C., and Tai, Y. C. (1995) Improved Micro Thermal Shear Stress Sensors, presented at IEEE Instrumentation and Measurement Conference, Waltham, MA.

20. Hsiai, T., I. M., Navab, M., R. S., and Ho, C. M. (2002) Microsensors to characterize shear stress regulating inflammatory responses in the arterial bifurcations. Presented at Proceedings of the Second Joint Meeting of the IEEE Engineering in Medicine and Biology and the Biomedical Engineering Society, Huston, Tx.
21. Soundararajan, G., Mahsa Rouhanizadeh, M., Yu, H., Kim, E. S., and Hsiai, T. K. (2005) MEMS sensors for microcirculation. *Sensors and Actuators* **118**, 25–32.
22. Hsiai, T., Cho, S. K., Navab, H. S. M., Demer, L. L., and Ho, C. M. (2002) Endothelial cell dynamics under pulsating flow: significance of high- vs. low shear stress slew rates. *Annals of Biomedical Engineeing* **30**, 646–656.
23. Ho, C. M., and Tai, Y. C. (1996) MEMS and its Applications for Flow Control. *Journal of Fluids Engineering* **118**, 437–447.
24. Chandrasekaran, V., Cain, A., Nishida, T., Cattafesta, L. N., and Sheplak, M. (2001) Characterization of a Micromachined Thermal Shear Stress Sensor. Presented at 39th Aerospace Sciences Meeting & Exhibit, Reno, NV.
25. Huang, J. B., Tung, S., Ho, C. M., Liu, C., and Tai, Y. C. (1996) Micro Therma Shear Stress Sensors. presented at IEEE Trans. on Instrumentation and Measurement.
26. Rouhanizadeh, M., Lin, T. C., Arcas, D., Hwang, J., and H. TK. (2005) Spatial variations in shear stress in a 3-d bifurcation model at low reynolds numbers. *Ann Biomed Eng* **33**, 1360–1374.
27. Zarins, C. K., Giddens, D. P., Bharadvaj, B. K., Sottiurai, V. S., and Mabon, R. F. (1983) Carotid bifurcation of plaque localization with flow velocity profiles and wall shear stress. *Circulaton Research* **53**, 502–514.
28. Ai, L. S., Yu, H. Y., Takabe, W., Paraboschi, A., Yu, F., Kim, E. S., Li, R. S., and Hsiai, T. K. (2009) Optimization of intravascular shear stress assessment *in vivo*. *Journal of Biomechanics* **42**, 1429–1437.
29. Yu, H., Ai, L., Rouhanizadeh, M., Patel, D., Kim, E. S., and Hsiai T. K. (2008) Flexible polymer sensors for *In Vivo* intravascular shear stress analysis. *IEEE/ASME J MEMS* **17** 1178–1186.
30. Hwang, J., M, I., A, S., Lassegue, B., Griendling, K. K., M, N., A, S., and Hsiai, T. K. (2003) Pulsatile vs. Oscillatory Shear Stress Regulates NADPH oxidase system: Implication for Native LDL Oxidation. *Circ Res* **93**, 1225–1232.
31. Hsiai, T. K., Hwang, J., Barr, M. L., Correa, A., Hamilton, R., Alavi, M., Rouhanizadeh, M., Cadenas, E., and Hazen, S. L. (2007) Hemodynamics influences vascular peroxynitrite formation: Implication for low-density lipoprotein apo-B-100 nitration. *Free Radic Biol Med* **42**, 519–529.
32. Ai, L., Rouhanizadeh, M., Wu, J. C., Takabe, W., Yu, H., Alavi, M., Li, R., Chu, Y., Miller, J., Heistad, D. D., and Hsiai, T. K. (2008) Shear stress influences spatial variations in vascular Mn-SOD expression: Implication for LDL nitration. *Am J Physiol Cell Physiol* **294**, C1576–1585.
33. Feintuch, A., Ruengsakulrach, P., Lin, A., Zhang, J., Zhou, Y. Q., Bishop, J., Davidson, L., Courtman, D., Foster, F. S., Steinman, D. A., Henkelman,

R. M., and Ethier, C. R. (2007) Hemodynamics in the mouse aortic arch as assessed by MRI, ultrasound, and numerical modeling. *Am J Physiol Heart Circ Physiol* **292**, H884–892.

34. Shahcheraghi, N., Dwyer, H. A., Cheer, A. Y., Barakat, A. I., and Rutaganira, T. (2002) Unsteady and three-dimensional simulation of blood flow in the human aortic arch. *J Biomech Eng* **124**, 378–387.

INDEX